T0264346

# Muscle Over-Activity in Upper Motor Neuron Syndrome: Assessment and Problem Solving for Complex Cases

*Editor*

MIRIAM SEGAL

## PHYSICAL MEDICINE AND REHABILITATION CLINICS OF NORTH AMERICA

www.pmr.theclinics.com

*Consulting Editor*
SANTOS F. MARTINEZ

August 2018 • Volume 29 • Number 3

**ELSEVIER**

1600 John F. Kennedy Boulevard ● Suite 1800 ● Philadelphia, Pennsylvania, 19103-2899

http://www.theclinics.com

**PHYSICAL MEDICINE AND REHABILITATION CLINICS OF NORTH AMERICA** Volume 29, Number 3
August 2018 ISSN 1047-9651, ISBN 978-0-323-61408-5

Editor: Lauren Boyle
Developmental Editor: Meredith Madeira

*Reprints.* For copies of 100 or more of articles in this publication, please contact the Commercial Reprints Department, Elsevier Inc., 360 Park Avenue South, New York, NY 10010-1710. Tel.: 212-633-3874; Fax: 212-633-3820; E-mail: reprints@elsevier.com.

*Physical Medicine and Rehabilitation Clinics of North America* (ISSN 1047-9651) is published quarterly by Elsevier Inc., 360 Park Avenue South, New York, NY 10010-1710. Months of issue are February, May, August, and November. Business and Editorial Offices: 1600 John F. Kennedy Blvd., Suite 1800, Philadelphia, PA 19103-2899. Customer Service Office: 3251 Riverport Lane, Maryland Heights, MO 63043. Periodicals postage paid at New York, NY and additional mailing offices. Subscription price per year is $294.00 (US individuals), $571.00 (US institutions), $100.00 (US students), $351.00 (Canadian individuals), $752.00 (Canadian institutions), $210.00 (Canadian students), $427.00 (foreign individuals), $752.00 (foreign institutions), and $210.00 (foreign students). Foreign air speed delivery is included in all *Clinics* subscription prices. All prices are subject to change without notice. **POSTMASTER:** Send address changes to *Physical Medicine and Rehabilitation Clinics of North America*, Customer Service Office: Elsevier Health Sciences Division, Subscription Customer Service, 3251 Riverport Lane, Maryland Heights, MO 63043. **Customer Service: 1-800-654-2452 (US). From outside of the United States, call 314-447-8871. Fax: 314-447-8029. E-mail: JournalsCustomer Service-usa@elsevier.com (for print support); JournalsOnlineSupport-usa@elsevier.com (for online support).**

*Physical Medicine and Rehabilitation Clinics of North America* is indexed in *Excerpta Medica, MEDLINE/PubMed (Index Medicus), Cinahl,* and *Cumulative Index to Nursing and Allied Health Literature.*

# Contributors

## CONSULTING EDITOR

### SANTOS F. MARTINEZ, MD, MS

Diplomate of the American Academy of Physical Medicine and Rehabilitation, Certificate of Added Qualification Sports Medicine, Assistant Professor, Department of Orthopaedics, Campbell Clinic Orthopaedics, The University of Tennessee, Memphis, Tennessee

## EDITOR

### MIRIAM SEGAL, MD

Attending Physician, Physical Medicine and Rehabilitation, Program Director, Brain Injury Medicine Fellowship, Drucker Brain Injury Center, MossRehab, Albert Einstein Medical Center, Elkins Park, Pennsylvania

## AUTHORS

### ANNE FELICIA AMBROSE, MD, MS

Vice Chair of Education and Residency Program Director, Associate Professor, Department of Rehabilitation Medicine, Burke Rehabilitation Hospital, Montefiore Medical Center, White Plains, New York

### KEITH BALDWIN, MD, MPH, MSPT

Assistant Professor, Department of Orthopaedic Surgery, Children's Hospital of Philadelphia, University of Pennsylvania, Philadelphia, Pennsylvania

### WESLEY CHAY, MD

Staff Physiatrist, Department of Physical Medicine and Rehabilitation, Shepherd Center, Assistant Professor (Adjunct), Department of Rehabilitation Medicine, Emory University School of Medicine, Atlanta, Georgia

### ERNESTO CRUZ, MD

Professor, Department of Physical Medicine and Rehabilitation, Lewis Katz School of Medicine, Temple University, Philadelphia, Pennsylvania

### CAROLIN DOHLE, MD

Assistant Clinical Director, Department of Neurology, Columbia University, Assistant Medical Director, Associate Director, Stroke Rehabilitation Program, Burke Rehabilitation Hospital, Montefiore Medical Center, White Plains, New York

### STEVEN ESCALDI, DO

Medical Director, Spasticity Management Program, Department of Rehabilitation Medicine, JFK Johnson Rehabilitation Institute, Edison, New Jersey; Clinical Associate Professor, Rutgers Robert Wood Johnson Medical School, Piscataway, New Jersey

**HAN-CHIAO ISAAC CHEN, MD**
Department of Neurosurgery, Hospital of the University of Pennsylvania, Perelman School of Medicine, University of Pennsylvania, Philadelphia, Pennsylvania

**ASHLEY M.F. JOHNSON, MD**
Department of Physical Medicine and Rehabilitation, Temple University Hospital, Philadelphia, Pennsylvania

**HEAKYUNG KIM, MD**
David Gurewitsch Professor of Rehabilitation Medicine and Pediatrics, Department of Rehabilitation and Regenerative Medicine, Vice Chair, Director, Pediatric Physical Medicine and Rehabilitation, Columbia University Irving Medical Center, Weill Cornell Medical College, NewYork-Presbyterian Hospital, New York, New York; Chief, Department of Physiatry, Blythedale Children's Hospital, Valhalla, New York

**SHIH-SHAN LANG, MD**
Department of Neurosurgery, Hospital of the University of Pennsylvania, Perelman School of Medicine, University of Pennsylvania, Division of Neurosurgery, Children's Hospital of Philadelphia, Philadelphia, Pennsylvania

**JOHN LIN, MD**
Staff Physiatrist, Department of Physical Medicine and Rehabilitation, Shepherd Center, Assistant Professor (Adjunct), Department of Rehabilitation Medicine, Emory University School of Medicine, Atlanta, Georgia

**PETER J. MADSEN, MD**
Department of Neurosurgery, Hospital of the University of Pennsylvania, Perelman School of Medicine, University of Pennsylvania, Philadelphia, Pennsylvania

**IAN B. MAITIN, MD, MBA**
Professor, Department of Physical Medicine and Rehabilitation, Lewis Katz School of Medicine, Temple University, Philadelphia, Pennsylvania

**MICHAEL H. MARINO, MD**
Physiatrist, Physical Medicine and Rehabilitation, MossRehab, Elkins Park, Pennsylvania; Medical Director, Physical Medicine and Rehabilitation, ReMed, Paoli, Pennsylvania

**NATHANIEL H. MAYER, MD**
Director, Motor Control Analysis Laboratory, Department of PM&R, MossRehab, Einstein Healthcare Network, Elkins Park, Pennsylvania; Emeritus Professor, Department of Rehabilitation Medicine, Temple University Health Sciences Center, Philadelphia, Pennsylvania

**KIMBERLY MICZAK, PT, NCS**
Physical Therapist, Drucker Brain Injury Center, MossRehab, Elkins Park, Pennsylvania

**DANIEL K. MOON, MD, MS**
Sheerr Gait and Motion Analysis Laboratory, Motor Control Analysis Laboratory, Department of Physical Medicine and Rehabilitation, MossRehab, Einstein Healthcare Network, Elkins Park, Pennsylvania

**JOSEPH PADOVA, OTR/L**
Occupational Therapist, MossRehab Outpatient Center, Elkins Park, Pennsylvania

**PREETI RAGHAVAN, MD**
Howard A. Rusk Associate Professor of Rehabilitation Research, Vice Chair Research Rusk Rehabilitation, NYU School of Medicine, New York, New York

**PETER RIEDEL, DO**
Physical Medicine and Rehabilitation, MossRehab, Elkins Park, Pennsylvania

**JENNIFER RUSSO, MD**
Physical Medicine and Rehabilitation Resident, Burke Rehabilitation Hospital, White Plains, New York

**MICHAEL SAULINO, MD, PhD**
Director of Neuromodulation, MossRehab, Elkins Park, Pennsylvania; Associate Professor, Department of Rehabilitation Medicine, Thomas Jefferson University, Philadelphia, Pennsylvania

**MIRIAM SEGAL, MD**
Attending Physician, Physical Medicine and Rehabilitation, Program Director, Brain Injury Medicine Fellowship, Drucker Brain Injury Center, MossRehab, Albert Einstein Medical Center, Elkins Park, Pennsylvania

**MI RAN SHIN, MD**
Chief Resident, Department of Physical Medicine and Rehabilitation, Johns Hopkins University, Baltimore, Maryland

**TANYA VERGHESE, MA**
Research Coordinator, Burke Rehabilitation Hospital, White Plains, New York

**THOMAS WATANABE, MD**
Clinical Director, MossRehab, Einstein Healthcare Network, Elkins Park, Pennsylvania; Associate Professor, Department of Physical Medicine and Rehabilitation, Lewis Katz School of Medicine, Temple University, Philadelphia, Pennsylvania

**MATTHEW T. WINTERTON, MD**
Resident Physician, Department of Orthopaedic Surgery, Children's Hospital of Philadelphia, Philadelphia, Pennsylvania

# Contents

**Muscle Overactivity in the Upper Motor Neuron Syndrome: Pathophysiology**   427

Miriam Segal

> The upper motor neuron syndrome is composed of negative, positive, and
> rheologic features. The positive features have to do with muscle overac-
> tivity, which results from abnormal signal processing in the spinal cord,
> from altered supraspinal inputs and/or dysfunctional segmental spinal
> modulatory mechanisms. The negative features are characterized by a
> reduction of muscle activity and loss of selective muscle control. Third
> are rheologic features characterized by changes in the physical properties
> of muscle. These 3 types of clinical features share perpetuating cause-
> and-effect relationships. This discussion highlights pathophysiology
> involved in muscle overactivity in the context of the upper motor neuron
> syndrome.

**Meaningful Assessment in Patients with Acquired Brain Injuries**            437

Thomas Watanabe

> There are several key components to the meaningful and comprehen-
> sive assessment of patients with acquired brain injuries with respect
> to management of the upper motor neuron syndrome. Type of brain
> injury, trajectory of recovery, relevant concomitant complications,
> development of appropriate goals, and an understanding of resources
> available for patients are all factors to assess when developing a
> treatment plan. Using appropriate outcome measures will help monitor
> the efficacy of interventions and guide ongoing management of
> spasticity.

**Special Considerations in Assessing and Treating Spasticity in Spinal Cord Injury**   445

John Lin and Wesley Chay

> The assessment and treatment of spasticity can be challenging in and of
> itself. The authors highlight some special considerations that may assist
> in the assessment and treatment approach of spasticity in individuals
> with spinal cord injury.

Pediatric spasticity management requires special consideration because of continuous growth and underlying medical complications due to upper motor neuron disease. Early intervention, regular follow-up, and management of spasticity are critical to improve function and prevent musculoskeletal complications, functional deterioration, and the development of pain. Thorough history taking along with comprehensive medical evaluation and physical examination by practitioners with knowledge about spasticity are important clues for spasticity management in addition to thorough history taking and review of current medications. This article reviews the rationale of early intervention and continuum of care, basic physical examination, and therapeutic options for spasticity management and spasticity's aggravating factors.

Multiple sclerosis is a progressive autoimmune neurologic disorder that may affect any region of the central nervous system. Spasticity in patients with multiple sclerosis can be debilitating and detrimental to the function and quality of life of patients. Treatment options include oral medications, chemodenervation, physical therapy, and modalities. Cannabinoids in the form of a delta-9-tetrahydrocannabinol/cannabidiol oro-mucosal spray has been shown to be effective in addressing spasticity in multiple sclerosis. Successful treatment of spasticity will be integrated, multimodal, and individualized.

Spasticity is a major physical complication of many neurologic and traumatic conditions of the brain and spine and can lead to muscle contracture, joint stiffness, reduced range of movement, skin breakdown, and pain. The management of spasticity includes a range of pharmacologic and nonpharmacologic interventions, often used in combination to optimize outcomes. However, it is important to identify and prioritize the patient's and clinician's goals, to create common attainable goals. These goals should be reviewed and revised at regular intervals.

Treatment of pathologic muscle overactivity associated with upper motor neuron syndrome can be multifaceted. One of the initial decisions to be made when formulating an overarching treatment plan is selecting a combination of strategies that is most applicable. Strategies may include physical interventions, such as stretching or splinting modalities, or surgery, whereas pharmacotherapeutic strategies encompass oral/systemic medications as well as agents, such as toxins and alcohols, used for focal chemodenervation. This article reviews the oral/systemic therapies as well as toxins that are used focally. Although medication can also be administered via intra-thecal pumps, this treatment approach is discussed elsewhere.

Steven Escaldi

 Video content accompanies this article at http://www.pmr.theclinics.com.

The key to the successful treatment of patients with spasticity is contin-gent on choosing appropriate interventions tailored to meet the needs, goals, and specific presentation of each patient. For the clinician attempt-ing to address the focal manifestations of hypertonia without surgical intervention, there have been 2 primary options: neurolysis or chemode-nervation. Before the introduction of the botulinum toxins, neurolysis was the only focal spasticity treatment option available to the previous gener-ation of physical medicine and rehabilitation practitioners.

Kimberly Miczak and Joseph Padova

The role of the physical or occupational therapist in addressing muscle hy-perexcitability is to carefully assess the implications that the abnormal tone has on function, especially active movement patterns. A thorough evalua-tion that includes neurologic and nonneurologic attributes allows the clini-cian to determine the most efficacious treatment interventions, especially when considering severity and chronicity of deficits. A holistic assessment that includes patient factors and resources guides the clinician's plan of care to allow for optimal functional outcomes.

Michael Saulino

Intrathecal baclofen therapy is a well-established technique for spasticity management. This article briefly reviews the pharmacology of intrathecal baclofen as well as customary approach for utilization of this targeted drug delivery concept. Following these descriptions, four unusual presentations are described, including the need for initial trialing, patient-directed boluses during chronic intrathecal baclofen therapy, use of medications other than baclofen for intrathecal therapy in spastic patients, and intraventricular bac-lofen delivery. These hypothetical cases are provided in an effort to expand the use of targeted drug delivery to larger population of spastic patients.

Peter J. Madsen, Han-Chiao Isaac Chen, and Shih-Shan Lang

Neurosurgery has long had a role in the treatment of disorders of muscle hyperactivity. This article discusses the use of selective peripheral neuro-tomy for the treatment of focal and multifocal spasticity, selective dorsal rhizotomy for alleviation of more generalized spasticity most often in the setting of cerebral palsy, dorsal root entry zone lesioning for cases of severe spasticity in a nonfunctioning limb, and deep brain stimulation for the treatment of dystonia. For each procedure, relevant pathophysiology and basic surgical anatomy and technique are addressed. In addition, relevant aspects of patient selection, efficacy data, and complications of these procedures are discussed.

Upper motor neuron disease or injury can lead to muscle spasticity or nonfunction throughout the body. Imbalance in muscle forces predisposes patients to development of functional deficiencies, contractures, pain, and poor hygiene. The approach to neuro-orthopedic patients is by necessity multidisciplinary, because a variety of nonsurgical and surgical options are available. In evaluating each patient, surgeons must consider the extent and quality of any deformity, potential for improvement in function, the ability to alleviate pain, and potential for improvement in hygiene and cosmesis. Surgical techniques include tendon lengthenings, releases, transfers, osteotomies, and bony fusions.

Consequences of an upper motor neuron syndrome (UMNS) include voluntary weakness or *paresis*, superimposed involuntary phenomena such as spastic cocontraction and associated reactions, and superimposed rheologic changes in affected muscles. This article describes the use of dynamic polyelectromyography to assess UMNS muscle overactivity and inform muscle selection for chemodenervation. Cases that involve spastic cocontraction, spastic dystonia, associated reactions, hyperextended wrist and finger flexor tenodesis, differentiating neural versus nonneural (rheologic) hypertonia, upper motor neuron weakness, muscle selection for chemodenervation, and electrical stimulation for muscle specific targeting are presented.

Lower limb dysfunction associated with upper motor neuron syndrome can be complex owing to interaction of muscle overactivity, weakness, impaired motor control, and contracture. Treatment should be goal directed and address the patient's passive and active functional impairments in addition to their symptoms. Therefore, a comprehensive, multidisciplinary team approach tailored to each patient's unique needs and functional goals is warranted. This article reviews the evaluation and management of issues related to lower limb muscle overactivity and how this approach was applied to 3 challenging cases.

Spasticity develops as a result of central nervous system injury; however, secondary changes within the muscles and connective tissue also contribute to muscle stiffness. The hyaluronan hypothesis postulates that the accumulation of hyaluronan promotes the development of muscle stiffness. Intramuscular injections of the enzyme hyaluronidase, which hydrolyzes long-chained hyaluronan polymers to smaller polymers, was shown to reduce muscle stiffness and increase passive and active range of motion in patients with spasticity. These results provide preliminary evidence of the hyaluronan hypothesis and suggest an emerging therapy to reduce muscle stiffness using the enzyme hyaluronidase.

# PHYSICAL MEDICINE AND REHABILITATION CLINICS OF NORTH AMERICA

## FORTHCOMING ISSUES

*November 2018*
**Value-Added Electrodiagnostics**
Karen Barr and Ileana M. Howard, *Editors*

*February 2019*
**Polytrauma Rehabilitation**
Blessen C. Eapen and David X. Cifu, *Editors*

*May 2019*
**Technological Advances in Rehabilitation**
Joel Stein and Leroy R. Lindsay, *Editors*

## RECENT ISSUES

*May 2018*
**Para and Adapted Sports Medicine**
Yetsa A. Tuakli-Wosornu and Wayne Derman, *Editors*

*February 2018*
**Interventional Spice Procedures**
Carlos E. Rivera, *Editor*

*November 2017*
**Promoting Health and Wellness in the Geriatric Patient**
David A. Soto-Quijano, *Editor*

---

### RELATED INTEREST

*Neurologic Clinics,* May 2018 (Vol. 2, Issue 4)
**Neuromuscular Junction Disorders**
Mazen M. Dimachkie and Richard J. Barohn, *Editors*
Available at https://www.neurologic.theclinics.com/

---

**VISIT THE CLINICS ONLINE!**
Access your subscription at:
www.theclinics.com

# Erratum

An error was made in the May 2017 issue of *Physical and Medicine and Rehabilitation Clinics* (Volume 28, Issue 2) in the article, "Chronic Traumatic Encephalopathy: Known Causes, Unknown Effects," by Diego Iacono, Sharon B. Shively, Brian L. Edlow, and Daniel P. Perl.

The Figure 2 legend on page 306 should read, "Fig. 2. Histopathologic appearance of a case of CTE in a 66-year-old former professional American football player, A-F. (A) Hemispheric section showing severe abnormal tau deposition (NFTs) in amygdala, parahippocampal cortex, and insular cortex (AT8/cresyl violet immunostain). (B) Severe hippocampal and parahippocampal abnormal tau (NFTs) accumulation. (C) High-power photomicrograph of NFTs in neocortex (AT-8 immunostain). (D) Insular cortex showing severe layer II/III NFT formation (AT-8/cresyl violet immunostain). (E) Higher power view of D. (F) Electron microscopy details of hippocampal NFT showing (arrows) paired helical filaments (ultrastructural appearance of an NFT). (*Courtesy of Ann McKee, MD, Boston University School of Medicine*.)"

The authors gratefully thank Dr. Ann McKee for sharing the histologic slides from this case of CTE, as well as tissue samples from which they prepared the electron micrograph.

The online version of the article has been corrected.

# Foreword

# Let's Get the Train Back on the Tracks

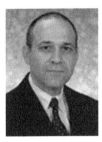

Santos F. Martinez, MD, MS
*Consulting Editor*

We have become a society with a fixation on efficiency, where each task is expected to carry on a predictable and synchronized sequence. What happens, however, when the train no longer follows the conductor's commands? This is the scenario of this issue of *Physical Medicine and Rehabilitation Clinics of North America*, where a host of medical and neurologic conditions have robbed one's ability to control mobility, resulting in considerable functional limitations. Through a sensitive, well-informed approach, the rehabilitation specialist utilizes the time-proven, multidisciplinary approach: utilizing the talents of a team provides a better solution than can be achieved by any single individual.

The practitioner's perception of the perceived challenge is the critical entry point, whether this be detected through the patient's history, physical examination, or functional assessment. Such perception may be obtained by an auditory clue, a visual or palpable perception, or more sophisticated tools such as peripheral electromyographic or gait laboratory resources. This basic interpretation provides the foundation for all our treatment modalities, whether the solution be noninvasive or surgical in nature. It is hoped that we can fine tune the body's motor control circuitry to assist mobility and control in a more predictable fashion, in order to yield a satisfactory outcome for the patient and their family.

I would like to thank Dr Segal and the authors, who carried us through this process and reacquainted the reader with some underutilized traditional approaches, and brought us to date with more current novel treatment options. I would like to thank

Moss Rehabilitation for spearheading this issue, and the decades' long tradition of providing a fertile climate for educating future leaders in our field.

Santos F. Martinez, MD, MS
American Academy of Physical
Medicine and Rehabilitation
Campbell Clinic Orthopaedics
Department of Orthopaedics
University of Tennessee
Memphis, TN 38104, USA

*E-mail address:*
smartinez@campbellclinic.com

# Preface

# Muscle Over-Activity in Upper Motor Neuron Syndrome: Assessment and Problem Solving for Complex Cases

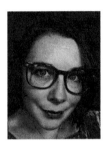

Miriam Segal, MD
*Editor*

It is a great pleasure and an honor to serve as guest editor of *Physical Medicine and Rehabilitation Clinics of North America*. Muscle overactivity results in a great number and variety of functional problems faced by our patients with upper motor neuron syndrome. As physiatrists, managing these problems has long been an integral part of our practice. Most of us are comfortable in the evaluation and treatment of problems related to muscle overactivity, whether it be the stroke patient with gait dysfunction, the child with cerebral palsy with skin compromise, the brain injury patient unable to open the hand, or the spinal cord injury patient with problematic spasms. We routinely manage these issues, and for the sake of convenience, our casual parlance involves known misnomers, such as "spasticity," in reference to all types of muscle overactivity. This issue was titled deliberately, in order to evoke a step back from this language of convenience and broad generalizations and encourage more thoughtful and precise descriptions of phenomena which we observe.

The objective of this issue is not to provide a general overview or an exhaustive review of the various phenomena of muscle overactivity seen in the upper motor neuron syndrome, but rather to discuss important and novel facets within this topic. We start with a discussion of the different phenomena of muscle overactivity and their underlying pathophysiology. This provides some of the foundation for discussions of how to focus our view of problems related to muscle overactivity in different disease states and conditions. The authors were encouraged to discuss difficult cases that required more sophisticated problem solving in order to give the reader more nuanced

Phys Med Rehabil Clin N Am 29 (2018) xvii–xviii
https://doi.org/10.1016/j.pmr.2018.05.001
1047-9651/18/© 2018 Published by Elsevier Inc.

pmr.theclinics.com

perceptions of what may be the presenting functional problem. We then proceed to unpack the toolbox of treatment options, including some new and emerging therapies.

It is my hope that the reader will take away from this issue a more thoughtful understanding of the phenomena of muscle overactivity, what is causing them, how they are impacting function, and how to approach treatment.

Miriam Segal, MD
MossRehab
Einstein Medical Center
60 Township Line Road
Elkins Park, PA 19027, USA

*E-mail address:*
segalmir@einstein.edu

# Muscle Overactivity in the Upper Motor Neuron Syndrome: Pathophysiology

Miriam Segal, MD

## KEYWORDS

- Spasticity • Muscle over-activity • Upper motor neuron syndrome • Hypertonia

## KEY POINTS

- The positive signs of the upper motor neuron syndrome, including spasticity, all involve muscle overactivity. Of these, some are stretch medicated and some are not—the so-called efferent" phenomena.
- The positive signs, including spasticity, clonus, flexor and extensor spasms, associated reactions, cocontraction and spastic dystonia, do not necessarily co-occur and may vary in their pathophysiology.
- Muscle activity is modulated by descending motor pathways, both inhibitory and excitatory.
- Muscle overactivity in the upper motor neuron syndrome results from abnormal signal processing in the spinal cord because of altered supraspinal inputs and/or dysfunction of segmental spinal modulation.
- Rheologic features of the upper motor neuron syndrome involve changes in the physical properties of muscle and can also affect and be affected by weakness and hypertonia.

## INTRODUCTION: ALL THAT GLISTENS IS NOT GOLD; ALL THAT CONTRACTS IS NOT SPASTICITY

Patients with upper motor neuron (UMN) syndrome often develop abnormal patterns of muscle activity as expressed clinically is negative signs (muscle underactivity) and positive signs (muscle overactivity). Although negative signs underlie clinical paresis of voluntary movement, positive signs present as a variety of involuntary phenomena, the most familiar of which are spastic stretch reflex behaviors. In day-to-day practice, clinicians often used the term, *spasticity*, as a catch-all term to describe the overlapping phenomena of muscle overactivity that is observed in patients with UMN syndrome.

---

Disclosure Statement: The author has nothing to disclose.
Physical Medicine and Rehabilitation, Brain Injury Medicine Fellowship, Drucker Brain Injury Center, MossRehab, Albert Einstein Medical Center, 60 Township Line Road, Elkins Park, PA 19027, USA
*E-mail address:* segalmir@einstein.edu

Phys Med Rehabil Clin N Am 29 (2018) 427–436
https://doi.org/10.1016/j.pmr.2018.04.005

The term, spasticity, however, is defined narrowly as "velocity dependent increase in tonic stretch reflexes with exaggerated tendon jerks, resulting from hyperexcitability of the stretch reflex, as one component of the upper motor neuron syndrome."[1] This definition only applies to a subset of the phenomena to which the term, spasticity, is often casually applied. These phenomena are perhaps more accurately discussed as the so-called positive features of the UMN syndrome. Pitfalls exist with this language as well, because it groups mechanistically different phenomena together that do not necessarily co-occur and may vary with respect to treatment. Additionally, this also implies that all of these features result directly from dysfunction of the upper motor neuron or pyramidal tracts. This is not entirely the case, because the pathology can have a much broader basis, from circuits which modulate the pyramidal tracts to plastic changes in the spinal reflex circuitry as well as pathologic changes in muscles themselves.[2,3] Semantics aside, in this article, the term, *muscle overactivity*, is preferred to understand and describe the presentation of the UMN within a larger pathophysiologic context.

## CHARACTERISTICS OF THE UPPER MOTOR NEURON SYNDROME

Characteristics of the UMN syndrome have been described in terms of the duality of negative and positive signs but some investigators have also suggested that changes in the viscoelastic properties of muscle, also known as rheologic changes, should be considered a third sign[4] (**Table 1**). This article focuses primarily on the positive signs, which all involve increased muscle activity and mostly involve exaggerated spinal reflexes. The negative, positive, and rheologic signs, however, interact with one another, often in a perpetuating manner.[2,5]

### Spasticity

As defined by Lance in 1980 (see above), spasticity refers to a velocity dependent increase in the tonic stretch reflex.[1] At velocities used to test tone in normal, relaxed muscle, tonic stretch reflexes do not contribute to muscle tone but rather tone is generated by the viscoelastic properties of muscle. In contrast, muscles of hemiparetic stroke patients demonstrate electromyographic activity in linear proportion to the stretch velocity imposed.[6] Of note however, spasticity is also a length dependent phenomenon, with a tendency toward an increase at longer lengths in the lower extremity and at shorter lengths in the upper extremity.[7-9] It has also been shown that there is an interaction between the length and velocity variables. For example, the

| Table 1 Characteristics of the upper motor neuron syndrome | |
| --- | --- |
| **Negative** | **Positive** |
| Weakness | Hyperreflexia and reflex irradiation |
| Loss of Dexterity | Clonus |
| Fatigue | Spasticity |
| Impaired motor planning | Positive babinski and other primitive reflexes |
| Impaired motor control | Extensor spasms |
| | Flexor spasms |
| | Positive support reaction |
| | Co-contraction |
| | Associated reactions (Sykinesis) |
| | Spastic dystonia |

finger flexors show greater velocity dependence at longer lengths and increased dependence on length at faster stretches.[9]

## Clonus

Clonus is a rhythmic contraction which can be seen electromyographically as alternating bursts of activity alternating between flexors and extensors. It is generated by a rapid stretch and hold of a muscle group.[5] While it has been suggested that the eliciting and maintaining of clonus lies in the skill and technique of the examiner,[10] clonus may be triggered during a voluntary movement or by various cutaneous stimuli.[5] Clonus and spasticity are considered a result of increased "gain" of the stretch reflex.[11] Gain modulation is defined as a change in the sensitivity of a neuronal response to one set of inputs that depends on the activity of a second set of inputs.[12]

## Flexion Withdrawal/Flexor Spasms

The various sensory afferents involved in the flexion withdrawal reflex are referred to as flexor reflex afferents (FRAs) and transmit touch, pressure, temperature and pain.[3] Activation of these polysynaptic reflexes excites flexor and inhibits extensor motor neurons.[10] A good case has been made for supraspinal modulation of these reflexes and in the UMN syndrome they are exaggerated and desynchronized.[13] Patients with UMN syndrome can exhibit flexor spasms that can at times appear without any apparent stimulus, but we can attribute these to occult stimuli such as pressure ulcers or visceral distention.[14]

## Extensor Reflexes/Extensor Spasms

These can be stimulated by cutaneous stimulation of the groin, buttock and posterior leg as well as proprioceptive input from the hip.[3] The flexor withdrawal response sometimes involves contralateral extension. It should be mentioned that an extensor posture can sometimes offer a functional advantage in the lower limbs for stability in weight bearing.

## Associated Reactions

This has also been referred to as synkinesia, and refers to the involuntary activity in one limb that is, associated with a voluntary movement effort made in the other limbs,[3,5] for example, flexion of the elbow with walking. These types of reactions can also occur with automatic activity such as yawning and sneezing. One theory, is that associated reactions are due to a disinhibited spread of voluntary motor activity into a limb affected by the UMN syndrome.[5] The specific mechanism has not been elucidated but is believed to be supraspinally mediated.[3]

## Co-contraction

In healthy individuals, simultaneous activation of agonist and antagonist muscles can act on a joint to increase stiffness in response to, or in preparation for, environmental instabilities or to stabilize a joint for tasks requiring a high degree of accuracy.[15] In this sense, co-contraction is normal and beneficial. Being able to modulate the amount of co-activation helps us respond to changes in environmental mechanics, to catch a ball for example, Pathologic or dysfunctional co-contraction is seen as a part of the UMN syndrome, usually with spastic dystonia.[3] In such patients, contraction and hence shortening of an agonist muscle can generate stretch and consequently elicit a hyperactive stretch reflex in its antagonist, this may appear grossly like co-contraction. We should distinguish this from actual co-contraction which by definition is *simultaneous* contraction of agonists and antagonist muscles. This can be extremely difficult to perceive grossly, particularly in the context of spasticity and rheologic changes. The timing of agonist/antagonist contraction can be discerned using electromyography.[5] In the UMN syndrome, pathologic co-contraction is thought to result from circumstances which lead to impairment of Ia reciprocal inhibition in the spinal cord.[3] This pathology may originate from dysregulation of supraspinal and other segmental inputs.[3] From both animal and human studies, it has been suggested that there is a separate population of co-contraction specific corticospinal neurons in the motor cortex.[16–18] Others have proposed an oligosynaptic descending pathway that diverges at segmental levels to innervate agonist–antagonist pairs.[19] Both lines of evidence are suggestive of an alternative descending control strategy from supraspinal centers to facilitate movements requiring co-contraction. There is some debate regarding the degree to which dysfunction of co-contraction contributes to impaired volitional movement in the UMN syndrome.[3]

### Dystonia

This term has evolved since it was first introduced in 1911 by German neurologist Hermann Oppenheim.[20] In 2013, an international panel proposed a revised definition: "Dystonia is a movement disorder characterized by sustained or intermittent muscle contractions causing abnormal, often repetitive, movements, postures, or both. Dystonic movements are typically patterned, twisting, and may be tremulous. Dystonia is often initiated or worsened by voluntary action and associated with overflow muscle activation."[21] While dystonia syndromes can occur in a variety of conditions, in the context of the UMN syndrome, we primarily focus on spastic dystonia as described by Denny-Brown as a 'persistent posture maintained by muscular contraction'.[22] He examined the postural reactions of monkeys after cortical ablations and, using emg, he demonstrated the continuous nature of the muscle contraction involved in maintaining these postures. By transecting the dorsal roots and finding that the phenomenon was unchanged, he also showed that this was not dependent on sensory afferent input at the level of the spinal reflexes.[22] In Nathaniel Mayer's article of this edition, he refers to UMN dystonia as activity of a muscle "at rest" that is, no triggering stretch reflex, no voluntary effort, no sensory trigger or other obvious trigger, again reflecting Denny-Brown's work that this continuous muscle contraction was caused by cortical damage and was not abolished by dorsal root section. This is why spastic dystonia is often described as an efferent phenomenon.[3,22] As a side note however, spastic dystonia is sensitive to stretch, and prolonged stretching can reduce it.[3,22]

## SUPRASPINAL INFLUENCES ON MUSCLE TONE

The descending motor pathways occupy a large amount of real estate, not only because large amount of cortex is occupied by the motor areas but also due to the fact that the motor pathways extend from the cortex to the spinal cord (**Fig. 1**). As a result, injury to these pathways is common.[23] Often, we think of injuries to the descending motor pathways as involving the pyramidal tracts, the main conduit of motor control, but *isolated* lesions of the pyramidal tract fibers, from the primary motor cortex (Brodmann's area 4), cerebral peduncle, basis pontis, medullary pyramids, all the way to the lateral corticospinal tract do not actually result in "spasticity". If they are truly focal and limited just to these areas, these lesions result in weakness and hypotonia.[24] Spasticity is produced when lesions extend further out to involve fibers of or originating from the premotor cortex, Brodmann's area 6.[3] These fibers travel near the pyramidal tracts and have been referred to as para-pyramidal.[3]

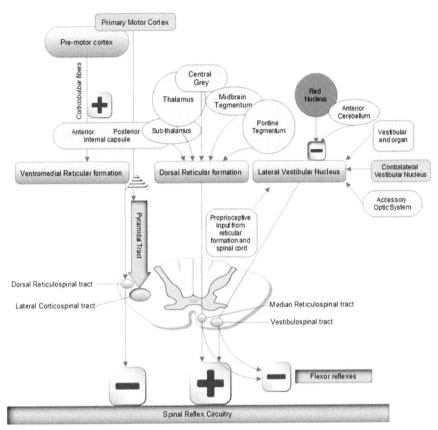

**Fig. 1.** Supraspinal influences on the spinal reflex circuitry.

An important inhibitory system arises in the premotor cortex, where these "para-pyramidal" fibers project to the *ventromedial reticular formation* which descends via the *dorsal reticulospinal tract* in the dorsolateral funiculus in close proximity to the lateral corticospinal tract.[3] This inhibitory pathway travels in anatomic parallel to the pyramidal pathway. Stimulation of the ventromedial reticular formation, which lies immediately behind the pyramids, results in suppression of muscle activity, including stretch reflex activity.[2] As one can imagine, lesions of this pathway result in exaggerated stretch reflex and muscle activity by virtue of the loss of inhibition.

In contrast to this inhibitory system, an excitatory system (see **Fig. 1**) exists which does not appear to originate in the motor areas or get very much cortical input but rather a broad variety of subcortical inputs, including the subthalamus, thalamus, and central gray, pontine and midbrain tegmentum.[25] These project to the *dorsal reticular formation*, descending in the spinal cord as the *median reticulospinal tract* in the ventromedial cord.[25] Through early animal studies involving stimulation and lesioning of these areas, we have come to understand that this pathway is a facilitator of muscle tone and spinal stretch reflexes, but at the same time an *inhibitor* of flexor reflexes and spasms.[25]

Originating in the *lateral vestibular nucleus* (also known as Deiter's nucleus) and traveling in the ventral spinal cord as the *lateral vestibulospinal tract*, is another excitatory pathway, acting on alpha and gamma motor neurons associated with muscles of the antigravity extensor system in the proximal limbs.[21,22] The lateral vestibular nucleus receives inhibitory inputs from the red nucleus and anterior cerebellum, which when lesioned, result in decerebrate posturing.[26] Afferent input is also received from bilateral vestibular end organs, accessory optic system, contralateral vestibular nucleus as well as proprioceptive feedback from the spinal cord and reticular formation.[27] Parenthetically, there is also an analogous medial vestibulospinal tract which arises from the medial vestibular nucleus and has a similar role in the neck and trunk musculature.[26] Similarly, to the medial reticulospinal tract, the vestibulospinal pathway is generally excitatory but *inhibits* flexor reflex afferents.[25] Some authors have suggested that the vestibulospinal pathways only play a minor role in maintaining spastic hypertonia.[2,3,25] This is based on the finding that isolated lesions of the lateral vestibular nucleus had little effect on spasticity in cats but did enhance the effects of bulbopontine tegmentum (medial reticulospinal tract) lesions[3,25] and that lesions of the vestibulospinal tracts performed to decrease spasticity had only a temporary effect.[3] More recently however, the importance of vestibulospinal pathways in spastic hypertonia has reemerged.[28–30]

Because of all of this, cerebral lesions which damage the corticobulbar fibers originating in the premotor cortex tend to result in spasticity due to resultant loss of descending inhibitory stimulus from the ventromedial reticular formation. This includes lesions of the anterior limb of the internal capsule were these fibers travel. Keep in mind that isolated lesions of the pyramidal fibers, including lesions of the *posterior* limb of the internal capsule where pyramidal tract fibers are fairly segregated, do not result in spasticity. In the spinal cord, incomplete injuries which involve the dorsal reticulospinal tract but spare the more ventral reticulospinal and vestibulospinal tracts result in spasticity with a predominating extensor pattern as the intact ventral excitatory pathways still exert inhibitory influence on the flexor reflexes. In the case of complete spinal cord lesions however, this inhibition of the flexors is lost as well and flexor spasm can predominate.[3]

## SPINAL SEGMENTAL INFLUENCES ON MUSCLE TONE
### Ia Presynaptic Inhibition

This involves the modulation of the monosynaptic reflex between Ia afferents from muscle spindles and alpha motoneuron efferent neurons. Release of neurotransmitter at the Ia afferent pre-synaptic terminal is inhibited by GABA mediated, axo-axonal connections with Ia afferent collaterals from the same and other muscles[31] (**Fig. 2**). While corticospinal and cutaneous influences have been demonstrated, modulation of presynaptic inhibition is not well understood.[32] Additionally, while it has been shown that presynaptic inhibition of Ia afferents is reduced in spastic limbs[33,34] it is unclear how significantly this contributes overall to the clinical picture of hypertonia in the UMN syndrome.

### Post Synaptic Inhibition

#### Ia reciprocal inhibition
This occurs when Ia afferents inhibit alpha motor neurons of antagonist muscles by means of a Ia inhibitory interneuron in a disynaptic pathway.[24] Impaired reciprocal inhibition is thought to be the underlying cause of pathologic co-contraction.[3]

#### Ib non-reciprocal inhibition
Ib afferents from the muscle's golgi tendon organ act on the alpha motoneuron in a diasynaptic pathway involving Ib interneurons. This mechanism acts to inhibit

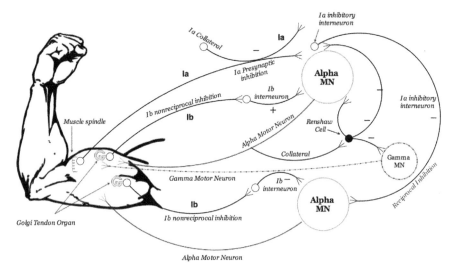

**Fig. 2.** Spinal segmental influences.

extensor and excite flexor motoneurons, therefore dysfunction or reduction in this mechanism would serve to favor extensor tone.[3]

### Renshaw cell inhibition

Alpha motoneuron collaterals synapse onto renshaw cells which then send inhibitory projections back to the alpha motoneuron (recurrent inhibition) preventing excessive output[35] hence serving as modulators of alpha motoneuron excitability. They also synapse with the associated gamma motoneuron and Ia interneuron responsible for reciprocal inhibition of the antagonist.[36] Renshaw cells may be considered components of a system uniting alpha motoneurons of a pool into a synergy, stabilizing the output of the pool.[36] Renshaw cell activity is influenced by descending motor pathways but the its role in the upper motor neuron syndrome is uncertain.[3]

### Post Activation Depression

This term refers to the reduction of neurotransmitter release from Ia afferents with repetitive activation.[37] In contrast to presynaptic inhibition, this is an intrinsic property of the Ia afferent neuron and has also been referred to as homosynaptic post activation depression.[37] This is independent of supraspinal control. A reduction of post activation depression has been demonstrated in patients with spasticity of various etiologies and is strongly correlated to the severity of spasticity.[38,39] There is also strong evidence that this reduction in post activation depression occurs as a result of limb immobilization (caused by negative features of UMN syndrome) and that exercise can help to mitigate this.[2,40,41] A recent study by Kawashi and colleagues[40] demonstrated that post activation depression can be partially normalized after rehabilitation in patients with subacute stroke.

## BIOLMECHANICAL INFLUENCES ON MUSCLE TONE

Changes in the viscoelastic properties of muscle that is, rheologic changes, can increase muscle tone independent of stretch reflexes.[3] This may be difficult to discern clinically, especially when biomechanical (non-reflex) hypertonia and neural hypertonia exist together, but since the treatments are different, it is an important distinction. Biomechanical hypertonia is best addressed with mechanical treatments such as stretching, splinting and casting.[3] Perhaps the most evident of the rheologic signs is contracture. The term contracture refers to physical shortening of muscle length, and it is often accompanied by physical shortening of other soft tissues such as fascia, nerves, blood vessels, and skin.[42] The treatment for contracture is often surgical. As mentioned above, the negative, positive and rheologic features of the UMN syndrome are all intimately related and perpetuate each other in many ways.[2–5,23]

## REFERENCES

1. Lance J. The control of muscle tone, reflexes, and movement: Robert Wartenberg lecture. Neurology 1980;30:1303–13.

2. Trompetto C, Marinelli L, Peosin E, et al. Pathophysiology of spasticity: implications for neurorehabilitation. Biomed Res Int 2014;2014:354906.

3. Sheean G. Neurophysiology of spasticity. In: Barnes MP, Johnson GR, editors. Upper motor neurone syndrome and spasticity clinical management and neurophysiology. 2nd edition. New York: Cambridge University Press; 2008.

4. Mayer NH. Clinicophysiologic concepts of spasticity and motor dysfunction in adults with an upper motoneuron lesion. Muscle Nerve Suppl 1997;6:S1–13.

5. Mayer NH, Herman RM. Phenomenology of muscle overactivity in the upper motor neuron syndrome. Eura Medicophys 2004;40(2):85–110.

6. Thilmann AF, Fellows SJ, Garms E. The mechanism of spastic muscle hypertonus. Variation in reflex gain over the time course of spasticity. Brain 1991;114:233–44.

7. Meinders M, Price R, Lehmann JF, et al. The stretch reflex response in the normal and spastic ankle: effect of ankle position. Arch Phys Med Rehabil 1996;77:487–92.

8. Burke D, Gillies JD, Lance JW. The quadriceps stretch reflex in human spasticity. J Neurol Neurosurg Psychiatry 1970;33:216–23.

9. Li S, Kamper DG, Rymer WZ. Effects of changing wrist positions on finger flexor hypertonia in stroke survivors. Muscle Nerve 2006;33:183–90.

10. Burke D. Spasticity as an adaptation to pyramidal tract injury. In: Waxman SG, editor. Functional recovery in neurological disease (Advances in neurology), vol. 47. New York: Raven Press; 1988. p. 401–23.

11. Rack PMH, Ross HF, Thilmann AF. The ankle stretch reflexes in normal and spastic subjects: the response to sinusoidal movement. Brain 1984;107:637–54.

12. Brozovic M, Abbot LF, Andersen RA. Mechanism of gain modulation at single neuron and network levels. J Comput Neurosci 2008;25:158–68.

13. Meinck HM, Benecke R, Conrad B. Spasticity and the flexor reflex. In: Delwaide PJ, Young RR, editors. Clinical neurophysiology in spasticity. Amsterdam: Elsevier Science Publishers; 1985. p. 39–54.

14. Whitlock JA. Neurophysiology of spasticity. In: Glen MB, Whyte J, editors. The practical management of spasticity in children and adults. Philadelphia: Lea and Febiger; 1990. p. 8–33.

15. Lewis GN, MacKinnon CD, Trumbower R, et al. Co-contraction modifies the stretch reflex elicited in muscles shortened by a joint perturbation. Exp Brain Res 2010;207(1–2):39–48.

16. Humphrey DR, Reed DJ. Separate cortical systems for control of joint movement and joint stiffness: reciprocal activation and co-activation of antagonist muscles. Adv Neurol 1983;39:347–72.
17. Nielsen J, Kagamihara Y. The regulation of presynaptic inhibition during co-contraction of antagonistic muscles in man. J Physiol 1993;464:575–93.
18. Johannsen P, Christensen LO, Sinkjær T, et al. Cerebral functional anatomy of voluntary contractions of ankle muscles in man. J Physiol 2001;535:397–406.
19. Humphrey DR. Separate cell systems in the motor cortex of the monkey for the control of joint movement and of joint stiffness. Electroencephalogr Clin Neurophysiol 1982;36:393–408.
20. Newby RE, Thorpe DE, Kempster PA, et al. A history of dystonia: ancient to modern. Mov Disord Clin Pract 2017;4:478–85.
21. Albanese A, Bhatia K, Bressman SB, et al. Phenomenology and classification of dystonia: a consensus update. Mov Disord 2013;28(7):863–73.
22. Mayer NH. Spasticity and other signs of the upper motor neuron syndrome. In: Brashear A, editor. Spasticity diagnosis and management. New York: Demos Medical Publishing; 2011. p. 17–32. McGuire JR.
23. Purves D, Augustine GJ, Fitzpatrick D, et al. Damage to descending motor pathways: the upper motor neuron syndrome. In: Purves D, Augustine GJ, Fitzpatrick D, et al, editors. Neuroscience. 2nd edition. Sunderland (MA): Sinauer Associates; 2001.
24. Mukherjee A, Chakravarty A. Spasticity mechanisms – for the clinician. Front Neurol 2010;1:149.
25. Brown P. Pathophysiology of spasticity. J Neurol Neurosurg Psychiatry 1994; 57(7):773–7.
26. Felten DL, O'Banion MK, Maida MS. Chapter 15: motor systems. In: Netter FH, Perkins JA, Carlos AG, et al, editors. Netter's atlas of neuroscience. 3rd edition. Philadelphia: Elsevier; 2016. p. 402.
27. Cornell BD, Musallam S. Vestibulospinal system and eye-head/neck movement. In: Squire LR, Bloom FE, Spitzer NC, et al, editors. Encyclopedia of neuroscience. 1st edition. Oxford (OK): Academic Press; 2009. p. 147–54.
28. Miller DM, Rymer WZ. Sound-evoked biceps myogenic potentials reflect asymmetric vestibular drive to spastic muscles in chronic hemiparetic stroke survivors. Front Hum Neurosci 2017;11:535.
29. Miller DM, Baker JF, Rymer WZ. Ascending vestibular drive is asymmetrically distributed to the inferior oblique motoneuron pools in a subset of hemispheric stroke survivors. Clin Neurophysiol 2016;127:2022–30.
30. Miller DM, Klein CS, Suresh NL, et al. Asymmetries in vestibular evoked myogenic potentials in chronic stroke survivors with spastic hypertonia: evidence for a vestibulospinal role. Clin Neurophysiol 2014;125:2070–8.
31. Iles JF. Evidence for cutaneous and corticospinal modulation of presynaptic inhibition of Ia afferents from the human lower limb. J Physiol 1996;491(Pt 1): 197–207.
32. Rudomin P, Schmidt RF. Presynaptic inhibition in the vertebral spinal cord revisited. Exp Brain Res 1999;129(1):1–37.
33. Iles JF, Roberts RC. Presynaptic inhibition of monosynaptic reflexes in the lower limbs of subjects with upper motoneuron disease. J Neurol Neurosurg Psychiatry 1986;49(8):937–44.
34. Morita H, Crone C, Christenhuis D, et al. Modulation of presynaptic inhibition and disynaptic reciprocal Ia inhibition during voluntary movement in spasticity. Brain 2001;124:826–37.

35. Fahn S, Janovic J. Principles and practice of movement disorders. Motor control [Chapter 2]. 2nd edition. Churchil Livingstone; 2011.

36. Latash ML. Fundamentals of motor control. Neurophysiological Structures [Chapter 10]. Academic Press; 2012. p. 176–8.

37. Hultborn H, Illert M, Nielsen J, et al. On the mechanism of the post-activation depression of the H-reflex in human subjects. Exp Brain Res 1996;108:450–62.

38. Lamy JC, Wargon I, Mazevet D, et al. Impaired efficacy of spinal presynaptic mechanisms in spastic stroke patients. Brain 2009;132(3):734–48.

39. Achache V, Roche N, Lamy JC, et al. Transmission within several spinal pathways in adults with cerebral palsy. Brain 2012;133(5):1470–83.

40. Kawaishi Y, Matsumoto N, Nishiwaki T, et al. Postactivation depression of soleus H-reflex increase with recovery of lower extremities motor functions in patients with subacute stroke. J Phys Ther Sci 2017;29(9):1539–42.

41. Trompetto C, Marinelli L, Mori L, et al. Postactivation depression changes after robotic-assisted gait training in hemiplegic stroke patients. Gait Posture 2013; 38:729–33.

42. Mayer NH, Esquenazi A. Upper limb skin and musculoskeletal consequences of upper motor neuron syndrome. In: Jankovic J, Albanese A, Atassi MZ, et al, editors. Botulinum toxin. Philadelphia: Saunders; 2009. p. 131–47.

# Meaningful Assessment in Patients with Acquired Brain Injuries

Thomas Watanabe, MD[a,b],*

## KEYWORDS

- Upper motor neuron syndrome • Acquired brain injury • Spasticity • Goal setting
- Physical examination

## KEY POINTS

- Knowledge of the implications of the type and severity of the acquired brain injury is important to developing a treatment strategy for patients with upper motor neuron syndrome (UMNS).
- Spasticity is often not the main factor limiting joint function or range of motion after acquired brain injuries; assessment of other components of the UMNS or other neuromedical complications is essential to optimize outcomes.
- Ongoing access to care must be considered when choosing specific interventions for patients with UMNS.
- Determination of a treatment plan should be based on the identification of relevant and attainable goals, with input from, as appropriate, the rehabilitation team, patients, and families.

Acquired brain injuries (ABIs) take many different clinical forms. Not surprisingly, spasticity, or perhaps more appropriately termed the *upper motor neuron syndrome* (UMNS), also presents in quite a varied fashion in different patients with ABI. Additionally, the clinician must consider other factors when assessing patients with ABI with respect to management of spasticity. This article primarily considers the similarities and differences between traumatic brain injuries (TBIs) and hypoxic-ischemic brain injury (HIBI) when addressing the cause. Relevant objective measures of spasticity and other elements of the UMNS are discussed. The impact of severity, prognosis, and chronicity of the ABI on assessment and treatment planning also needs to be considered. Variables related more specifically to the presentation of spasticity,

Disclosure Statement: The author has nothing to disclose.
[a] MossRehab at Elkins Park, Einstein Healthcare Network, Elkins Park, PA, USA; [b] Department of Physical Medicine and Rehabilitation, Temple University School of Medicine, Philadelphia, PA, USA
* MossRehab at Elkins Park, 60 Township Line Road, Elkins Park, PA 19027.
*E-mail address:* Watanabt@einstein.edu

such as extent, severity, complications that limit function, resources available, and appropriate goals, are also important to consider in the assessment and to formulate a management plan.

## TYPE OF BRAIN INJURY

TBIs may be relatively focal or more diffuse. The extent and location of cerebral injury will affect the presentation of spasticity and its functional implications. HIBI is always diffuse, although certain areas of the brain are more susceptible to hypoxic injury than others, such as the hippocampus, basal ganglia cortex, and cerebellum.[1] HIBI also tends to lead to other movement disorders that might be confused with spasticity but may require significantly different management strategies, such as dystonia, rigidity, ataxia, and myoclonus, although these problems may also be seen after TBIs. Some of these disorders may have a delayed presentation.[2] Of course, patients who sustain TBIs may also have elements of HIBI depending on the complications associated with their traumatic injury. Careful examination including an evaluation of functional activities may help the clinician to differentiate among various movement disorders. When assessing passive range of motion (ROM), rigidity or cogwheeling will present with resistance to ROM that is not velocity dependent. Dystonic movements will be present even in the absence of ranging a joint. Another movement disorder that sometimes is seen after ABIs, especially HIBI, is myoclonus. Myoclonus may worsen with activity or be present at rest. Positive myoclonus results from sudden muscle contractions and may be brought on by stimuli, including movement.[3]

The difference in causes may also affect clinical decision-making because of the effects on long-term prognosis. This concern is especially relevant for patients with more severe injuries. It is known that the likelihood for significant functional recovery is worse for patients with HIBI relative to those with TBIs.[4] The choice of interventions should be based in part on the goals identified. Patients with, for example, disorders of consciousness, will likely benefit more from goals such as ease of passive care rather than more cognitively and motorically complex functional activities. Treatment options based on goals of active function might be favored if the anticipation is that further neurologic recovery is to be expected.

The contrasts in the likelihood of meaningful functional recovery for these two types of ABIs is exemplified by older literature that used the terms *persistent* versus *permanent* vegetative state.[5] Permanence was said to be determined if there was no recovery of consciousness after 3 months in a nontraumatic injury and 12 months after a TBI. One does not, of course, need to wait for these specific time points to guide decisions regarding the types of goals and interventions for spasticity. These definitions help in the description and prognostication of more severe ABIs. Other functional goals will demand different degrees of preservation of cognitive function, and management of the UMNS should be guided to a large degree by the likelihood that patients will have the cognition necessary to achieve such goals. This point is just one of several examples of why spasticity management must be individualized.

## MEASURES OF SPASTICITY AND OTHER ELEMENTS OF UPPER MOTOR NEURON SYNDROME

The UMNS is often described as having positive and negative signs. Positive signs include heightened muscle stretch reflexes, spastic cocontraction, dystonia, and muscle spasms. Negative signs include weakness and loss of selective muscle control.[6] As part of the assessment, it is useful to incorporate measures that quantify some of these elements as a way to characterize the specific patient's condition and to evaluate the efficacy of the treatments rendered. The goal of spasticity management is often not specifically to quantitatively improve results based on scales, but improvement in the scales is often correlated with meaningful clinical outcomes. Such outcomes may be beneficial for patients regardless of their functional level. For example, improvement in passive ROM (PROM) may lead to improved ease of care, increased comfort, and/or functional gains. PROM is usually measured with a goniometer. Strength is another important functional measure and is most commonly assessed using the Medical Research Council Scale for Muscle Strength.[7] Spasticity, classically defined as velocity-dependent resistance to ROM, is most commonly described by using the Modified Ashworth Scale, although this scale actually does not have a velocity-dependent component. Another limitation of this scale is that it is difficult to accurately reproduce the results because of the limb positioning and changes in the soft tissues that may affect both ROM and stiffness. Nevertheless, it has reasonably good inter-rater reliability.[8] An outcome scale that does have a velocity-dependent component is the Tardieu Scale.[9]

Depending on the clinical conditions that are being targeted for intervention, other outcome measures may be useful. Spasms can be quantified using the Penn Spasm Frequency Scale.[10] Quantifying spasms may be clinically relevant, as they often interfere with function and can be uncomfortable. Evidence supporting the ability of standardized functional scales to quantify improvement related to spasticity intervention is lacking.[11] The Disability Assessment Scale, which assesses upper extremity function, has been used to demonstrate efficacy in the management of upper extremity spasticity.[12] The Goal Attainment Scale has also been used to assess treatment effects for patients who have undergone upper extremity spasticity management.[13] In the lower extremity, efficacy of botulinum toxin has been demonstrated quantitatively using measures obtained from gait laboratory analysis.[14]

## NEUROMUSCULOSKELETAL CONDITIONS THAT ARE RELATED TO SPASTICITY

Patients with ABIs often have neuro-medical complications that may lead to loss of function and/or ROM. An important aspect of assessment of patients with ABIs is to consider what conditions other than spasticity may be compromising extremity function. For example, heterotopic ossification (HO) or other orthopedic problems including fractures may be a primary factor in loss of ROM of a joint.[15,16] Radiographs and/or triple-phase bone scan can be considered if either of these complications are suspected. On examination, a warm or swollen joint with a firm end field may suggest HO. A painful joint due to other causes (eg, trauma or infection) may also appear clinically similar to spasticity, as a patient may guard against passive movement of the affected joint.

Hypertonia for patients with ABIs may also occur as part of a condition termed paroxysmal sympathetic hyperactivity. This condition has been referred to by different names over the years, but one of the main features is the presence of increased motor activity, including spasticity, posturing, and/or dystonia.[17] This condition is relevant in the discussion of patient assessment because the accurate diagnosis and treatment is important to prevent many of the complications that are seen with inadequately managed spasticity. Other important clinical features of this syndrome are the paroxysmal nature and evidence of increased sympathetic activity, including elevated heart rate, blood pressure, and temperature.[18] Although this condition presents with aspects of spasticity, management (pharmacologic and nonpharmacologic) is based more on pharmacologic treatment of the sympathetic elements with, for example, propranolol. Noxious stimuli are thought to be triggers, so identifying and eliminating sources of pain or addressing pain pharmacologically with narcotic analgesics is also a common treatment approach. Gabapentin and clonidine are also commonly used. To address the dystonia/hypertonia, dantrolene may also be used.[19] Intrathecal baclofen has also been used for refractory cases.[20]

Lower motor neuron injuries may be present as well. Pressure-induced mononeuropathies, plexopathies, and radiculopathies can all contribute to motor dysfunction, contractures, and pain. Any or all of these complications should be considered depending on the nature of the underlying injury and any preexisting conditions. Spasticity that leads to excessive wrist flexion may predispose patients to carpal tunnel syndrome.[21] Electrodiagnostic studies will aid in the identification of these injuries and provide some information regarding prognosis.

## ASSESSING THE SPASTIC JOINT

Assessment of active joint function is very important for patients who have functional goals. Close observation of motor control in general and the ability to perform specific tasks will also guide the clinician in the determination of what interventions to consider. Although spasticity may be present, the primary barrier to effective movement may be something else, such as weakness, orthopedic/soft tissue restrictions, apraxia, ataxia, sensory deficits, neglect, poor initiation, or movement disorders related to ABIs.[22] A thorough assessment of strength, active and PROM, sensation, and coordination, if possible, is very important. If functional goals are appropriate from a neurologic standpoint, it may important for the treatment team to generate hypotheses regarding what the main barriers are and to establish an evaluation and treatment plan related to determining whether the hypotheses are correct. For example, a trial of carbidopa/levodopa may be indicated if there are features such as freezing or bradykinesia. If efficacy is not noted, the medication dose can be altered or discontinued and another hypothesis tested.

Another challenge when assessing joints with restricted ROM is to determine whether underlying contracture is part of the UMNS. Shortening of muscles and tendons can occur when joints are not regularly stretched. Typically, there is less of a firmness at the limit of ROM compared with orthopedic restrictions, but it is hard to make a determination based on this alone. Diagnostic blocks with an anesthetic agent (eg, bupivacaine) can be useful, as a properly performed nerve block can abolish activity of the muscles in question, effectively eliminating hypertonicity as a cause of the restricted ROM. If orthopedic issues can also be ruled out, then soft tissue contracture would be the most likely cause for the loss of ROM. Response to interventions that provide that provide prolonged passive stretch of the joint, such as serial casting, can also help determine whether soft tissue contracture is present and amenable to nonsurgical intervention. The loss of ROM in the joint may lead to skin maceration or breakdown as well as breakdown of overly stretched skin. Avoiding these complications may provide a rationale for spasticity intervention.

Obtaining an accurate history about any prior functional limitations is also helpful. Patients may have had preexisting arthritis, tendinopathies, or other joint pathology. Trauma or immobility may have worsened these conditions. A review of medications may also be useful, as some medications have side effects that may impact movement, such as dystonia. Examples of such drugs include antipsychotic and anticholinergic medications.

Spasticity may also be of assistance to function at some stages in the recovery process. It is well known that some patients may use their spasticity and that loss of spasticity may contribute to functional weakness. This concern is especially true of lower extremity spasticity, whereby a relatively stiff leg can be used for standing and transfers. Evaluating the functional impact of spasticity is another situation in which diagnostic nerve blocks may be helpful in treatment planning. This is also true regarding intrathecal baclofen therapy, where preimplant trials, including continuous infusion trials with external pumps, may help determine the functional implications of the intervention.[23]

When assessing the function of a joint, consideration must often be given as to how alteration of the position of one joint may affect related joints. One example of this is the interplay between the wrist and finger position. A flexed wrist with flexed fingers is a common pattern of muscle overactivity seen in the upper limb after ABIs. Moving the wrist from a flexed to a more neutral position may worsen the flexion of the fingers, as wrist extension stretches the long finger flexors (tenodesis). Therefore, it may be important to address the muscles of the forearm and hand that are contributing to the excessive finger flexion. One must consider not only the long finger flexors (flexor digitorum superficialis and profundus) but perhaps also the lumbricals and interossei, which are flexors at the metacarpophalangeal joint. Alternatively, correction of excessive wrist extension may lead to a loss of finger flexion power, which may also have functional implications.

## ASSESSMENT IN THE CONTEXT OF RECOVERY

The initial assessment of spasticity should also take into account the anticipated natural history of the ABI. As mentioned previously, some movement disorders may evolve in the subacute period, especially after HIBI. Frank spasticity may also evolve over time, in part because this upper motor neuron process may be dampened by critical illness neuropathy. As the name implies, this lower motor neuron process is typically seen in patients who have several medical complications during their acute hospitalization, especially prolonged mechanical ventilation.[24] Symmetric hypotonicity and depressed muscle stretch reflexes in this clinical context are suggestive of this condition. As patients recover medically, the peripheral nerves and the muscles innervated by the damaged nerves may also recover and then the upper motor neuron condition may predominate.

The trajectory of recovery must be taken into account. Where spasticity is rapidly evolving, shorter-acting interventions or perhaps no intervention may be considered. More expensive (eg, intrathecal baclofen) or longer-term (eg, phenol nerve blocks) should be reserved for cases whereby longer-term problematic spasticity is anticipated.

## CONSIDERATION OF SIDE EFFECTS OF INTERVENTIONS

Patient assessment is also crucial when considering pharmacologic intervention and choice of medication, and some consideration of patient-specific goals is necessary to guide this intervention. Many of the medications used to address spasticity are sedating, which may have a deleterious effect on some but not all patients. Not surprisingly, patients with higher levels of cognition tend to tolerate the cognitively suppressing side effects better than those who are more impaired. At the other end of the spectrum in terms of severity, sedation may not have as much of a negative impact for patients with severe cognitive deficits with less anticipation of neurologic recovery. There may be a role for specific medications based on their side effect profile and the needs of the patients. For example, dantrolene sodium, which decreases the force of muscle contraction, acts peripherally, and may have a better side effect profile regarding cognition. However, it may cause generalized weakness, hindering function in some patients.[25]

Similarly, an evaluation of patients' needs may alter the choice of botulinum toxin. For example, the relatively greater anticholinergic effects of rimabotulinumtoxin B could be used to positive benefit for patients who have significant sialorrhea when treating cervical dystonia.[26] However, if dysphagia is a concern, patients given this serotype of botulinum toxin may be more prone to this complication.[27]

## PSYCHOSOCIAL ASSESSMENT

To effectively manage spasticity for patients with ABIs, a psychosocial evaluation must also be included in the assessment. This evaluation is especially important for long-term planning, especially outside of the acute hospital or acute inpatient rehabilitation levels of care. Many interventions will require follow-up and interventions other than just injections or medication prescription. Patients with intrathecal baclofen pumps must be able to consistently make follow-up appointments for refills to avoid the potentially life-threatening baclofen withdrawal syndrome.[28] They must also have access to specialized care in case of pump malfunction. Focal spasticity management (nerve blocks and botulinum toxin injections) often requires postinjection therapies, which may not be available to some patients based on factors such as relative geographic isolation and barriers related to transportation or cost. Some therapy interventions require a significant amount of expertise and monitoring to avoid complications, for example, serial casting, which may not be available. Lack of insurance coverage or high copays may make aspects of spasticity management financially untenable. Even fairly simple pharmacologic interventions may become problematic if, for example, the availability of blood draws to monitor for adverse effects of medications is not consistently available.

## ASSESSING AND DEVELOPING APPROPRIATE AND MEANINGFUL GOALS

The earlier discussion highlights how the appropriate assessment of patients will guide the management plan to address the UMNS. The treatment team must understand the goals and expectations of the patients and families as part of the assessment process. The team must also take into account variables such as prognosis, severity of neurologic deficits, barriers to access to care, comorbidities that affect recovery and function, and others. It is not uncommon for the clinician to be faced with unrealistic goals from patients and families and at times members of the treatment team. It is important to be able to articulate the factors that may affect the outcome. It is also important to listen to the patients and families, as they may have goals that have not been considered but may be obtainable. Although rehabilitation teams often focus on functional goals, other goals, such as pain relief and ease of care, may be more relevant in certain situations.[29] Goal setting may involve some degree of compromise; awareness of potential adverse effects will allow the clinician to consider potential trade-offs, such as overall comfort and ease of care, at the expense of alertness. ABI is not a static condition; goals that were appropriate previously may no longer be relevant. Assessment of the response to prior treatments may also guide subsequent interventions. The prognosis may become clearer as the trajectory of recovery is defined over time. Frequent discussion with the patients and families may provide opportunities for education and further their understanding of their condition. It will also allow them to adjust goals and expectations.

## SUMMARY

A comprehensive assessment of patients with ABIs is crucial for the development of an appropriate treatment plan to address elements of the UMNS. This assessment should include an understanding of the nature and extent of injury, prognosis, awareness of relevant past medical and functional history, and evaluation of current neuro-medical and musculoskeletal conditions. Patients and families (as able and appropriate) need to participate in the assessment and development of the treatment plan by helping to identify possible challenges of access to care as well as sharing goals and expectations. Appropriate outcome measures should be used to evaluate the efficacy of interventions. Assessment is a dynamic process, as these factors will change during the recovery from ABIs and in response to rehabilitation interventions.

## REFERENCES

1. Caine D, Watson JDG. Neuropsychological and neuropathological sequelae of cerebral anoxia: a critical review. J Int Neuropsychol Soc 2000;6:86–99.
2. Scott BL, Jankovic J. Delayed-onset progressive movement disorders after static brain lesions. Neurology 1996;46(1):68–74.
3. Frucht S, Fahn S. The clinical spectrum of posthypoxic myoclonus. Mov Disord 2000;15(S1):2–7.
4. Katz DI, Polyak M, Coughlan D, et al. Natural history of recovery from brain injury after prolonged disorders of consciousness: outcome of patients admitted to inpatient rehabilitation with 1–4 year follow-up. Prog Brain Res 2009;177:73–88.
5. Multi-Society Task Force on PVS. Medical aspects of the persistent vegetative state. N Engl J Med 1994;330(21):1499–508.
6. Thibaut A, Chatelle C, Ziegler E, et al. Spasticity after stroke: physiology, assessment and treatment. Brain Inj 2013;27(10):1093–105.
7. Medical Research Council. Aids to the examination of the peripheral nervous system, memorandum no. 45. London: Her Majesty's Stationery Office; 1981.
8. Brashear A, Zafonte R, Corcoran M, et al. Inter-and intrarater reliability of the Ashworth scale and the disability assessment scale in patients with upper-limb post-stroke spasticity. Arch Phys Med Rehabil 2002;83(10):1349–54.
9. Tardieu G, Shentoub S, Delarue R. Research on a technic for measurement of spasticity. Rev Neurol (Paris) 1954;91(2):143–4 [in French].
10. Penn RD, Savoy SM, Corcos D, et al. Intrathecal baclofen for severe spinal spasticity. N Engl J Med 1989;320(23):1517–21.
11. Hinderer SR, Gupta S. Functional outcome measures to assess interventions for spasticity. Arch Phys Med Rehabil 1996;77(10):1083–9.
12. Brashear A, Gordon MF, Elovic E, et al. Intramuscular injection of botulinum toxin for the treatment of wrist and finger spasticity after a stroke. N Engl J Med 2002;347(6):395–400.
13. Turner-Stokes L, Baguley IJ, De Graaff S, et al. Goal attainment scaling in the evaluation of treatment of upper limb spasticity with botulinum toxin: a secondary analysis from a double-blind placebo-controlled randomized clinical trial. J Rehabil Med 2010;42(1):81–9.
14. Esquenazi A, Sale P, Moon D, et al. Poster 290 spatiotemporal changes in gait performance due to onabotulinumtoxina injection to lower limb muscles in patients with upper motor neuron syndrome. PM R 2014;6(9):S286.
15. Simonsen LL, Sonne-Holm S, Krasheninnikoff M, et al. Symptomatic heterotopic ossification after very severe traumatic brain injury in 114 patients: incidence and risk factors. Injury 2007;38(10):1146–50.
16. Garland DE, Bailey S. Undetected injuries in head-injured adults. Clin Orthop Relat Res 1981;155:162–5.

17. Perkes I, Baguley IJ, Nott MT, et al. A review of paroxysmal sympathetic hyperactivity after acquired brain injury. Ann Neurol 2010;68(2):126–35.
18. Baguley IJ, Perkes IE, Fernandez-Ortega JF, et al, Consensus Working Group. Paroxysmal sympathetic hyperactivity after acquired brain injury: consensus on conceptual definition, nomenclature, and diagnostic criteria. J Neurotrauma 2014;31(17):1515–20.
19. Choi HA, Jeon SB, Samuel S, et al. Paroxysmal sympathetic hyperactivity after acute brain injury. Curr Neurol Neurosci Rep 2013;13(8):370.
20. Cuny E, Richer E, Castel JP. Dysautonomia syndrome in the acute recovery phase after traumatic brain injury: relief with intrathecal baclofen therapy. Brain Inj 2001;15(10):917–25.
21. Orcutt SA, Kramer WG, Howard MW, et al. Carpal tunnel syndrome secondary to wrist and finger flexor spasticity. J Hand Surg 1990;15(6):940–4.
22. Krauss JK, Trankle R, Kopp KH. Post-traumatic movement disorders in survivors of severe head injury. Neurology 1996;47(6):1488–92.
23. Bleyenheuft C, Filipetti P, Caldas C, et al. Experience with external pump trial prior to implantation for intrathecal baclofen in ambulatory patients with spastic cerebral palsy. Neurophysiol Clin 2007;37(1):23–8.
24. van Mook WN, Hulsewé-Evers RP. Critical illness polyneuropathy. Curr Opin Crit Care 2002;8(4):302–10.
25. Zafonte R, Elovic EP, Lombard L. Acute care management of post-TBI spasticity. J Head Trauma Rehabil 2004;19(2):89–100.
26. Albanese A, Abbruzzese G, Dressler D, et al. Practical guidance for CD management involving treatment of botulinum toxin: a consensus statement. J Neurol 2015;262(10):2201–13.
27. Comella CL, Jankovic J, Shannon KM, et al, Dystonia Study Group. Comparison of botulinum toxin serotypes A and B for the treatment of cervical dystonia. Neurology 2005;65(9):1423–9.
28. Coffey RJ, Edgar TS, Francisco GE, et al. Abrupt withdrawal from intrathecal baclofen: recognition and management of a potentially life-threatening syndrome. Arch Phys Med Rehabil 2002;83(6):735–41.
29. Ward AB, Kadies M. The management of pain in spasticity. Disabil Rehabil 2002;24(8):443–53.

# Special Considerations in Assessing and Treating Spasticity in Spinal Cord Injury

John Lin, MD[a,b], Wesley Chay, MD[a,b],*

## KEYWORDS

- Spasticity • Assessment • Treatment • Management • Spinal cord injury

## KEY POINTS

- The effects of spasticity after spinal cord injury may be easier to understand when looking at functional neurologic levels.
- The assessment of spasticity should include both subjective descriptions from the individual and objective findings of the examiner.
- Spasticity treatment should be guided by the presence or absence of problems/difficulty stemming from the effects of spasticity on the individual.

## SPINAL CORD INJURY AND SPASTICITY

Spinal cord injury (SCI) is a condition that affects the spinal cord either by trauma or intrinsic pathologic conditions, such as multiple sclerosis or compressive epidural abscess. As the SCI has multi-organ sequelae, one of the more functionally disabling consequences is the compromise onto the musculoskeletal system. When the corticospinal tract is affected, upper motor neuron syndrome ensues. The incidence of spasticity affecting persons with SCI may approach 80%.[1] The incidence is affected by timing after injury as well as level and severity of injury. In general those with tetraplegic SCI report more difficulties with spasticity.[2] Those with incomplete tetraplegia have the highest incidence of spasticity.[3] Although spasticity can affect activities of daily living (ADLs) in individuals with SCI[4] with an associated decrease in quality of life[5] in no small part due to pain and insomnia for some,[6] it has also been observed to decrease life expectancy.[7]

Disclosure Statement: The authors have no commercial or financial conflicts of interest or any funding sources to disclose.
a Department of Physical Medicine and Rehabilitation, Shepherd Center, 2020 Peachtree Street Northwest, Atlanta, GA 30309, USA; b Department of Rehabilitation Medicine, Emory University School of Medicine, 2020 Peachtree Road Northwest, Atlanta, GA 30309, USA
* Corresponding author. Shepherd Center, 2020 Peachtree Street, Northwest, Atlanta, GA 30309.
E-mail address: Wes_Chay@Shepherd.org

Phys Med Rehabil Clin N Am 29 (2018) 445–453
https://doi.org/10.1016/j.pmr.2018.03.001

Many define spasticity as "a motor disorder characterized by a velocity-dependent increase is tonic stretch reflexes with exaggerated tendon jerks, resulting from hyperexcitability of the stretch reflex, as one component of the upper motor neuron syndrome."[8] Others may ascribe to a modified definition, whereby various components of spasticity are separated into subdefinitions: "(1) intrinsic tonic spasticity: exaggeration of the tonic component of the stretch reflex (manifesting as increased tone), (2) intrinsic phasic spasticity: exaggeration of the phasic component of the stretch reflex (manifesting as tendon hyper-reflexia and clonus), and (3) extrinsic spasticity: exaggeration of extrinsic flexion or extension spinal reflexes."[9]

Special considerations in the pathophysiology of spasticity in SCI should be noted. As with other causes of upper motor neuron syndromes, the spinal reflexes below the neurologic level unaffected by injury are intact. However, at the level of injury, affected motor neuron and spinal roots may lead to denervation of corresponding muscles and consequent flaccidity. That is, at the affected spinal segments, spinal reflexes may be abated and spasticity mitigated. For incomplete injuries, at the level, the muscles may be unaffected with volitional activity or partially affected with some mild tone. However, depending on the muscles involved, the volitional muscles, although unaffected by increased tone, may be functionally affected by the antagonist muscle having unopposed and uncoordinated muscular hyperactivity. For example, elbow flexion by biceps brachii and brachialis muscles may be impeded by spasticity of the elbow extension muscle of the triceps.

For persons with SCI, spasticity may have both a positive and negative impact on their lives. Incomplete injuries, with some preserved sensations, may experience spasticity as uncomfortable and painful.[10] It is commonly noted that spasticity may adversely affect ambulation. Additionally, a decrease in daily activity functional independence, especially in transfers, is commonly observed.[4] Nonintuitively, spasticity has been observed to have either no impact[11] or a negative impact on bone mineral density preservation for persons with SCI[12] just as hemiplegic stroke survivors.[13] Similarly, arterial insufficiency is noted with concordant limb spasticity.[14]

Although nocturnal spasticity is often reported, it can generally be secondary to 3 causes. Nocturnal spasticity that occurs when a person first goes to bed into the supine or recumbent position is primarily due to extension of the flexed muscles, for example, hip flexors, from the sitting to the supine position, exciting the reflex arc. This spasticity often triggers a flexor response and is often transient, although recurrent, depending on the body position in bed and has been noted to correlate with insomnia.[6] For those with the inability to spontaneously reposition different parts of the limbs, a second contributing factor to increased nocturnal spasticity is prolonged recumbency in one position leading to otherwise undetectable discomfort, that is, increased nociceptive stimuli, resulting in increased reflex activity and spasticity. Shorter-acting half-life of medications, such as baclofen and tizanidine, may reach subtherapeutic levels by mid to late portions of sleep with manifestations of increased spasticity hours before completion of intended restful sleep. Lastly, subjectively reported spasticity refractory to all attempts at antispasmodic medication titration may need to have a differential diagnosis broadened to include considerations for periodic limb movements (Levy).

On the other hand, spasticity has beneficial effects for persons with SCI. Muscle mass maintenance is noted with those with increased spasticity.[11] By association, there is noted improvement in lipid profile and glucose metabolism with increased spasticity.[15] Interestingly, although spasticity has been noted to improve standing posture for some,[2] others use spasticity as sentinel for tissue injury or pathological condition below the neurological level, such as urinary tract infection, stool impaction/constipation, or ingrown toenail.[10] In addition, rostral extension of spinal cord pathology, for example, postoperative epidural hematoma, subacute posttraumatic ascending myelopathy, syringomyelia, and so forth, can be correlated with increased spasticity,[16] those serving as an adjunctive tool to facilitate early diagnosis.

## SEGMENTAL MANIFESTATION OF SPINAL CORD INJURY–RELATED SPASTICITY

Spasticity as it pertains to spinal cord pathology typically follows the injury level, although the manifestation is protean, especially when the injury is incomplete or progressive. Each neurologic level has a unique set of muscle spasms that affect physiology and function of the individual affected. Injuries affecting the sacral spinal segments are not typically affected by upper motor neuron syndrome, as involvement of the segmental motor neurons leads to motor denervation and flaccidity. In addition, the lack of any further caudal spinal levels means that all muscles still have either volitional control by intact motor neurons or are flaccid because of denervation. This is typical of the SCI syndrome of conus medullaris and cauda equina.

Although the incidence of the L5 SCI level is not high among all spinal injuries, lack of motor control of the caudal S1 spinal level means that the corresponding muscles may be affected by increased spasticity and tone. These muscles include gastrocnemius, soleus, tibialis posterior, flexor digitorum longus/brevis, and plantaris. As most of these patients are ambulatory, increased tone of the intrinsic and extrinsic toe flexors can lead to skin abrasion along the dorsum of the interphalangeal joints. Ankle inversion due to hyperactive tibialis posterior and medial gastrocnemius leads to ankle instability on initial contact in addition to skin abrasion at the lateral malleolus against rigid orthosis, for example, ankle-foot orthosis and shoe. Over time, varus deformity and contracture at the ankle ensue leading to ground reaction force exerting asymmetric and nonphysiologic load on the ankle joints resulting in neuropathic degeneration, for example, Charcot arthropathy. Similarly, increased tone of the gastrocnemius-soleus complex leads to effective limb-length discrepancy during the swing phase of the gait cycle, decreasing limb clearance and increasing the risk of fall. As the tone overpowers the smaller muscle strength of the ankle dorsiflexors and the intrinsic stability of the orthosis, compensatory strategies used to increase limb clearance, for example, hip hiking, result in gait inefficiency and easy fatigability. Gait instability also results, as the limb's initial contact is not made with the heel strike. Lastly, the phasic nature of spasticity is exacerbated during weight bearing, as these muscles undergo stretch leading to increased excitability of the Golgi tendons and clonic activations of the ankle plantar flexors. Gait and standing balance are compromised.

At the L4 neurologic level, muscles that may be spastic with the L5 neurologic level are still present. In addition, the L5 innervated muscles become autonomous with spasticity. The most prominent of these is the extensor hallucis longus. Increased spasticity of the extensor hallucis longus leads to the phenomenon of hitchhiker toe that may abrade against the inside of the shoes leading to skin abrasion at the distal phalanx of the great toe. Without proper spasticity treatment, considerations must be given to shoes with a larger toe box.

With an L3 SCI level, the primarily L4 innervated tibialis anterior has spasticity that affects dorsiflexion of the ankles. This spasticity usually presents more as a phasic, rather than tonic, spasticity leading to clonic dorsiflexion of the ankle. While at rest in a seated position, this clonic dorsiflexion may not pose any significant functional compromise. However, standing balance and gait stability are affected when the dorsiflexed ankle allows the ground reaction force to shift anterior of the knee leading to knee flexion and compromised limb stability. Some hand control using drivers may note the ankle dorsiflexion spasticity to dangerously interfere with the accelerator or brake pedal actions necessitating installation of pedal guards.

With neurologic levels at and above L2, there is an increasing reliance on a manual wheelchair as a more dominant mode of mobility. Therefore, spasticity of the primarily S1 innervated muscles would have a different functional compromise compared with predominant ambulators. For a wheelchair user, ankle inversion from tibialis posterior and medial gastrocnemius spasticity exposes the lateral malleolus to increased risk of skin compromise. Ankle plantar flexion from the spastic gastrocnemius and soleus muscles allows the feet to slide off the foot plate and endangers the feet as they slide under the foot plate while the wheelchair is in forward motion. Not being protected on the foot rest, the toes and the feet are in danger to bump against an object as the wheelchair moves. Ankle clonus from the phasic spasticity of the gastroc-soleus muscles may in addition lead to skin abrasion on the posterior side against the leg strap and on the posterolateral sides against the wheelchair frame.

Furthermore, other muscles compromised by spasticity at the L2 neurologic level include the predominantly L3 innervated adductors longus, brevis, and magnus. Spasticity of these muscles leads to adduction at the hip and scissoring gait. At the seated position in a wheelchair, knock-knee syndrome may lead to abrasion of the medial aspect of the knee against the contralateral knee. Urethral catheterization becomes difficult, especially for women. For those who have spasticity of these muscles but whose neurologic impairment at higher levels necessitate dependence on perineal hygiene, spasticity of the adductors makes it exceedingly difficult to provide optimal hygiene.

Additionally, the other primary L3 innervated muscles are the quadriceps femoris muscles, which account significantly for lower extremity extension tone, which has been noted to be the most common type of lower limb spasticity affecting individuals with SCI.[10] When involuntarily activated, quadriceps femoris extend the knee, which decreases the effective limb clearance during ambulation in addition to endangering the distal lower extremity in the seated position while the wheelchair is in motion. Also, some report spasticity of the quadriceps to affect functional transfers.[17] However, although deleterious as it may be, spasticity can be of functional use, especially when it can be triggered or reliably expected. Such is the case with the quadriceps, which some can be triggered by tapping the muscle itself, as in invoking a muscle stretch reflex. Others trigger its activation with hip extension, presumably extending the muscle belly and the Golgi tendons of the rectus femoris to initiate the spasticity interneuron excitation. This activation may aid in standing initiation or stability, such as during a car transfer onto a seat higher than the wheelchair.

Although a person with an L1 neurologic injury level may have increasing reliance on wheelchairs for mobility, at the seated position, spasticity of the L2 spinal cord level predominant muscle of iliopsoas usually does not pose functional compromise at the mild to moderate degree because the iliopsoas is already at a flexed position. With a severe degree of spasticity, phasic activation of the iliopsoas, whether provoked or not by the vibration of the mobile wheelchair, can lead to flexion of the hips, with resultant forward translation of the ischium, sacral sitting posture, and ultimately undue pressure on the sacrum. Involuntary hip flexion can to lead to safety compromise during transfers. Bed positioning is affected as well, increasing the risk of decubitus. Chronic hip flexion tone can lead to contractures making ambulation and standing even more difficult.

For thoracic-level SCIs, all the aforementioned muscle spasms still prevail. The higher the level of thoracic injuries, the more likely muscles of the trunk may lose supraspinal control leading to increased spasticity. These muscles may involve the abdominal rectus and obliques that are more often tonic than clonic. As the muscles fatigue, the tonic contractions may abate. However, during the height of the involuntary muscle contractions, affected individuals may experience significant dyspnea with compromised inspiration as the outward abdominal excursion, to accommodate downward descending diaphragm with inspiration, is affected.

Spasticity of other trunk muscles, for example, para-spinalis and quadratus lumborum, may affect trunk stability in extension and make wheelchair operation and propulsion difficult. Asymmetric excitation of these muscles of the trunk contributes to the lateral lean while in the seated position. For those not having reached skeletal maturity, the lateral leaning posture may exacerbate any preexisting propensity for idiopathic scoliosis.

Although possible, spasms of the intercostal muscles do not affect respiratory function to the same degree as the abdominal muscles.

Those patients with lower tetraplegic spinal cord injuries may not exhibit significant functional difficulties related to upper extremity spasticity. If spasticity is moderate to severe, complaints of hand cramping or clenching of the fist may be noted. At this level, pain from muscle spasms may predominate over fine motor hand functional compromise.

At the C6 spinal cord neurologic level, the predominant C7, C8, and distally innervated muscles leading to clinical concern are primarily finger flexors, for example, flexor digitorum superficialis/profundus, flexor pollicis longus, and so forth. These flexors may present as finger flexion with compromised extension range of motion posing difficulty in palmar hygiene maintenance and nail trimming. Further progression may see skin compromise from the growing nails entrenched into the skin of the palm.

Although at the C6 neurologic level the radial nerve innervated extensor muscles, for example, triceps, can be affected with muscle spasms, the incidence and severity are much less relatively severe compared with the flexion-based muscle spasms. Patients who spend most of the day in bed with elbow extended may experience extension contracture due to triceps muscle hypertonicity compounded by lack of flexion range of motion.

Of special consideration at this neurologic level of C6, care must be taken not to treat some resting hand muscle tone or position too aggressively. The act of tenodesis grasp requires some degrees of thumb in the adducted position and the index finger in the flexed position, especially at the metacarpal phalangeal joint. Overzealous range of motion of these fingers above physiologic state may render the use of this passive tension grasp nonfunctional.

A person with a C5 SCI level is reliant on power wheelchair for mobility and has the assistance of aides for most of the ADLs. At this level, palliation of spasticity aims to improve resting posture, maintain range of motion, and minimize pain induction. The primarily C6 innervated pronator teres may keep the forearm in a pronated position on the arm rests of the power wheelchair. The wrists may be flexed because of overactive flexor carpi radialis. Prevention of loss of range of motion and contraction at the wrists is important to preserve potentially functional tenodesis as patients recover to the C6 neurologic level during the subacute injury period.

With tetraplegic SCI at and above the C4 level, elbow flexion spasticity is predominant along with shoulder adduction and internal rotation. In bed, patients often assume the position of elbow flexion and shoulder abduction resembling the chicken wing posture. In the seated position, elbow flexion (due to activation of brachialis and biceps brachii) is often coupled with shoulder adduction and internal rotation (due to hyperactive pectoralis major). Such shoulder positioning makes the prospect of upper extremity power wheelchair operation even more difficult should patients recover to improved volitional motion to allow goal-post joystick operation. Dependent hygiene and upper body dressing are compromised, as shoulder abduction range of motion is affected. If elbow flexion contractures are set in, recovering patients are not able to use either gravity or balanced forearm orthosis for elbow extension in order to make hand-to-mouth activities functional.

## ASSESSING SPASTICITY IN SPINAL CORD INJURY

Assessing spasticity in an individual may be approached both subjectively (what the patients/caregivers describe) and objectively (physical examination, spasticity scale).

In exploring one's history of spasticity, questions that may be helpful in identifying problems associated with spasticity may include the following: Do you find your spasticity/spasms to make it difficult to manage your ADLs, transfers, or mobility? Does your spasticity/spasms cause any pain? Does your spasticity/spasms make it difficult to sleep? Have you had any skin breakdown because of your spasticity/spasms? Do you have difficulty with positioning (in wheelchair or bed) because of spasticity/spasms? When you get spasms, do they make it difficult to breathe? Additionally, it can be helpful to identify if there are any patterns related to spasticity (time of day, specific positions/activities, environment).

It is also worth noting that many individuals with SCI may use spasticity to assist with ADLs (tapping leg causing extension to thread leg through pans/shorts), transfers, and ambulation (providing support in the lower extremities for such activities). However, if spasticity is uncontrolled/uncontrollable, it can also hinder such activities.

Additionally, in individuals with SCI, although it may be normal for spasticity to change with the course of SCI, it is not unusual that an acute change in spasticity is associated with some underlying issue, such as painful/noxious stimulus; bladder issue, such as cystitis; bowel issue, such as constipation; or skin issue, such as pressure injury or ingrown toenail. Additionally, other complications of SCI, such as heterotopic ossification or syringomyelia, can result in changes in spasticity as well.

On physical examination, observing how transfers are performed or how positional changes affect spasticity/spasms may shed light on how spasticity may be adversely affecting the individual. Also, one can look at the different spasticity patterns elicited with passive range of motion versus active movement and evaluation of stretch reflexes. There are many spasticity scales that have been described (and modified), including the Ashworth Scale, Modified Ashworth Scale, Modified Tardieu Scale, Penn Spasm Frequency Scale, the self-reported Spasm Frequency Scale, and the Pendulum Test, to name a few. As beneficial as it is to be familiar with each of these spasticity scales, it may be worth stating the obvious, that no single spasticity scale encapsulates all of what individuals affected by spasticity may experience. In other words, in assessing and eventually treating spasticity, one should not be treating a number on a scale unnecessarily but, rather, focus on the impact of spasticity on function and quality of life of the individual.

## SPECIAL CONSIDERATIONS IN APPROACHING TREATMENT OF SPASTICITY IN SPINAL CORD INJURY

In assessing spasticity, one should seek to identify whether or not spasticity is causing/contributing to problems experienced by patients: succinctly put, treat spasticity if it bothers patients, not you. The presence of spasticity does not necessitate the treatment of it. However, one would likely benefit from treatment if spasticity: causes pain; negatively affects ADLs; negatively affects transfers/mobility; negatively affects positioning in bed/wheelchair; negatively affects sleep; or causes skin breakdown/irritation.

In approaching spasticity management, in general, it is appropriate to start with more conservative treatment options before pursuing more invasive measures. Non-medication options may include stretching, which usually yields only short-term benefits, and heat/cold modalities which given sensory impairments may also put patients at risk for skin issues. Commonly initiated medications are baclofen, dantrolene (Dantrium), tizanidine, and diazepam. Baclofen is generally considered first line in SCI and can be very effective for tonic spasticity. Dantrium may be first line with somebody with a concomitant brain injury, given its peripheral (rather than central) mechanism of action, inhibiting the release of calcium at the level of the sarcoplasmic reticulum. Additionally, one should monitor liver function tests when using Dantrium (at the start of treatment and at least every 3 months while remaining on treatment). When using tizanidine, one needs to be cautious to not also prescribe ciprofloxacin for urinary tract infection. The interaction between ciprofloxacin and tizanidine results in a potentiation of the antihypertensive effect (tizanidine is a centrally acting alpha agonist), which can cause severe hypotension/orthostasis. Diazepam can be very effective in treating phasic spasticity, but one needs to consider the potentially sedating and cognitively impairing side effects. Other medications that sometimes may help decrease spasticity include cyproheptadine (also used as an appetite stimulant) and gabapentin (often used for neuropathic pain/sensations).

## CASES AND DISCUSSION
### Case 1

A 35-year-old right-hand dominant man presents with history of C7 American Spinal Injury Association Impairment Scale (AIS) A SCI after a rollover motor vehicle collision approximately 6 months prior. The patient reports no active finger movements still at this time, but he reports functional strength at his elbows and wrists. He and his wife report tightness of the fingers but deny any skin breakdown. He reports he saw his primary care physician (PCP), and the PCP was concerned that his fingers were going to get stuck in a closed position. He also notes some extensor spasms of his legs when he is stretched out at night in the bed but denies any problems with sleeping or positioning in the bed or wheelchair. He notes he has been taking baclofen 20 mg 3 times a day since discharge from the rehab hospital, and his PCP had suggested adding some other medications or pursuing botulinum toxin (Botox) injections. He and his wife are looking for recommendations for treatment.

### Discussion

Based on the level of injury (and function) and description of spasticity, one should consider that, although the individual certainly describes some spasticity, it does not seem to be functionally limiting him at this time. Specifically, regarding the concern of his fingers getting stuck in a closed position, one should consider counseling the patient and wife that there may be a functional benefit to allowing the fingers to be tighter and in a more flexed position in order to use a tenodesis grasp. With tenodesis, wrist extension results in shortening of the finger flexors, which leads to finger flexion that can be used for gross grasping of objects. Conversely, wrist flexion can help the fingers extend/open and release items. In general, when trying to maximize upper extremity function and make use of tenodesis, it is important to not overstretch the finger flexors and, thereby, preclude tenodesis. In this case, spasticity may actually be helpful with function (gaining gross grasp); if one were to overstretch or inject botulinum toxin into his finger flexors, he would be losing potential function that otherwise he could use.

### Case 2

A 52-year-old right-hand dominant woman presents with a history of C5 AIS D SCI status after a ground-level fall around 9 months ago. She reports she has progressed well in outpatient therapy but has been having some challenges walking. She notes that her legs tend to cross when she tries to advance each leg forward, and it is difficult for her to get her heel down to make contact with stepping and keep her heel on the ground. She reports occasionally her foot/ankle rolls inward, but she has not fallen. She reports her gait improves when using the ankle foot orthosis, but she develops red spots when wearing it because of how her foot/ankle pushes against the brace. She reports she is frustrated by her legs because she thinks she could be doing better. She notes she has tried taking baclofen, tizanidine, and diazepam; but they have all made her too tired. She reports she tried taking Dantrium, but her liver enzymes increased. She inquires what can be done to help her with her situation.

### Discussion

In this individual with incomplete tetraplegia and ambulatory dysfunction, she describes typical spasticity patterns in the hip adductor muscles that result in a scissoring gait, the ankle plantar flexors (gastrocnemius and soleus muscles), and ankle inverter (posterior tibialis muscle). Of note, in assessing spasticity of the lower extremity, one can assess with passive range of motion as well as observing ambulation. Also, in order to tease out whether only one or both of the gastrocnemius muscles and/or soleus muscle is involved, one can assess passive dorsiflexion of the ankle with the knee bent (isolating soleus) or knee straight (gastrocnemius muscle). Additionally, one could consider referral to a gait laboratory if available/necessary.

Management strategies in light of prior trialing and failure of multiple medications would likely warrant further options, such as botulinum toxin and/or phenol injections and an intrathecal baclofen pump trial if warranted. One could also consider performing phenol blocks to the obturator nerves in order to preserve/maximize dosing of botulinum toxin to the gastrocnemius/soleus muscles and posterior tibialis muscles.

In this case, spasticity is limiting function and progress with therapy; in order to prevent skin breakdown and maximize rehabilitation gains and improve functional gait, offering spasticity management is appropriate.

### REFERENCES

1. Maynard FM, Karunas RS, Waring WP 3rd. Epidemiology of spasticity following traumatic spinal cord injury. Arch Phys Med Rehabil 1990;71(8):566–9.
2. Mahoney JS, Engebretson JC, Cook KF, et al. Spasticity experience domains in persons with spinal cord injury. Arch Phys Med Rehabil 2007;88:287–94.
3. Taricco M, Pagliacci MC, Telaro E, et al. Pharmacological interventions for spasticity following spinal cord injury: results of a Cochrane systematic review. Eura Medicophys 2006;42(1):5–15.
4. Bravo-Esteban E, Taylor J, Abián-Vicén J, et al. Impact of specific symptoms of spasticity on voluntary lower limb muscle function, gait and daily activities during subacute and chronic spinal cord injury. NeuroRehabilitation 2013;33:531–43.
5. Westercam D, Saunders LL, Krause JS. Association of spasticity and life satisfaction after spinal cord injury. Spinal Cord 2011;49:990–4.

6. Little JW, Micklesen P, Umlauf R, et al. Lower extremity manifestations of spasticity in chronic spinal cord injury. Am J Phys Med Rehabil 1989;68(1):32–6.
7. Krause JS, Carter RE, Pickelsimer E. Behavioral risk factors of mortality after spinal cord injury. Arch Phys Med Rehabil 2009;90:95–101.
8. Lance JW. The control of muscle tone, reflexes, and movement: Robert Wartenberg lecture. Neurology 1980;30:1303–13.
9. Decq P. Pathophysiology of spasticity. Neurochirurgie 2003;49:163–84.
10. Fleuren JF, Voerman GE, Snoek GJ, et al. Perception of lower limb spasticity in patients with spinal cord injury. Spinal Cord 2009;47(5):396–400.
11. Löfvenmark I, Werhagen L, Norrbrink C. Spasticity and bone density after a spinal cord injury. J Rehabil Med 2009;41(13):1080–4.
12. Kostovski E, Hjeltnes N, Eriksen EF, et al. Differences in bone mineral density, markers of bone turnover and extracellular matrix and daily life muscular activity among patients with recent motor-incomplete versus motor-complete spinal cord injury. Calcif Tissue Int 2015;96(2):145–54.
13. de Brito CM, Garcia AC, Takayama L, et al. Bone loss in chronic hemiplegia: a longitudinal cohort study. J Clin Densitom 2013;16(2):160–7.
14. Dhindsa MS, Merring CA, Brandt LE, et al. Muscle spasticity associated with reduced whole-leg perfusion in persons with spinal cord injury. J Spinal Cord Med 2011;34(6):594–9.
15. Gorgey AS, Chiodo AE, Zemper ED, et al. Relationship of spasticity to soft tissue body composition and the metabolic profile in persons with chronic motor complete spinal cord injury. J Spinal Cord Med 2010;33:6–15.
16. Rekand T, Hagen EM, Grønning M. Spasticity following spinal cord injury. Tidsskr Nor Laegeforen 2012;132(8):970–3.
17. Tibbett J, Widerström-Noga EG, Thomas CK, et al. Impact of spasticity on transfers and activities of daily living in individuals with spinal cord injury. J Spinal Cord Med 2018;1–14 [Epub ahead of print].

# Special Considerations in Pediatric Assessment

Heakyung Kim, MD[a,b,*], Mi Ran Shin, MD[c]

## KEYWORDS

- Spasticity • Pediatric • Cerebral palsy • Secondary complication • Prevention
- Physical examination

## KEY POINTS

- Children's growth should be taken into consideration when assessing and managing spasticity.
- Early and regularly repeated aggressive, comprehensive spasticity management can prevent musculoskeletal complications and functional deterioration and improve function and quality of life.
- Comprehensive history taking and systematic physical examination are critical in the assessment for spasticity treatment.

## INTRODUCTION

Cerebral palsy (CP) is the most common (90%) condition associated with spasticity in children and young people.[1] In CP, spasticity results from a dysregulated reflex-arc from upper motor neurons of the medullary pyramid to the motor end plate of the limb musculatures.[2] It is caused by an intricate change along different interdependent pathways.[2,3] Unlike the disease processes in adults whose motor system was already developed at the time of injury, for instance, like stroke, children with a prenatal brain abnormality are affected by reorganization of supraspinal input and impaired motor maturation.[2] Children with CP may have concomitant extrapyramidal involvement causing additional movement disorders, including dystonia (10%–15%), ataxia, flaccidity, and athetosis.[1] Other causes of spasticity in children

Disclosure: The authors have nothing to disclose.
[a] Department of Rehabilitation and Regenerative Medicine, Pediatric Physical Medicine and Rehabilitation, Columbia University Irving Medical Center, Weill Cornell Medical College, New-York-Presbyterian Hospital, 180 Fort Washington Avenue, Harkness Pavilion Suite 165, New York, NY 10032, USA; [b] Department of Physiatry, Blythedale Children's Hospital, Valhalla, NY 10595, USA; [c] Department of Physical Medicine and Rehabilitation, Johns Hopkins University, 600 North Wolfe Street Phipps 160, Baltimore, MD 21287, USA
* Corresponding author. Pediatric Physical Medicine and Rehabilitation, Columbia University Medical Center, 180 Fort Washington Avenue, New York, NY 10032.
E-mail addresses: hk2641@cumc.columbia.edu; Kheakyung@blythedale.org

Phys Med Rehabil Clin N Am 29 (2018) 455–471
https://doi.org/10.1016/j.pmr.2018.03.002
1047-9651/18/© 2018 Elsevier Inc. All rights reserved.

include traumatic brain injury, stroke, spinal cord injury, and inherited disorders, such as Wilson disease, Hallervorden-Spatz disease, and hereditary spastic hemiparesis.[4]

The difference between adult and children in terms of spasticity management is the fact that children grow. In growing children, their muscles and bones grow at the same ratio. However, in children with spasticity, their muscles are shorter, smaller,[2] and cannot catch up with their bone growth. Such length discrepancy between bones and spastic muscles gets worse during children's growth spurts; close follow-up throughout children's growth is critical to prevent secondary complications. Aggressive stretching of spastic muscles will help minimize the length discrepancy between bone and spastic muscles despite its short effect. Early physical therapy and repeated spasticity management treatments, ie chemoneurolysis with botulinumtoxin and/or alcohol injections, are critical components in reducing the need for multiple orthopedic surgeries, ie muscle tendon lengthening or skeletal procedures, and promote functional improvement and delay functional deterioration as they get older.[5]

## DIAGNOSIS
### Clinical Presentation

Spasticity is defined as velocity-dependent increased resistance to passive muscle stretch.[6] Spasticity can affect the entire body or certain body parts. Most children with CP can be classified according to which body area is affected: hemiplegia, diplegia, and tetraplegia.[7] If a child has spasticity in trunk muscles, the spasticity can cause postural and gait impairments. If there is bulbar involvement, it can cause dysphagia and dysarthria. Other functional impairments include difficulty in movement, sitting, transfers, hygiene, and dressing.

### Secondary Complications

Management of spasticity becomes very important because of its complications, especially when not treated. Spasticity causes shortening of muscles, which hampers normal muscle lengthening during children's growth and contributes to muscles and soft tissue contractures, and functional limitation.[2] Spasticity, for example, prevents normal derotation of the femur that results in coxa valga of the femur.[8] In addition, spasticity of the muscles around the hip contributes to hip subluxation, especially in nonambulatory children.[9] In return, hip subluxation can cause pain in the hip area. Prolonged postures in flexion or extension of joints or continuous involuntary movements can cause peripheral neuropathy.[10] Such pain and musculoskeletal complications from spasticity can further disturb sleep, present major difficulties for care workers, and deteriorate children's function.[11]

### Assessment

- Assessment of children with spasticity needs to be considerate and systematic.
  - Detailed history taking and thorough review of system and medications review
  - Observation of children in the most comfortable setting and throughout the encounter
  - Thorough static and dynamic examination

Spasticity will be most notable through physical examination: reflexes are brisk and can have accompanying upper motor neuron signs, such as extensor plantar signs and clonus.[2] It is important to know if the present spasticity of children is their baseline because any noxious stimulation or discomfort can increase spasticity. The most common pain sources that aggravate spasticity by systems are summarized in **Table 1**.

Medication should also be reviewed. Selective serotine reuptake inhibitors, antiemetics, or anxiolytics can cause movement disorders, such as dystonia or dyskinesia[12]; prolonged use of anticholinergics causes mucous plugging or bladder retention; antispastic drugs, such as baclofen, can cause severe constipation and bladder retention, which in return can cause worsening of spasticity.

### Physical Examination

To assess children well, they should be relaxed and comfortable. They should not be undressed yet, to observe for any posturing, signs of contractures, hip subluxation, or primitive reflexes without making them upset. Examination at rest can give clues to underlying pathology for worsening spasticity.

Gastrointestinal-related findings: When children with spastic quadriplegia show intermittent severe trunk arching with increased spasticity in the extensors of limbs and if the trunk arching and limb spasticity get better with an upright sitting position, this trunk arching is most likely gastroesophageal reflux disease

| Table 1 Spasticity aggravating factors | |
|---|---|
| Gastrointestinal | • Gastroesophageal reflux disease<br>• Formula intolerance<br>• Severe constipation due to neurogenic bowel, immobilization, medications, or spasticity around anal sphincter or its surrounding muscles<br>• Gaseous abdominal distention possibly due to severe spasticity in the anal sphincter or its surrounding muscles<br>• Gall stones<br>• Superior mesenteric artery syndrome, especially after a spinal surgery |
| Musculoskeletal | • Hip and shoulder subluxation/dislocation<br>• Pathologic fracture<br>• Postoperative muscular pain<br>• Arthritis<br>• Myelopathy due to cervical spinal stenosis<br>• Knee pain caused by hamstring tightness, especially during growth spurt<br>• Frequent ankle sprains due to foot deformities |
| Respiratory | • Mucous plugging<br>• Recurrent aspiration pneumonia from dysphagia<br>• Headache due to prolonged accumulation of carbon dioxide from the global hypoventilation in the setting of hypotonic trunk |
| Genitourinary | • Bladder retention due to detrusor/sphincter dyssynergia<br>• Spastic bladder wall could cause vesicoureteral reflux that results in kidney damage<br>• Frequent urinary tract infection<br>• Kidney stones |
| Neurologic | • Shunt malfunction in children with hydrocephalus |
| Skin | • Fungal infections or skin irritation after applying splints/orthoses to severe sweating hands and feet<br>• Pressure injury due to spastic muscles |
| Dental | • Dental decay due to poor oral hygiene or drooling due to poor oral-motor skill<br>• Temporomandibular joint pain due to trismus |
| Endocrine | • Severe osteopenia causing bony pain |

(GERD) rather than increased muscle tone, such as severe spasticity or dystonia. If a child has severe opisthotonic posture without a significant history of neurologic disorders that could cause dystonia or spasticity in the trunk, clinicians need to rule out Sandifer syndrome from severe GERD, esophagitis, or presence of hiatal hernia.

Indications of a posterior lateral hip subluxation include the patients' hip in an externally rotated position with knee flexion. If moved out of this position, particularly in hip internal rotation, they will likely experience pain and may indicate by crying or grimacing.

Musculoskeletal examination is an important component of the physical assessment of the child with spasticity. Clinicians should be familiar with the techniques of the musculoskeletal examination. The examination process should be done in a systemic fashion.

### Static examination
If a child has ATNR, the arm and leg of the side where the child is faced become extended and the other arm and leg become flexed. Therefore, the child's head should be in the middle to avoid provoking ATNR during examination to assess spasticity of limbs correctly. Severely increased leg extensor tone causes difficulty with examining both legs because legs cannot be flexed. Clinicians can use the Marie-Foix reflex to flex legs with severe extensor tone. The Marie-Foix maneuver is a manipulation for exciting a flexion reflex in all joints in the lower extremities by a passive and slow flexion of the toes and feet (**Fig. 1**).

**Muscle tone evaluation** Before the evaluation of range in each limb, the severity of spasticity needs to be assessed because mobilizing joints multiple times will decrease spasticity.

- The spasticity evaluation tools that are commonly used are the Modified Ashworth Scale (MAS) and the Modified Tardieu scale. A more quantifiable measurement for spasticity was developed by Tardieu and may benefit more than MAS by better differentiation of contractures from spasticity.[13]
- To differentiate hypertonicity between spasticity versus dystonia versus rigidity, the Hypertonia Assessment Tool (HAT) is used frequently.[14] HAT's advantages are in its simplicity and clarity.[15]

**Range-of-motion evaluation** It is important to perform range of motion of each joint to know the available range, degree of stiffness, and presence of pain. This information will help clinicians plan spasticity management based on the findings on physical examination and treatment goals. Upper extremity examination includes shoulder internal rotation and external rotation, abduction; elbow extension and flexion; wrist extension and flexion; active and passive forearm supination; presence of cortical

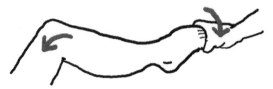

**Fig. 1.** Marie-Foix reflex: In the supine position, apply passive and slow flexion of toes and feet.

thumb; and fisted hands. Lower extremity examination includes the Thomas test and rotational profiles for the gait pattern including (1) hip internal rotation to assess the degree of femoral anteversion, (2) hip external rotation, (3) thigh-foot angle for tibial torsion, (4) hip abduction with the knee flexed and extended (5), knee extension with hip extension, (6) popliteal angle, (7) ankle dorsiflexion with the knee extended for gastrocnemius tightness and with the knee flexed for soleus tightness, and (8) the Ely test for rectus femoris of the quadriceps tightness (**Fig. 2**).

**Thomas test** This test is performed with the child lying supine on the examination table and the examiner bringing the child's contralateral knee to the chest until the child's lordosis disappears. If there is no hip flexion contracture, then the opposite hip will completely extend. If there is a hip flexion contracture, there will be a limitation of hip extension on the nonflexed side (opposite side). The amount of hip flexion contracture is quantified as the amount of hip flexion on the side being tested (**Fig. 3**). When the child's knee is contracted, the child' knee should be placed below the examination table to measure only the hip flexor contracture.

**Hip internal rotation** In typically developing children, there is a rotation of the femur between the hip and the knee joints. Spasticity prevents normal derotation of femur. The child without spasticity has approximately 15° to 20° of femoral anteversion. In child with spasticity, this approximation may be abnormally increased or occasionally decreased. An abnormal amount of femoral rotation may affect his or her gait pattern. Increased femoral anteversion causes intoeing gait. A child can be positioned on her or his back. The hip and the knee will be flexed at 90° to be internally rotated (**Fig. 4**). The prone position test can also be useful to quantifying the amount of femoral anteversion (**Fig. 5**). An increased angle of internal rotation of the thigh can be consistent with an increased femoral anteversion (see **Fig. 5**).

**Hip external rotation** A child can be in the prone or supine position. The hip and knee will be flexed at 90°, and the hip will be externally rotated (**Fig. 6**).

**Hip abduction with knee extended and knee flexed** Hip abduction on supine position can be measured in two ways. To assess for tightness in the hip adductors, a one joint muscle, we measure abduction with knees flexed. To assess for tightness in the gracilis, a two joint muscle, we measure abduction with knees extended (**Fig. 7**). A hip at risk for hip subluxation or dislocation is defined as one in which abduction is limited to less than 45° or one in which asymmetries of abduction exist on the clinical examination[16] (**Fig. 8**).

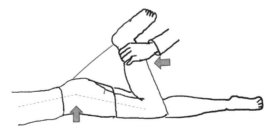

**Fig. 2.** Ely test: The child lies prone in a relaxed state. The examiner is standing next to the child, at the side of the leg that is being tested. One hand should hold the leg at the heel and passively flex the knee in a rapid fashion until the heel touches the buttocks. The test is positive when the heel cannot touch the buttocks, the hip of the tested side rises from the table, and the child feels pain or tingling in the back or legs.

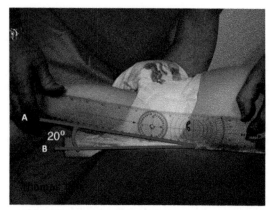

**Fig. 3.** Thomas test. The child is in the supine position. The child's femur is 20° from full extension. Bring the child's contralateral knee to the chest until the child's lordosis disappears. If there is no hip flexion contracture, then the opposite hip will completely extend. If there is hip flexion contracture, there will be a limitation of hip extension on the non-flexed side (opposite side).

**Popliteal angle** To measure hamstring tightness, with the child lying in a supine position on the examination table, the examiner flexes the child's hip and knee being examined until they reach 90°. Once the knee gets stretched to the end range, the degree of extension from full extension will be measured, as in **Fig. 9**. In order to eliminate any confusion as to the reference for the degree measurement, the popliteal angle is communicated as *X degrees from full extension*. To differentiate between knee contracture and hamstring tightness from spasticity, place the hip in the extension position to relax the hamstring. Any inability to fully extend the knee is a sign of contracture of the deep posterior soft tissues of the knee, such as the knee capsule and cruciate ligament.

**Ankle dorsiflexion with knee extended** Gastrocnemius contracture is evaluated by quantifying the maximum amount of ankle dorsiflexion with the knee extended because the gastrocnemius muscle is two joint muscle. The angle of the ankle will

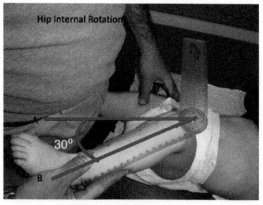

**Fig. 4.** Hip internal rotation: A child can be positioned on her or his back. Then the hip and knee will be flexed at 90° to be internally rotated.

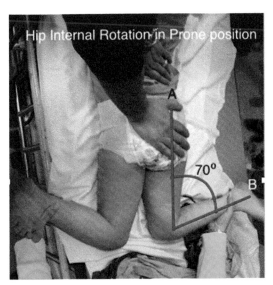

**Fig. 5.** Hip internal rotation in prone position: In prone position, internally rotate the hip.

be measured by the amount of angle between neutral to plantar flexion of the ankle (**Fig. 10**). To measure the soleus, which is one joint muscle, the knee will be flexed during ankle dorsiflexion.

**Thigh-foot angle** To assess tibial torsion, the thigh-foot angle needs to be assessed. A child will be placed in the prone position on the examination table. The examiner notes the axis of the child's foot (between the middle of heel and the second and third toes) with the axis of the child's femur (**Fig. 11**). This thigh-foot angle can be diagnosed as either internal, contributing to intoeing, or external, contributing to outtoeing. **Figs. 11** and **12** show the cause of right intoeing during walking is most likely due to right tibial torsion. Intoeing can be caused by various etiologies such as femoral anteversion and/or metatarsus adductus. It is important that the clinician measure the hip internal rotation and thigh foot angle to determine the source of intoeing.

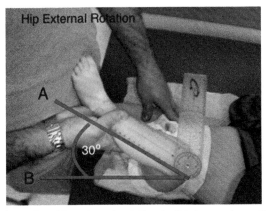

**Fig. 6.** Hip external rotation: Hip external rotation in this image shows 30° (angle between points A and B).

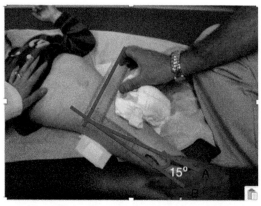

**Fig. 7.** Hip abduction with knee extended to measure gracilis.

### Dynamic examination

For dynamic evaluation, you can have children use their own body. To assess upper extremity function you can have children do actions, such as holding a spoon, palm up to see forearm supination, high 5 for shoulder flexion and elbow extension, and scratching the back of their head or lower back to see shoulder rotation. We need to observe children's movement on a mat to see their trunk control, sitting, crawling, or kneeling. Gait can be assessed with and without orthoses and walk aides.

### TREATMENT
#### Decision-Making Process for Pediatric Spasticity Management

Management of spasticity is challenging, and no standard approach exists. There are special considerations for pediatric spasticity management (**Fig. 13**):

1. Underlying diagnosis, static versus progressive: If the underlying disease that causes spasticity is progressive, intrathecal baclofen (ITB) could be the best option because the dose of baclofen can be easily adjusted and eventually it prevents patients from multiple invasive procedures for spasticity management as the disease progresses. Chemoneuroloysis can begin early on in the disease progress and can be continued until surgical decision has been made.

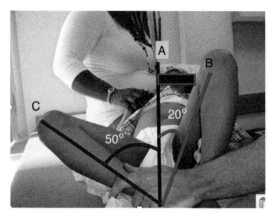

**Fig. 8.** Hip abduction with knee flexed: to measure hip adductors. Left hip at risk for hip subluxation due to abduction <45°.

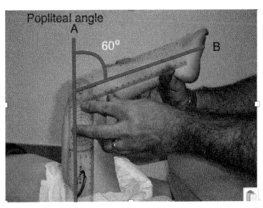

**Fig. 9.** Popliteal angle: Position the child in a supine position with the hip and knee flexed to 90°. Examiner stretches the knee into extension and the popliteal angle value is the angle of the knee from full extension.

2. Timing of spasticity management
   - Physical therapy: Physical therapy is conventionally physiotherapy, mostly stretching exercises, using orthotics, and braces and started any time spasticity is found.[17]
   - Chemoneurolysis: There has been no consensus for the timing of chemoneurolysis including botulinum toxin (BTX) injections and alcohol motor nerve blocks at this time. Most clinicians are comfortable treating spasticity with BTX before 2 years of age. Phenol or alcohol motor point or nerve blocks are rarely used to control spasticity. Despite the low cost, rapid onset of action, and potency, phenol and alcohol are less popular than BTX because of the possibility of unintended effects, such as dysesthesia, need for sedation due to pain during injections, and the requirement for administration by a skillful clinician.[18]
   - Orthopedic surgery: Orthopedic surgery is usually postponed until children reach 4 years of age or older because of the rapid growth of the musculoskeletal system. By 4 years of age, their muscles double their birth length; by the time they

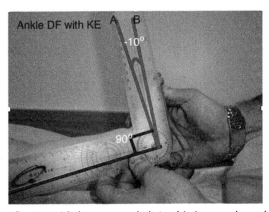

**Fig. 10.** Ankle dorsiflexion with knee extended: In this image, the ankle is 10° short of neutral. DF, dorsiflexed; KE, knee extended.

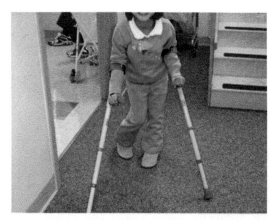

**Fig. 11.** Dynamic gait evaluation. The child should be asked to walk if possible, with and without an assistive device. In this gait, right intoeing is obvious during walking.

reach adulthood, their muscles will be doubled in length again. Muscles lengthening before 4 years of age will frequently need lengthening again at a later stage.[19]

- Selective dorsal rhizotomy (SDR): SDR is a classic indication for around 4- to 5-year-old patients with diplegic CP with severe spasticity. A recent publication indicates that SDR can be performed as early as 2 years of age.[20]
- ITB pump: There is no age limitation but child's body size. Contraindications of ITP pump placement could be insufficient body size for an implantable pump, implant depth greater than 2.5 cm below skin, or in the presence of spinal anomalies.[21]

3. Diffuse versus focal spasticity: When the child's spasticity is focally involved, chemoneurolysis, especially BTX, has been recommended. For diffuse spasticity, more systemic therapy options, such as oral antispastic drugs, ITB pump, or single-event multilevel chemoneurolysis (SEMLC) with BTX and phenol or alcohol

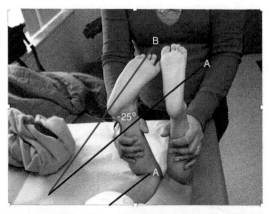

**Fig. 12.** Thigh-foot angle: A child will be placed in prone position on the examination table. Examiner notes the axis of the child's foot (between middle of heel and second and third toes) with the axis of the child's femur. In this image, right tibial torsion is evident with thigh-foot angle of −25°.

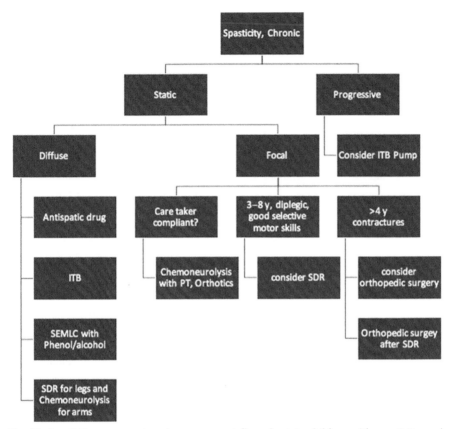

**Fig. 13.** Spasticity assessment and management flow chart. In children with spasticity, multiple factors should be considered to optimize management. PT, physical therapy.

blocks, are considered. Oral antispastic medications and use of an ITB pump are recommended when a generalized antispastic effect is desired, whereas chemoneurolysis is used for localized or segmental spasticity.[22]

4. Severity of spasticity: Neurosurgical interventions are usually considered for children with severe and diffuse spasticity, such as ITB pump or SDR.

5. Goals of spasticity management: Frequent spasticity management goals are to improve walking, dressing, ease of care, and prevent musculoskeletal complications. The ITB pump is an option for patients who have diffuse and severe spasticity that cannot be adequately controlled by oral baclofen and BTX-A injection only.[23] However, generalized reduction of spasticity, including extensor spasticity, may compromise ambulatory and transfer abilities in ambulant persons.[23] This potential compromise is one of the main reasons for hesitation in ITB pump placement, in addition to a concern about possible complications from an invasive procedure.[24] The SEMLC approach has been developed because CP is a nonfocal condition, and several overactive muscle groups (ie, multiple levels [such as hip, knee, and ankle levels] of a single limb) may need to be targeted in a single session to achieve a specific goal during treatment.[25] The advantages of using SEMLC, as opposed to oral medications and ITB, include selectively addressing problematic muscles with different doses of

chemoneurolytic agent according to the severity of spasticity and avoiding the adverse effects of oral antispastic medications.

BTX and phenol/ethanol have difference properties that help to guide treatment decisions. The mechanism of BTX is such that is diffuses to the neuromuscular junction. This known diffusion property is beneficial for abnormal anatomy due to chronic spasticity and muscles whose motor points can be difficult to identify for phenol or alcohol injections, such as iliopsoas and hamstrings.[26] We must also consider the adverse effects that could occur with diffusion of BTX when doing injections in muscles such as the hip adductors and sternocleidomastoid muscle. Diffusion in these areas may affect the nearby bladder or neck muscles causing bladder incontinence or dysphagia.[27]

6. Child's intelligence and attention span: If the goal is to improve function that requires training by therapists, the child needs to be trainable and has enough attention span to work with therapists. When the child has a significantly impaired attention span, a child developmental medicine specialist can be consulted for further evaluation and management.

7. Compliance of care takers: The spasticity management will not be beneficial if there is no continuum of care. Children with toe walking due to hemiplegic CP may have benefit after BTX injections with ability to ambulate with flat foot. However, if there is not appropriate follow up and repeat injections are not performed in a timely manner, they may develop ankle contracture and will not have as much benefit from repeat injections. In children with an ITB pump, if caretakers forget the refill dates, patients can be in danger of rebound rigidity from withdrawal of ITB that results in critical medical conditions, such as neuroleptic malignant syndrome.

8. Geographic limitation/resources: When we introduce the ITB pump for refill or chemoneurolysis for regular repeat injections, there should be at least 1 or 2 hospitals where they can offer these services to promote compliance of patient care and to prevent significant complications by traveling far to get to the institution where they can have those services. SDR can be a good option for children with severe spasticity in lower limbs who do not have access to nearby specialists in spasticity management or are not able to attend frequent clinic appointments.

## *Treatment Options*

1. Pharmacologic treatment

    Oral medications are used when a generalized antispasticity effect is desired.[28] Diazepam ($\gamma$-aminobutyric acid [GABA]$_a$ agonist), dantrolene (sarcoplasmic reticulum), baclofen (GABA$_b$ agonist), and tizanidine (alpha agonist) are the most-studied medications.[29–32] Diazepam is effective in treating spasticity for the short-term. Different adverse effects should be closely monitored for each drug.

2. Chemodenervation

    Chemodenervation is used for focal spasticity. BTX, which is a neuromuscular junction blocking agent, is considered effective and generally safe. The only 2 preparations of BTX-A with published evidences of efficacy in children with CP are onabotulinumtoxinA and abobotulinumtoxinA.[33] Receiving BTX-A at an earlier age (<5 years) has a greater response in changes in spasticity of the ankle plantar flexor in spastic CP.[34] Starting early (<6 months) with physical therapy can also be beneficial to improve function as an adjunct.[35] A more focused approach needs to be established to improve function and motor development and to prevent adverse compensations and contractures.[18]

Safety: Adverse effects of BTX can be divided into the following categories: generalized, focal distant, focal local, and procedural.[25] Phenol and alcohol are other agents used for neurolysis, and there is insufficient evidence to support or refute their use to treat spasticity in children with CP. The main side effect is dysesthesia if sensory nerves are damaged. However, a recent retrospective review of the effectiveness and safety of SEMLC did not result in dysesthesia.[36]

Successful outcome determinant factors: The intensity of physical therapy, postinjection casting, and frequency of using orthoses could be crucial factors for a successful outcome. The advantages of using SEMLC, as opposed to oral medications and ITB, include selectively addressing problematic muscles with different doses of a chemoneurolytic agent according to the severity of spasticity and avoiding the adverse effects of oral antispastic medications.

3. ITB

A Cochrane review that evaluated 6 studies showed that longer-term study found a small improvement in gross motor function and also in domains of health-related quality of life.[37] ITB pump is also considered to be a cost-effective method to treat severe spasticity.[38] Safety: One of the concerns with ITB is its complications, which include infection, cerebrospinal fluid leak, catheter problem, and pump problems. The most common problem was catheter associated, which most frequently happened during the first year after the implant.[39] There were case reports that were concerned about possible development of scoliosis after ITB placement; however, retrospective chart review of 107 patients who underwent ITB therapy with a matched cohort did not have a significant effect on curve progression, pelvic obliquity, or the incidence of scoliosis.[40,41]

4. Orthopedic surgeries

Surgical options include tenotomy, tendon lengthening, osteotomy, and dorsal spinal cord/muscle stimulation. One patient may undergo multiple surgical procedures, and the decisions should be made in a multidisciplinary setting.[42] Musculotendinous lengthening can functionally elongate the muscle and decrease the spasticity by interrupting the Golgi receptors for a short period.

5. Selective dorsal rhizotomy

SDR involves single-level or multilevel osteoplastic laminectomies exposing the L2-S1 nerve roots. Children who are 3 to 8 years of age with spastic diplegia, minimal upper limb involvement, minimal contractures, and good selective motor skills are good candidates. Positive predictors include the ability to rise from a squatted position with minimal support or the ability crawl on hands and knees. If performed before 5 years of age, 35% of children may avoid other surgeries. Long-term complications include sensory dysfunction, bladder/bowel dysfunction, and back pain.[43] Long-term outcomes of childhood SDR showed positive effects on quality of life and ambulation without late complications 20 to 28 years after SDR.[44]

6. Serial casting

Serial casting for spastic ankle plantar flexion has been used in conjunction with BTX and physical therapy.[45]

7. Treatment controversies

There are a few studies that show a cell transplant can improve function and spasticity in children with incurable neurologic disorders.[46] However, much remains to be understood regarding its safety, feasibility, and efficacy.[47] Vibration therapy,[48] shock wave therapy,[49] and horseback riding therapy[50] are also being studied for their effectiveness. Myofascial release may improve gait quality in children with CP who are less than 4 years of age.[51] Neuromodulation therapy, such as deep anterior cerebellar stimulation, that was chronically applied in 13 young patients with CP with dystonia showed a significant reduction of spasticity in the upper extremities and lower extremities. Focal dystonia symptoms were also reduced.[52]

## SUMMARY

In pediatric spasticity management, factors such as the goals of treatment, current functional status, degree and location of spasticity, age, weight, caregiver's compliance, intelligence, and speed of growth, in addition to thorough history taking and examination need to be considered for successful spasticity management. The difference in managing spasticity between adults and children is the growth in children. The basic principle of pediatric spasticity management is to equalize the growth between bone and spastic muscle until their growth is done. Spasticity in growing children impacts on their bones and muscles. Musculoskeletal complications, such as joint contractures, foot deformity, hip dislocation, pain, or functional deterioration, can occur with and without spasticity management because of the discrepancy of the growth ratio between bones and spastic muscles. Therefore, early intervention, continuum of care, and understanding the special considerations in pediatric spasticity management should be considered to prevent or minimize musculoskeletal complications and functional deterioration and improve quality of life.

## REFERENCES

1. Van Naarden Braun K, Doernberg N, Schieve L, et al. Birth prevalence of cerebral palsy: a population-based study. Pediatrics 2016;137(1). https://doi.org/10.1542/peds.2015-2872.
2. Bar-On L, Molenaers G, Aertbelien E, et al. Spasticity and its contribution to hypertonia in cerebral palsy. Biomed Res Int 2015;2015:317047.
3. Mukherjee A, Chakravarty A. Spasticity mechanisms - for the clinician. Front Neurol 2010;1:149.
4. Levitt M, Browd S. Spasticity. In: Ellenbogen R, editor. Principles of neurological surgery. 3rd edition. Philadephia: Elsvier; 2012. p. 757–63.
5. Hagglund G, Andersson S, Duppe H, et al. Prevention of severe contractures might replace multilevel surgery in cerebral palsy: results of a population-based health care programme and new techniques to reduce spasticity. J Pediatr Orthop B 2005;14(4):269–73.
6. Lance JW. The control of muscle tone, reflexes, and movement: Robert Wartenberg lecture. Neurology 1980;30(12):1303–13.
7. O'Shea TM. Cerebral palsy in very preterm infants: new epidemiological insights. Ment Retard Dev Disabil Res Rev 2002;8(3):135–45.
8. Copley LA, Dormans JP. Cervical spine disorders in infants and children. J Am Acad Orthop Surg 1998;6(4):204–14.
9. Terjesen T. The natural history of hip development in cerebral palsy. Dev Med Child Neurol 2012;54(10):951–7.
10. Alvarez N, Larkin C, Roxborough J. Carpal tunnel syndrome in athetoid-dystonic cerebral palsy. Arch Neurol 1982;39(5):311–2.
11. Barnes MP. Management of spasticity. Age Ageing 1998;27(2):239–45.
12. Gerber PE, Lynd LD. Selective serotonin-reuptake inhibitor-induced movement disorders. Ann Pharmacother 1998;32(6):692–8.

13. Patrick E, Ada L. The Tardieu scale differentiates contracture from spasticity whereas the Ashworth scale is confounded by it. Clin Rehabil 2006;20(2):173–82.
14. Knights S, Datoo N, Kawamura A, et al. Further evaluation of the scoring, reliability, and validity of the hypertonia assessment tool (HAT). J Child Neurol 2014;29(4):500–4.
15. Albright L, Andrews M. Development of the hypertonia assessment tool (HAT). Dev Med Child Neurol 2010;52(5):411–2.
16. Sharrard WJ, Allen JM, Heaney SH. Surgical prophylaxis of subluxation and dislocation of the hip in cerebral palsy. J Bone Joint Surg Br 1975;57(2):160–6.
17. Matthews DJ, Balaban B. Management of spasticity in children with cerebral palsy. Acta Orthop Traumatol Turc 2009;43(2):81–6.
18. Strobl W, Theologis T, Brunner R, et al. Best clinical practice in botulinum toxin treatment for children with cerebral palsy. Toxins (Basel) 2015;7(5):1629–48.
19. Gage JR, Fabian D, Hicks R, et al. Pre- and postoperative gait analysis in patients with spastic diplegia: a preliminary report. J Pediatr Orthop 1984;4(6):715–25.
20. Center for cerebral palsy spasticity. Available at: http://www.stlouischildrens.org/our-services/center-cerebral-palsy-spasticity/patient-selection. Accessed December 29th, 2017.
21. About the therapy intrathecal baclofen therapy with lioresal intrathecal (baclofen injection). Medtronic Web site. Available at: https://www.medtronic.com/us-en/healthcare-professionals/therapies-procedures/neurological/intrathecal-baclofen-therapy/education-training/about-the-therapy.html. Updated 2017. Accessed December 29th, 2017.
22. Balaban B, Tok F, Tan AK, et al. Botulinum toxin a treatment in children with cerebral palsy: its effects on walking and energy expenditure. Am J Phys Med Rehabil 2012;91(1):53–64.
23. Pin TW, McCartney L, Lewis J, et al. Use of intrathecal baclofen therapy in ambulant children and adolescents with spasticity and dystonia of cerebral origin: a systematic review. Dev Med Child Neurol 2011;53(10):885–95.
24. Ghosh D, Mainali G, Khera J, et al. Complications of intrathecal baclofen pumps in children: experience from a tertiary care center. Pediatr Neurosurg 2013;49(3):138–44.
25. Heinen F, Desloovere K, Schroeder AS, et al. The updated European consensus 2009 on the use of botulinum toxin for children with cerebral palsy. Eur J Paediatr Neurol 2010;14(1):45–66.
26. Van Campenhout A, Verhaegen A, Pans S, et al. Botulinum toxin type A injections in the psoas muscle of children with cerebral palsy: muscle atrophy after motor end plate-targeted injections. Res Dev Disabil 2013;34(3):1052–8.
27. Tilton AH. Injectable neuromuscular blockade in the treatment of spasticity and movement disorders. J Child Neurol 2003;18(Suppl 1):S50–66.
28. Whelan MA, Delgado MR. Practice parameter: pharmacologic treatment of spasticity in children and adolescents with cerebral palsy (an evidence-based review): report of the quality standards subcommittee of the American Academy of Neurology and the practice committee of the Child Neurology Society. Neurology 2010;75(7):669.
29. Joynt RL, Leonard JA Jr. Dantrolene sodium suspension in treatment of spastic cerebral palsy. Dev Med Child Neurol 1980;22(6):755–67.
30. Pinder RM, Brogden RN, Speight TM, et al. Dantrolene sodium: a review of its pharmacological properties and therapeutic efficacy in spasticity. Drugs 1977;13(1):3–23.

31. Dantrolene. New indication. Cerebral palsy in children: uncertain clinical benefit. Prescrire Int 2008;17(98):237.
32. Quality Standards Subcommittee of the American Academy of Neurology and the Practice Committee of the Child Neurology Society, Delgado MR, Hirtz D, et al. Practice parameter: pharmacologic treatment of spasticity in children and adolescents with cerebral palsy (an evidence-based review): report of the quality standards subcommittee of the American Academy of Neurology and the practice committee of the Child Neurology Society. Neurology 2010;74(4):336–43.
33. Carraro E, Trevisi E, Martinuzzi A. Safety profile of incobotulinum toxin A [xeomin((R))] in gastrocnemious muscles injections in children with cerebral palsy: randomized double-blind clinical trial. Eur J Paediatr Neurol 2016;20(4):532–7.
34. Alcaraz J, Oliver A, Sanchez JM. Platelet-rich plasma in a patient with cerebral palsy. Am J Case Rep 2015;16:469–72.
35. Ronan S, Gold JT. Nonoperative management of spasticity in children. Childs Nerv Syst 2007;23(9):943–56.
36. Ploypetch T, Kwon JY, Armstrong HF, et al. A retrospective review of unintended effects after single-event multi-level chemoneurolysis with botulinum toxin-A and phenol in children with cerebral palsy. PM R 2015;7(10):1073–80.
37. Hasnat MJ, Rice JE. Intrathecal baclofen for treating spasticity in children with cerebral palsy. Cochrane Database Syst Rev 2015;(11):CD004552.
38. Saulino M, Guillemette S, Leier J, et al. Medical cost impact of intrathecal baclofen therapy for severe spasticity. Neuromodulation 2015;18(2):141–9 [discussion: 149].
39. Motta F, Antonello CE. Analysis of complications in 430 consecutive pediatric patients treated with intrathecal baclofen therapy: 14-year experience. J Neurosurg Pediatr 2014;13(3):301–6.
40. Sansone JM, Mann D, Noonan K, et al. Rapid progression of scoliosis following insertion of intrathecal baclofen pump. J Pediatr Orthop 2006;26(1):125–8.
41. Senaran H, Shah SA, Presedo A, et al. The risk of progression of scoliosis in cerebral palsy patients after intrathecal baclofen therapy. Spine (Phila Pa 1976) 2007;32(21):2348–54.
42. Lynn AK, Turner M, Chambers HG. Surgical management of spasticity in persons with cerebral palsy. PM R 2009;1(9):834–8.
43. Steinbok P. Selective dorsal rhizotomy for spastic cerebral palsy: a review. Childs Nerv Syst 2007;23(9):981–90.
44. Park TS, Liu JL, Edwards C, et al. Functional outcomes of childhood selective dorsal rhizotomy 20 to 28 years later. Cureus 2017;9(5):e1256.
45. Newman CJ, Kennedy A, Walsh M, et al. A pilot study of delayed versus immediate serial casting after botulinum toxin injection for partially reducible spastic equinus. J Pediatr Orthop 2007;27(8):882–5.
46. Sharma A, Gokulchandran N, Chopra G, et al. Administration of autologous bone marrow-derived mononuclear cells in children with incurable neurological disorders and injury is safe and improves their quality of life. Cell Transplant 2012;21(Suppl 1):S79–90.
47. Zali A, Arab L, Ashrafi F, et al. Intrathecal injection of CD133-positive enriched bone marrow progenitor cells in children with cerebral palsy: feasibility and safety. Cytotherapy 2015;17(2):232–41.
48. Cheng HY, Yu YC, Wong AM, et al. Effects of an eight-week whole body vibration on lower extremity muscle tone and function in children with cerebral palsy. Res Dev Disabil 2015;38:256–61.

49. Wang T, Du L, Shan L, et al. A prospective case-control study of radial extracorporeal shock wave therapy for spastic plantar flexor muscles in very young children with cerebral palsy. Medicine (Baltimore) 2016;95(19):e3649.
50. Alemdaroglu E, Yanikoglu I, Oken O, et al. Horseback riding therapy in addition to conventional rehabilitation program decreases spasticity in children with cerebral palsy: a small sample study. Complement Ther Clin Pract 2016;23:26–9.
51. Loi EC, Buysse CA, Price KS, et al. Myofascial structural integration therapy on gross motor function and gait of young children with spastic cerebral palsy: a randomized controlled trial. Front Pediatr 2015;3:74.
52. Sokal P, Rudas M, Harat M, et al. Deep anterior cerebellar stimulation reduces symptoms of secondary dystonia in patients with cerebral palsy treated due to spasticity. Clin Neurol Neurosurg 2015;135:62–8.

# Special Considerations and Assessment in Patients with Multiple Sclerosis

Ian B. Maitin, MD, MBA*, Ernesto Cruz, MD

## KEYWORDS

- Multiple sclerosis • Spasticity • Botulinum toxin • Cannabinoids

## KEY POINTS

- Multiple sclerosis is a progressive neurologic autoimmune disorder that may cause demyelinating lesions anywhere in the central nervous system.
- Spasticity is a symptom of multiple sclerosis that causes an increase in muscle tone, hyperreflexia, spasms, and pain.
- Spasticity in patients with multiple sclerosis can have profound functional implications that influence the quality of life for patients.
- Treatment objectives for spasticity in patients with multiple sclerosis should be clearly defined and individualized.
- Treatment of spasticity may include pharmacologic agents, physical therapy, botulinum toxin, cannabinoids, and modalities.

## INTRODUCTION

Multiple sclerosis (MS) is an autoimmune disorder associated with demyelination, axonal damage, neurodegeneration, and astrogliosis.[1] It is a progressive disease that can cause damage anywhere in the central nervous system (CNS). Spasticity is a symptom of MS, which is part of the upper motor neuron syndrome and is typified by increase in tone, muscle hyperactivity, spasms, and stiffness, among other complications. Spasticity is a disabling symptom of MS in more than 80% of patients, often leading to decreased function, pain, contractures, and skin breakdown.

## PATHOPHYSIOLOGY

The process of demyelination and remyelination, with exacerbation and remission, adds a dynamic component to the MS disease process. The pathology is unpredictable

Disclosures: The authors have nothing to disclose.
Department of Physical Medicine and Rehabilitation, Lewis Katz School of Medicine, Temple University, 3401 North Broad Street, Philadelphia, PA 19140, USA
* Corresponding author.
E-mail address: Ian.Maitin@tuhs.temple.edu

Phys Med Rehabil Clin N Am 29 (2018) 473–481
https://doi.org/10.1016/j.pmr.2018.03.003
1047-9651/18/© 2018 Elsevier Inc. All rights reserved.

and individualized; accordingly, the associated spasticity can change significantly over time. The chronically damaged neurons of patients with MS are vulnerable to metabolic changes, stress, or inflammatory signals accounting for dynamic changes seen in patients with MS.[2] Similarly, the burden of the disease and function of patients can change. Continual reevaluation of the approach to treating spastic patients with MS by physicians, therapists, and patients based on individualized symptoms is critical to maintaining function, activities of daily living (ADLs), and quality of life.[3]

In the setting of central autoimmune damage in MS with neuroplasticity, there is a shift that increases the excitatory inputs to alpha motor neurons with disinhibition of reflexes. With compromise of the myelin sheath, there is ephaptic spread among axons of the action potentials distributing the excitation.

Patterns of spasticity in MS can vary and may be restricted to one limb or one side of the body. Alternatively, the spasticity can be more diffuse or assume a para or tetra pattern. A change in balance of the excitation and inhibition of alpha motor neurons can cause spasticity change throughout the day. A para-spastic pattern involving the lower limbs has important ramifications for transfers and ambulation.

## EPIDEMIOLOGY

The prevalence of spasticity in MS was studied looking at patient data from the North American Research Committee on Multiple Sclerosis (NARCOMS).[4] They found that 74% of relapsing remitting patients were spastic with 55% mild and 19% moderate or severe, and 90% of secondary progressive patients were spastic with 48% mild and 43% moderate to severe. The primary progressive group of patients revealed 80% spasticity with 50% mild and 30% moderate to severe. Men were more likely than women to be severely spastic, and the spasticity symptoms worsened with age and duration of MS. Risk factors for the development of spasticity included pain, motor impairment, and bladder dysfunction.[5]

## ASSESSMENT

Illomei and colleagues,[6] in 2017, published a report on the use of muscle elastography to evaluate spasticity in patients with MS. Elastography is real-time ultrasound that evaluates muscle fiber status and changes with treatment. Working with the understanding that the Ashworth scale has limitations in that it does not correlate well with disability and is not sensitive to change, they developed a muscle elasticity MS score. This scale is a muscle fiber rigidity imaging scale, which has strong correlation with the Ashworth scale, serving as an objective means to evaluate MS spasticity.

## TREATMENT

Detrimental effects of spasticity include decreased function, pain, increased burden of care, contractures, skin breakdown, and pressure wounds. This point is not to say that all spasticity needs to be treated. One must consider the negative effects of reducing tone, for example, patients who rely on stiff, spastic lower limbs for stability during transfers and standing. Immunotherapy and spasticity medications may have a negative effect on the MS disease process by increasing spasticity (immunotherapy) and by decreasing autoimmunity (spasticity meds).[7] Sometimes transient short-term treatment of spasticity is required, as when symptoms are worsened by a urinary tract infection or decubitus ulcer.

Treatment objectives and therapeutic targets should be clearly defined. The treatment protocol is most successful when multimodal, integrated, and individualized.

An ambulating patient with tight adductors clearly will have differing objectives from a bedbound immobile patient with painful spasms and high burden of care due to spastic limbs. Control of MS disease progression will reduce spasticity, but frequently additional treatment focused on spasticity is required.

Treatment with intrathecal steroids can be effective for controlling leg spasticity.[8] Steroids may decrease neuronal excitability and may interrupt excitatory signals from immune cells to neurons. Steroids change the excitatory calcium and sodium currents and reduce intracellular calcium in hippocampal neurons.[8]

Beta-interferon may worsen spasticity.[9] It has a direct effect on neuronal function, membrane conductance, and synaptic currents of cortical and subcortical neurons. Worsening spasticity with beta-interferon may necessitate change of medications. Glatiramer acetate shows no evidence of excitatory properties.[10] Natalizumab has little influence on spasticity.

Many patients with MS are not adequately treated for their spasticity-related symptoms. Side effects of the medications and unfamiliarity with appropriate medication treatment are some of the reasons. A survey of patients with MS by NARCOMS showed that increased spasticity is associated with higher MS-related disability and lower quality of life.[11] Bethoux and Marrie[11] conducted a cross-sectional survey of more than 15,000 NARCOMS participants examining the influence of spasticity on ADLs, the bother of spasticity symptoms, and the level of treatment of such. Thirty-five percent reported a moderate or great bother from stiffness, spasms, or pain, primarily in the lower limbs. Greater spasticity was associated with worse disability, mobility, bladder function, and fatigue. Spasticity was reported to most frequently interfere with stair climbing, walking, and sleep. Most patients reported being treated for spasticity, but less than half were satisfied with their current treatment.

Vermersch and Trojano[12] in 2014 published a study examining the burden of MS spasticity in European Union countries. They reviewed charts of 281 patients and surveyed the patients and their physicians. MS spasticity was found to frequently restrict daily activities and cause problems with mobility and usual activities while causing pain and discomfort. Forty-eight percent of physicians and 34% of patients were at least partially dissatisfied with the effectiveness of available pharmacotherapy options.

## MEDICATIONS

Oral medications are usually the first line of treatment of MS spasticity. When choosing an agent one must consider side effects, comorbidities, pattern of spasticity, cognition of the patients, and cost of the medication.

Baclofen is a $\gamma$-aminobutyric acid (GABA) receptor analogue with a low side-effect profile. Dosing is usually started at 5 mg 3 times a day and titrated up as tolerated to a maximum of 120 to 140 mg daily, though some clinicians may go to higher doses. Binding to $GABA_B$ receptors reduces primarily flexor spasticity. Fatigue or sedation may limit baclofen usefulness.

Tizanidine is an alpha-2 central agonist similar in structure to clonidine. Site of action is in the central alpha-2–adrenergic agonist in the brainstem and spinal cord. It presumably reduces spasticity by increasing presynaptic inhibition of the motor neurons. Studies have proven the efficacy of tizanidine in reducing MS spasticity with effects comparable with baclofen. Side effects include hypotension, sedation, and dry mouth. Dosing is started at 2 mg daily and can be titrated up to 36 mg a day.

Dantrolene sodium reduces muscle contraction by inhibiting the release of calcium from the sarcoplasmic reticulum. This peripheral effect ensures little cognitive influence; however, the drug may cause muscle weakness and may be hepatotoxic. Dosing starts at 25 mg daily and is titrated up to 400 mg a day.

Diazepam is a $GABA_A$ agonist that causes presynaptic inhibition of monosynaptic and polysynaptic reflexes. Unlike baclofen, it does not bind directly to GABA receptors. It binds near $GABA_A$ receptors promoting the presynaptic effects of GABA by facilitating sodium conductance. The dosing starts at 4 mg daily and is titrated up to 40 mg a day in divided doses. Diazepam can have central effects such as sedation and memory impairment and must be tapered off when discontinued. Tolerance and dependence are other adverse effects of concern.

## INTRATHECAL BACLOFEN

Intrathecal baclofen (ITB) is indicated for severely spastic patients with MS who have not responded to combination treatments of medications and chemodenervation. This treatment allows for direct infusion of baclofen into the cerebrospinal fluid (CSF). With a fraction of the systemic dose of other treatments, ITB can provide multiple strengths of medication. An ITB trial is performed before permanent pump placement, which entails a bolus infusion of 50 to 100 mcg of baclofen into the thecal sac. Patients are monitored in the hours afterward for the effect of the drug on muscle tone, specifically lower limb spasticity. After implantation, patients are monitored frequently and drug infusion rates are appropriately titrated. The ITB baclofen pump will require periodic refill by a health professional.

## CANNABINOIDS

Cannabinoids have been shown to be an effective treatment of MS spasticity and associated pain. The active component 9-tetrahydrocannabinol binds to CB1- and CB2-type receptors and can cause symptom relief. CB1 receptors are found in the basal ganglia, cerebellum, hippocampus, and cerebral cortex, whereas CB2 receptors are found in immune cells.[13] Endocannabinoids activating CB1 receptors inhibit neurotransmitter release, such as glutamate, which may influence MS spasticity. Experimental Authoimmune Encephalomyelitis models of MS in rats found the administration of delta-9-tetrahydrocannabinol (THC) can ameliorate disease progression and spasticity, whereas a CB1 antagonist worsens spasticity. This finding is likely due to decreased excitability of neuronal and glutamatergic excitatory pathways with inhibition of sodium and potassium currents.[14] In patients with MS, the beneficial effect of THC on disease progression is seen with patients having an expanded disability status scale of 5.5 or less.[14]

THC/cannabidiol (CBD) oro-mucosal spray is effective for moderate to severe spasticity in patients with MS who have not responded to other antispasmodic medications. THC has psychoactive effects, but CBD is nonpsychoactive. The combination reduces spasticity by inhibition of cortical and spinal pathways.[7]

The Mobility Improvement (MOVE) 2 study in Germany was published in 2014 as a prospective multicenter examination of the effects of THC/CBD on 335 patients with MS with moderate to severe spasticity. The response was evaluated at baseline, 1, and 3 months. At 1 month, 74.6% of patients had relief of spasticity with a mean numerical rating scale (NRS) decrease from 6.1 to 5.2. At 3 months, the mean NRS decreased by 25% from baseline. Significant improvement was maintained beyond the study at 12 months.[15]

Patti and colleagues,[16] in 2016, published results of a study on 1615 patients from the Italian Medicines Agency registry similarly using THC/CBD to treat MS spasticity. At 1 month, the NRS dropped from a mean of 7.5 to 5.9, with 70.5% of patients showing greater than 20% improvement and 28.5% showing greater than 30% improvement.[16] The NRS dropped to 5.1 and 4.8 at 3 and 6 months, respectively.

Carotenuto and colleagues,[17] in 2016, found that spasticity improved in patients with MS spasticity treated with THC/CBD for 12 months but did not correlate with changes in MRI or central motor conduction time.[17]

A study of 339 MS patients found that treatment with THC/CBD did not result in an increase in cognitive disorders.[18]

In addition to the oro-mucosal spray, THC is available in tablet form. Dronabinol and nabilone are used for chemotherapy-induced nausea, human immunodeficiency virus–related wasting, and glaucoma.[7] Most common side effects reported of oral THC include increased appetite, dry mouth, somnolence, and bowel disturbance.

The literature for other oral medications used as antispasmodics is limited. Gabapentin, cyproheptadine, progabide, carisoprodol, and threonine have been studied for efficacy in spasticity but results are inconclusive.

## CHEMODENERVATION

Intramuscular botulinum toxin is an effective treatment of MS spasticity, and benefits are maximized when associated with early mobilization and physical therapy treatment. Botulinum blocks the cholinergic neuromuscular synapse by preventing presynaptic release of acetylcholine, resulting in muscle weakness. The effect lasts 2 to 4 months in most cases. The benefit is not influenced by the type or location of the upper motor neuron lesion, and multiple studies support the efficacy of botulinum for MS spasticity.[19] Toxin is most effective for focal spasticity, such as found in the hip and shoulder adductors or with equinovarus and striatal toe.[20] It allows focused treatment of tone without the systemic risk associated with oral or intrathecal medications. There are no cognitive effects of toxin injection, and the effects of treatment are reversible.

There are multiple subtypes of botulinum toxin, but only types A (Onabotulinum, Abobotulinum, Incobotulinum) and B (Rimabotulinum) are approved for use in the United States.

The dosing protocols differ for each type of toxin, and they all carry a black box warning concerning the risk of distant spread of the drug with focal intramuscular injection. With patients with MS, it is recommended to start at the lowest effective dose to avoid contributing to fatigue and weakness.

Nerve blocks can be used effectively to treat focal muscle hyperactivity in lower-level patients whose spasticity has not resolved with other treatments. A 6% solution of phenol injected intramuscularly near a motor point, or perineural, can reduce tone adequately to reduce hygiene challenges or sometimes improve function. Dysesthesias are possible, so patient selection is imperative. Patients with MS treated with phenol have been shown to experience reduced skin breakdown and lower burden of care after injection. Some patients with a scissoring gait underwent an obturator phenol block and displayed an improved gait pattern after injection.[21] One of the benefits of nerve block is that you can affect multiple muscles with injection around one nerve. For example, block of the median nerve proximally in the axilla can reduce tone in the wrist flexors, pronators, and finger flexors.

## PHYSICAL THERAPY

Physical therapy can be effective in controlling MS spasticity while avoiding complications from hypertonia, such as contractures and skin breakdown. Range of motion of major joints with stretching of muscles crossing those joints is imperative. Some muscles, such as the elbow and knee flexors, gastrocnemius/soleus complex, hip flexors, and finger flexors, are particularly prone to developing spasticity and contractures. Slow sustained stretch through the entire range of motion for 30 seconds can reduce tone and avoid contracture if done twice daily. Patients and families can be instructed on the proper technique. Orthotics can be used to provide prolonged stretch and maintain joint posture when patients are sleeping or at rest. Serial casting can also provide sustained stretch and assist in lengthening developing contractures. Casts are bulky and time consuming to apply but remain very effective in correcting joint deformity due to spasticity.

Modalities are frequently used in therapy to reduce spasticity. Cooling has been found to be beneficial for MS fatigue and weakness, and muscle cooling has been found to reduce muscle stretch activity and clonus. The effects of muscle cooling and stretch on muscle spindle is secondary to a reduction in the sensitivity of the muscle spindle organ itself and is more likely the primary mechanism of action than the decrease in gamma motoneuron excitability.[22,23]

In addition, skin cooling at less than 10°F increases the pain threshold by reducing the receptor sensitivity of low-threshold afferents, which may contribute to spasticity reduction.[24,25] Cooling vests can reduce body temperature up to 1.8°F, which can alleviate some MS symptoms, including spasticity. Just like cold modality, superficial heat has an inhibitory effect to the nociceptive neurons at the spinal cord level and may result in increased pain threshold, which may eventually contribute to decreased spasticity.[25]

Both superficial heat and cooling modalities can reduce muscle spasms; however, cold is deemed more effective for decreasing spasticity in patients with upper motor lesion, particularly in MS.[25] Heat modalities and warm pools should be avoided in patients with MS.

Transcutaneous electrical nerve stimulation (TENS) has shown some evidence of reducing MS spasticity. Armutlu and colleagues[26] found reduced ankle plantar flexion spasticity after applying TENS for 20 minutes daily. Hans and colleagues[27] stated that the potential effect of TENS might be related to the production of beta-endorphin in the CSF, which may decrease the excitability of the motor neurons through the kappa opiate receptors, because the antispastic effect was partially reversed by a high dose of naloxone.[28]

Goulet and colleagues[29] found that TENS reduced spinal spasticity. Studies in healthy individuals before and after stimulation by TENS show that there are several neurohormonal effects recorded after stimulation, particularly the elevations in the CSF levels of beta-endorphin and serotonin and in the plasma levels of serotonin, GABA, beta-endorphin, and dehydroepiandrosterone, with accompanying decreased levels of tryptophan and cortisol.[28,30]

There is some evidence that functional electrical stimulation may influence spasticity in patients with MS.[31]

Low-amplitude, high-frequency vibratory stimulation to muscle may decrease tone and reduce fatigue symptoms in patients with MS.[20] Vibration induces presynaptic inhibition of IA afferents, which can alter the excitability of the corticospinal pathway by modulating intracortical inhibitory and facilitatory inputs to the primary motor cortex. Vibration reduces the stretch-related input and also has an influence on CNS inhibition.

## MASSAGE

Massage has been found to influence spasticity in patients with MS. Backus and colleagues[32] studied 24 spastic patients with MS who underwent massage therapy for 1 hour weekly for 6 weeks. Fatigue was reduced in 22 of the 24 patients, with a positive impact on pain and quality of life. There was no change in the modified Ashworth scale. Brouwer and de Andrade[33] showed that patients with MS had reduced spasticity immediately after massage therapy. The repetitive mechanical skin stimulation provides a sensory input that might reduce pain in a similar way to TENS techniques.[34]

The mechanism of the effects of massage may not be neurohormonal, as massage has not been shown to increase the level of endorphins and other endogenous opiates in healthy subjects. Studies showed that the continuous stretching of the skin with pressure activates the pacinian corpuscles, which are fast-adapting receptors and may inhibit muscle activity.[35]

Other reported nonpharmacologic treatments of spasticity in adults with MS are physical activity programs, transcranial magnetic stimulation, repetitive transcranial magnetic stimulation, electromagnetic therapy, and whole-body vibration.[30,36,37] However, in the 2013 review by Amatya and colleagues[38] all MS participants in the nonpharmacologic treatment group showed low level or no evidence of spasticity improvement.

## SUMMARY

Spasticity in patients with MS can have an immense impact on function and quality of life. If untreated, spasticity may cause pain and spasms, functional decline, contractures, and skin breakdown. With early recognition and a multimodal approach to treatment, the adverse impact of spasticity on the well-being of patients with MS can be minimized.

## REFERENCES

1. Junker A, Bruck W. Autoinflammatory grey matter lesions in humans: cortical encephalitis, clinical disorders, experimental models. Curr Opin Neurol 2012;25(3): 349–57.
2. Trapp BD, Bo L, Mork S, et al. Pathogenesis of tissue injury in MS lesions. J Neuroimmunol 1999;98(1):49–56.
3. Maitin IB, Shah AN. Spasticity due to multiple sclerosis. In: Brashear A, editor. Spasticity: diagnosis and management. 2nd edition. New York: Demos; 2015. p. 341–P356.
4. Rizzo MA, Hadjimichael OC, Preiningerova J, et al. Prevalence and treatment of spasticity reported by multiple sclerosis patients. Mult Scler 2004;10(5): 589–95.
5. Patejdl R, Zettl UK. Spasticity in multiple sclerosis: contribution of inflammation, autoimmune mediated neuronal damage and therapeutic interventions. Autoimmun Rev 2017;16(9):925–36.
6. Illomei G, Spinicci G, Locci E, et al. Muscle elastography: a new imaging technique for multiple sclerosis spasticity measurement. Neurol Sci 2017;38(3): 433–9.
7. Keating GM. Delta-9-tetrahydrocannabinol/cannabidiol oromucosal spray (sativex((R))): a review in multiple sclerosis-related spasticity. Drugs 2017;77(5): 563–74.
8. Rommer PS, Kamin F, Petzold A, et al. Effects of repeated intrathecal triamcinolone-acetonide application on cerebrospinal fluid biomarkers of axonal damage and glial activity in multiple sclerosis patients. Mol Diagn Ther 2014; 18(6):631–7.
9. Walther EU, Hohlfeld R. Multiple sclerosis: side effects of interferon beta therapy and their management. Neurology 1999;53(8):1622–7.

10. Meca-Lallana JE, Balseiro JJ, Lacruz F, et al. Sanchez spasticity improvement in patients with relapsing-remitting multiple sclerosis switching from interferon-b to glatiramer acetate: the Escala study. J Neurol Sci 2012;315(1–2):123–8.

11. Bethoux F, Marrie RA. A cross-sectional study of the impact of spasticity on daily activities in multiple sclerosis. Patient 2016;9(6):537–46.

12. Vermersch P, Trojano M. Tetrahydrocannabinol: cannabidiol oromucosal spray for multiple sclerosis-related resistant spasticity in daily practice. Eur Neurol 2016; 76(5–6):216–26.

13. Katchan V, David P, Shoenfeld Y. Cannabinoids and autoimmune diseases: a systematic review. Autoimmun Rev 2016;15(6):513–28.

14. Zajicek J, Ball S, Wright D, et al. Effect of dronabinol on progression in progressive multiple sclerosis (CUPID): a randomised, placebo-controlled trial. Lancet Neurol 2013;12(9):857–65.

15. Flachenecker P, Henze T, Zettl UK. Long-term effectiveness and safety of nabiximols (tetrahydrocannabinol/cannabidiol oromucosal spray) in clinical practice. Eur Neurol 2014;72(1–2):95–102.

16. Patti F, Messina S, Solaro C, et al. Efficacy and safety of cannabinoid oromucosal spray for multiple sclerosis spasticity. J Neurol Neurosurg Psychiatry 2016;87(9): 944–51.

17. Carotenuto A, Iodice R, Petracca M, et al. Upper motor neuron evaluation in multiple sclerosis patients treated with sativex ((R)). Acta Neurol Scand 2017;135(4): 442–8.

18. Langford RM, Mares J, Novotna A, et al. A double-blind, randomized, placebo-controlled, parallel-group study of THC/CBD oromucosal spray in combination with the existing treatment regimen, in the relief of central neuropathic pain in patients with multiple sclerosis. J Neurol 2013;260(4):984–97.

19. Dressler D, Bhidayasiri R, Bohlega S, et al. Botulinum toxin therapy for treatment of spasticity in multiple sclerosis: review and recommendations of the IAB-interdisciplinary working group for movement disorders task force. J Neurol 2017;264(1):112–20.

20. Paoloni M, Giovannelli M, Mangone M, et al. Does giving segmental muscle vibration alter the response to botulinum toxin injections in the treatment of spasticity in people with multiple sclerosis? A single-blind randomized controlled trial. Clin Rehabil 2013;27(9):803–12.

21. Jarrett L, Nandi P, Thompson AJ. Managing severe lower limb spasticity in multiple sclerosis: does intrathecal phenol have a role? J Neurol Neurosurg Psychiatry 2002;73(6):705–9.

22. Burke D, Skuse NF, Stuart DG. The regularity of muscle spindle discharge in man. J Physiol 1979;291:277.

23. Knutson E, Mattson E. Effects of local cooling on monosynaptic reflexes in man. Scand J Rehabil Med 1979;1:126.

24. Kunesh E, Schmidt R, Nordin M, et al. Peripheral neural correlates of cutaneous anesthesia induced by skin cooling in man. Acta Physiol Scand 1987;129:247.

25. Preisinger E, Quittan M. Thermo- and hydrotherapy. Wien Med Wochenschr 1994; 144:520.

26. Armutlu K, Meric A, Kirdi N, et al. The effect of transcutaneous electrical nerve stimulation on spasticity in multiple sclerosis patients: a pilot study. Neurorehabil Neural Repair 2003;17(2):79–82.

27. Hans JS, Chen XH, Yuan Y, et al. Transcutaneous electrical nerve stimulator for treatment of spinal spasticity. Chin Med J (Engl) 1994;107:6.

28. Liss S, Liss B. Physiological and therapeutic effects of high frequency electrical pulses. Integr Physiol Behav Sci 1996;31:88.
29. Goulet C, Arsenault AB, Bourbonnais D, et al. Effects of transcutaneous electrical nerve stimulation on H-reflex and spinal spasticity. Scand J Rehabil Med 1996;28: 169–76.
30. Mori F, Ljoka C, Magni E, et al. Transcranial magnetic stimulation primes the effects of exercise in multiple sclerosis. J Neurol 2011;258(7):1281–7.
31. Szecsi J, Schlick C, Schiller M, et al. Functional electrical stimulation-assisted cycling of patients with multiple sclerosis: biomechanical and functional outcome—a pilot study. J Rehabil Med 2009;41(8):674–80.
32. Backus D, Manella C, Bender A, et al. Impact of massage therapy on fatigue, pain, and spasticity in people with multiple sclerosis: a pilot study. Int J Ther Massage Bodywork 2016;9(4):4–13.
33. Brouwer B, de Andrade VS. The effects of slow stroking on spasticity in patients with multiple sclerosis: a pilot study. Physiother Theory Pract 1995;11(1):13–21.
34. Roberts BL. Soft tissue manipulation: neuromuscular and muscle energy techniques. J Neurosci 1997;29:123.
35. Cherry DB. Review of physical therapy alternatives for reducing muscle contracture. Phys Ther 1980;60:877.
36. Lappin MS, Lawrie FW, Richards TL, et al. Effects of a pulsed electromagnetic therapy on multiple sclerosis fatigue and quality of life: a double-blind, placebo controlled trial. Altern Ther Health Med 2003;9:38–48.
37. Schyms F, Paul L, Finley L, et al. Vibration therapy in multiple sclerosis: a pilot study exploring its effect on tone, muscle force, sensation and functional performance. Clin Rehabil 2009;23(9):771–81.
38. Amatya B, Khan F, La Mantia L, et al. Non pharmacological interventions for spasticity in multiple sclerosis. Cochrane Database Syst Rev 2013;(2):CD009974.

# Muscle Overactivity in the Upper Motor Neuron Syndrome

## Conceptualizing a Treatment Plan and Establishing Meaningful Goals

Anne Felicia Ambrose, MD, MS[a],*, Tanya Verghese, MA[a],
Carolin Dohle, MD[b], Jennifer Russo, MD[a]

### KEYWORDS

- Spasticity • Treatment goals • Goal setting • Muscle overactivity

### KEY POINTS

- Spasticity is a condition that presents in a variety of ways, and therefore its treatment must be equally multifaceted and specific to the individual.
- It is important to establish patient-centered goals, which are specific, attainable, measurable, relevant to the patient, and achievable within a specified time.
- Factors to be considered include gathering data regarding effectiveness of prior treatments and their side effects, identifying muscle(s) contributing to the impairment, and impact of proposed treatments.
- Previously, treatment recommendations focused on a stepwise progression.
- Current recommendations suggest combining multiple therapeutic options to optimize results, particularly when spasticity is present with other features of upper motor neuron dysfunction.

## INTRODUCTION

Spasticity is defined as a velocity-dependent increase in tonic stretch reflexes with exaggerated movements due to the hyperexcitability of stretch reflexes[1] and is a component of upper motor neuron syndromes.[2] It can be the result of acute injury to the central nervous system along the neural axis or of chronic neurologic conditions,

Disclosure Statement: The authors have nothing to disclose.
[a] Department of Rehabilitation Medicine, Burke Rehabilitation Hospital, Montefiore Medical Center, White Plains, NY 10605; [b] Department of Neurology, Montefiore Medical Center, Burke Rehabilitation Hospital, 785, Mamaroneck Avenue, White Plains Hospital, NY 10605, USA
* Corresponding author.
*E-mail address:* aambrose@burke.org

such as cerebral palsy, amyotrophic lateral sclerosis, and multiple sclerosis. Spasticity is sometimes classified according to its origin.[3] *Spinal spasticity* results from the removal or destruction of supraspinal control and leads to increased excitability of motor neurons. *Cerebral spasticity* stems from a loss of descending inhibition.[4]

Spasticity can result in pain, increased disability, and decreased quality of life.[5] It may interfere with the use of the affected extremity; affect mobility, dressing, and hygiene; and increase the burden on caregivers.[5] In the pediatric population, chronic severe spasticity can also impede normal bone growth, resulting in reduced bone length, joint distortion, or abnormal rotation. Left untreated, spasticity may lead to deformities, such as kyphoscoliosis and contractures, that require invasive interventions in order to be corrected.[2]

### Approach to Spasticity Management

Spasticity is a multifaceted condition that affects each patient in a unique way. Therefore, treatment must be tailored to the specific needs of the individual. When developing a treatment plan, the following questions should be considered.

### Gathering background information

1. What is the cause of the spasticity? Is it true spasticity?
   The patient's history should establish the underlying cause and determine the onset and progression of the condition. Spasticity is usually caused by lesions along the corticospinal tract and may be accompanied by weakness, hyperreflexia, and clonus.[2] The resistance encountered in the affected limb is velocity-dependent, frequently marked by a "catch" followed by release of the tension. When moving the affected joint, one direction is usually more profoundly affected; for example, in chronic stroke, spasticity is frequently more pronounced in the flexor than the extensor groups. *Spasticity* should be distinguished from rigidity, which is seen in extrapyramidal lesions, such as those within the rubrospinal or vestibulospinal tracts, and includes cogwheel (eg, Parkinson disease) and lead pipe rigidity (eg, neuroleptic malignant syndrome or stiff man syndrome).[6,7] This resistance to movement is uniform in all directions and is not velocity-dependent.
2. What are the factors that affect the patient's spasticity?
   The history should include details regarding the manifestation of spasticity and its progression. Patients often report that their symptoms may change according to temperature, emotional status, time of day, level of pain, body position, and the amount of prior stretching.
3. Which tool(s) are the most appropriate to evaluate the patient's physical findings?
   A thorough examination of the muscle groups to evaluate muscle strength, range of motion, tone, and reflexes is critical. Several examples of additional tools that can be used are given in **Table 1**.
4. What functional limitations are the results of the spasticity?
   Functional limitations may include tactile, proprioceptive, visual, auditory, vestibular, cognitive impairments, hemineglect, impaired learning, and procedural sequencing, which can further magnify the patient's disability.
5. What physical abnormalities are noted? Which muscles are affected? Do these muscles have any other function?
   Abnormal position of digits, joints, or limbs require careful examination for imbalance between agonist and antagonist muscles. These muscles should be examined for tone, coordination, and strength. Usually, examination of agonist and antagonist muscle groups shows that one group predominates

| Table 1 Spasticity tools | |
|---|---|
| **Test** | **Purpose** |
| Modified Ashford Scale[8] | Most commonly used scale for spasticity. Measures resistance during passive stretching of the affected muscle groups |
| Tardieu Scale[9] | Measures resistance to movement both at slow and fast speeds. A goniometer is required to measure the angle of muscle reaction |
| Bartels Index | Measures caregiver dependence in activities of daily living |
| Visual Analogue Pain Scale | Measures subjective pain perception |
| Action Research Arm test | Measures upper limb dexterity by assessing 19 items grouped in 4 categories: grasp, pinch, grip, and gross movement |

over the other. However, it is important not only to identify the spastic muscles but also to take into consideration the other actions that these muscles may have, because these functions may be affected as well once the muscle is injected. The following are some examples of common postural abnormalities:

a. Adducted, internally rotated shoulder: this can result in difficulty with axillary hygiene, skin maceration, and difficulty with upper body dressing. Muscles exhibiting overactivity may be
   i. Pectoralis major: adducts and medially rotates humerus, draws scapula anteriorly and inferiorly. When acting alone, the clavicular head flexes humerus, and the sternocostal head extends it
   ii. Teres major: adducts and medially rotates arm
   iii. Latissimus dorsi: extends, adducts, and medially rotates humerus, raises body toward arms during climbing
   iv. Subscapularis: medially rotates arm and adducts it. Helps to hold humeral head in glenoid cavity of scapula
   v. Long head of triceps: extends shoulder. Long head steadies the head of abducted humerus chief extensor of forearm
   vi. Coracobrachialis: forward flexes the shoulder

b. Flexed hip: may interfere with lower limb positioning and can be associated with hip and thigh spasm. Chronic flexion posturing can eventually lead to flexion contracture. A flexed hip affects gait. In bilateral hip flexion, patients will walk with a crouched gait pattern and may also have compensatory knee flexion and/or thigh abduction.
   i. Iliopsoas: flexes the torso and thigh with respect to each other
   ii. Rectus femoris: flexes the hip and extends the knee
   iii. Pectineus: adducts the thigh and flexes the hip joint
   iv. Adductor longus: adducts and flexes the thigh and helps to laterally rotate the hip joint
   v. Adductor brevis: adducts and flexes the thigh and helps to laterally rotate the thigh
   vi. Gluteus maximus: acts as the major extensor of the hip joint

c. Equinovarus foot: foot and ankle turn down and in; toe-curling or toe-clawing may be present. Skin breakdown over the fifth metatarsal may develop, especially along the lateral border if compressed against the mattress, bed rail, footrest, or floor. Patient may experience difficulty with donning and wearing braces and shoes. Knee swing during preswing is limited, and an early swing foot drag might develop.

   i. Medial gastrocnemius: powerful plantar flexor of ankle. Minor knee flexor

   ii. Lateral gastrocnemius: powerful plantar flexor of ankle

   iii. Soleus: plantar flexes foot

   iv. Tibialis anterior: dorsiflexes ankle

   v. Tibialis posterior: inverts and plantar flexes the foot

   vi. Flexor digitorum longus and brevis: flexes lesser toes

   vii. Extensor hallucis longus: extends the great toe, dorsiflexes ankle, and can invert foot

   viii. Flexor hallucis longus: flexes the great toe, plantar flexes the foot, and can invert foot

   ix. Peroneus longus: extends foot and plantar flexes ankle. Helps to support the transverse arch of foot

6. The timing or stage of motor recovery should be established. Some patients may be undergoing progression in their spasticity as described by the Brunnstrom staging, whereas others may have arrested at a particular stage.

7. What treatment options have already been attempted? What were the results and side effects?

   A list of all interventions and medications that have been tried individually and in combination should be obtained, including benefits, treatment failures, or side effects.

8. Are there any limitations to patient's ability to obtain the recommended prescription and attend appropriate follow-up care?

   Most patients have to have caregivers who are able to provide transport whenever necessary. This is especially critical in the case of baclofen pump management, when timely refill is critical to avoid potentially life-threatening adverse effects. Injections of botulinum toxin or baclofen pump refills may not be covered by the patient's insurance.

### Setting goals

When creating a treatment plan for spasticity patients and their caregivers, it is important to set clear objectives. Patients with spasticity frequently present with generalized complaints of loss of function, so it is important to manage expectations by creating clear and measurable goals. It is also vital to assess whether the patient would benefit from an aggressive spasticity intervention. Many spasticity treatments involve muscle weakening, and patients may use their spasticity to compensate for their lack of strength. In these patients, weakening of the affected muscles may negatively affect function. The following are examples of common goals.

1. Tone management: patients who have spasticity often have increased tone, which causes increased stiffness of their muscles making movements difficult to initiate or control.

2. Prevention of contractures: prolonged spasticity can result in shortening of muscles and contractures. Once contractures form, most nonsurgical interventions are not effective. It is therefore imperative to manage spasticity aggressively before muscles develop contraction.

3. Functional improvements: patients with moderate to severe spasticity can have "hidden" motor strength in a spastic limb. Once the spasticity is treated appropriately, the patient may be able to have some functional use of the limb. For example, a patient with a clenched fist may not use the hand for any functional

purposes. However, if the patient's finger flexors are relaxed, the hand may be used as a stabilizer for two-handed activities. But this has to be done judiciously. Patients sometimes use tone to their advantage. One example is when a patient with lower limb weakness and knee extensor spasticity uses it to maintain standing. Treating the tone too aggressively can be weight bearing and thus result in ambulation.

4. Pain management: chronic spasticity can cause muscle soreness and aching in addition to spasms. Patients also develop pain in joints where spastic muscles cause chronic subluxation, for example, subluxed shoulder poststrokes.
5. Improving tolerance of therapy, casts, orthotics, or braces and reducing pressure sores.
6. Reducing caregiver burden by easing transfers, dressing, donning and doffing of orthotics, and making hygiene activities easier.
7. Improvement of sitting and/or standing postures and correction of gait (eg, toe walking).
8. Improving control of neurogenic bladder.
9. Prevention of aspiration by reducing drooling.
10. Allow normal bone and muscle growth and prevent shortened or distorted limbs.

**Creating patient-centered treatment goals** Setting clear and realistic goals regarding the improvement a patient can expect at the beginning of treatment is imperative, because patients may have unrealistic expectation regarding functional improvements. This can lead to patient disappointment and physician frustration. It is therefore wise to explain the purpose of the interventions and set goals informally or formally before starting.

**Informal goals** These can be a description of what the physician expects, for example, "We will try to straighten your elbow" or "open your fingers out."

**Semiformal goals** Using more standardized measures of spasticity. For example, "Reduce spasticity in elbow flexors from Modified Ashford of 3 to 2."

**Standardized goals** This is done using tools such as Goal Attainment Scales.[10] Goal Attainment Scales (GAS) methodology consists of the following:

a. Defining a rehabilitation goal,
b. Choosing an observable behavior that reflects the degree of goal attainment,
c. Defining the patient's initial (ie, pretreatment) level with respect to the goal,
d. Defining five goal attainment levels (ranging from a "no change" to a "much better than expected outcome"),
e. Setting a time interval for patient evaluation,
f. Evaluating the patient after the defined time interval,
g. Calculating the overall attainment score for all the rehabilitation goals.

Goals should be SMART[10]:

a. Specific
b. Measurable, quantified by improvements in ROM, modified Ashford, etc.
c. Attainable
d. Relevant to the patient and caregiver and have meaningful results
e. Time-based (an expected time frame should be discussed with the patient)

Two additional goal characteristics have been suggested: reevaluate and revise.

### Treatment Strategies

Therapeutic selection for the treatment of spasticity is guided primarily by patient and caregiver goals. Therapeutic options are divided into the following categories: non-pharmacologic versus Pharmacologic and noninvasive versus invasive (**Table 2**). In addition, invasive procedures may be reversible or permanent. Often, multiple therapeutic options are combined to optimize results, particularly when spasticity is present with other features of upper motor neuron dysfunction, such as spasm, clonus, dystonia, extensor plantar responses, reduced dexterity, and weakness[11–17] (**Table 3**).

#### Pharmacologic management

**Noninvasive treatments: oral medications** Oral baclofen is the most commonly used oral spasmolytic, because of its effectiveness, price, and tolerability. Other common oral medications include tizanidine, gabapentin, dantrolene and benzodiazepines, such as diazepam[18,19] (**Table 4**).

Baclofen and benzodiazepines are centrally acting GABAergic medications that decrease spasticity by increasing inhibitory signals. Baclofen binds to the $GABA_B$ receptors to enhance inhibitory signals.[20–22] Although structurally similar to GABA, gabapentin has not been found to bind at either $GABA_A$ or $GABA_B$ receptors. Instead, gabapentin seems to act centrally at voltage-sensitive calcium channels.[23,24]

Tizanidine is an alpha-2 adrenergic agonist, which acts centrally to decrease spasticity through presynaptic inhibition of sensory afferents.[25] Tizanidine has been associated with severe hepatotoxicity, requiring regular monitoring of liver function test (LFT) results.[26] In addition, because of its action on alpha-2 receptors, tizanidine should be avoided in patients with hypotension. All centrally acting agents have the potential for causing drowsiness and sedation, which may be undesirable in patients experiencing impairments in attention or alertness secondary to traumatic brain injury or stroke.

Dantrolene, unlike other oral agents, is peripherally acting.[27–30] It works directly on skeletal muscle by inhibiting release of calcium from the sarcoplasmic reticulum. Common side effects include dizziness, drowsiness, fatigue, and muscle weakness. Hepatotoxic effects have been observed and careful monitoring of LFTs is required.[27] Usefulness of dantrolene as a first-line treatment is also limited by relative high cost compared with other available treatments.

**Table 2**
**Common pharmacologic and nonpharmacologic treatment options for spasticity management**

| Pharmacologic | | Nonpharmacologic | |
|---|---|---|---|
| Noninvasive | Invasive | Noninvasive | Invasive |
| • Baclofen | • Botulinum toxin | • Stretching | • Neurosurgery techniques, for example, dorsal rhizotomy, selective neurotomy, spinal cord stimulation |
| • Tizanidine | • Phenol | • Casting | |
| • Dantrolene | • Intrathecal baclofen | • Splints | |
| • Gabapentin | | • Orthotics | • Orthopedic techniques, such as tendon lengthening and transfer, derotational osteotomy surgery, scoliosis corrections, joint replacements |
| • Diazepam | | • FES | |
| • Nabiximols | | • TENS | |

*Abbreviations:* FES, functional electrical stimulation; TENS, transcutaneous electrical nerve stimulation.

**Table 3**
**Upper motor neuron syndrome**

| Positive Symptoms | |
| --- | --- |
| Enhanced Stretch Reflexes | Increased muscle tone<br>Exaggerated tendon reflexes<br>Clonus |
| Released Flexor Reflexes | Babinski response<br>Mass synergy patterns |
| Negative Symptoms | Weakness<br>Loss of dexterity<br>Reduced postural response |

No definitive evidence exists to support the choice of one oral agent over the others, and the selection of medication is often guided by the side-effect profile, tolerability, and secondary symptoms, such as mood disturbance, seizures, insomnia, spasms, and pain[19]. Tizanidine has antinociceptive effects that make it useful in the treatment of

**Table 4**
**Common oral medications for the treatment of spasticity**

| Drug | Dosage | Mechanism | Adverse Effects | Considerations |
| --- | --- | --- | --- | --- |
| Baclofen | 5–100 mg in divided doses 3 times per day | GABA analogue, binds to $GABA_B$ receptors | Drowsiness, sedation, weakness | Risk of seizure with abrupt withdrawal |
| Tizanidine | 2–36 mg daily in 3–4 divided doses | Alpha-2 receptor agonist | Hypotension, dry mouth, weakness, drowsiness | Hepatotoxicity— must monitor liver function regularly; risk of postural hypotension |
| Dantrolene | 25–400 mg daily in 4 divided doses | Blocks ryanodine receptors limiting $Ca^{2+}$ release from sarcoplasmic reticulum | Weakness, drowsiness, GI upset, rare fatal hepatotoxicity | Hepatotoxicity—rare fatal cases reported; must monitor liver function closely; expensive |
| Gabapentin | 100–3600 mg daily in 3 divided doses | GABA-ergic | Drowsiness | May be helpful with pain |
| Diazepam | 2–60 mg in 3–4 divided doses | Stimulation of $GABA_A$ receptors | Reduced attention, impaired memory, drowsiness | Risk of tolerance, dependence, and withdrawal; may be helpful with insomnia or seizures; avoid with cognitive impairment |
| Nabiximols | 1–12 sprays per day | Partial agonist CB1 and CB2 receptors | Psychotropic effects, dizziness, fatigue, cognitive blunting | Approved as add-on for MS-related spasticity |

*Abbreviations:* GI, gastrointestinal; MS, multiple sclerosis.

patients with spasticity-related pain.[11] Potential for physical dependence has limited the widespread use of benzodiazepines for the treatment of spasticity, but benzodiazepines may be useful for patients who experience other symptoms amenable to benzodiazepine treatment, such as anxiety, seizures, insomnia, or spasms.

The use of oral spasmolytics is particularly helpful in the treatment of generalized spasticity because the effects are systemic. In general, monotherapy is preferred, but multiple agents may be combined to achieve desired results or minimize side effects.

**Invasive pharmacologic treatments** Commonly used invasive pharmacologic treatments include intrathecal baclofen therapy (ITB), chemodenervation with local injection of botulinum toxin, and neurolysis with alcohol or phenol (**Table 5**).

ITB: this therapy has been shown to be effective in spinal cord injury, cerebral palsy, stroke, traumatic brain injury, and multiple sclerosis.[31,32] Baclofen crosses the blood-brain barrier poorly, and the high systemic doses needed to achieve the desired effect may result in sedation.[33] ITB allows use of much lower doses, because the medication is administered directly to the central nervous system (CNS) within the intrathecal space. Multiple factors must be considered before initiating treatment with ITB, including ability to attend regular follow-up appointments, family and financial support systems, availability of transportation, and commitment of caregivers.[34] Adverse events can be serious and may result from the medication itself or from the equipment used for administration. These include pump failure, breakage or migration, infection, and depletion. Abrupt cessation of therapy due to pump failure or reservoir depletion can result in serious side effects, including seizure, coma, and death.[35] Traditionally, ITB is reserved for use in those who have trialed oral therapy for 1 year, but recent literature supports earlier initiation in selected patients.[36]

Chemodenervation: Chemodenervation with botulinum toxin has become an increasingly common treatment for focal spasticity.[37] Botulinum works focally at the

**Table 5**
**Invasive pharmacologic therapies**

| Drug | Mechanism | Advantages | Disadvantages |
|------|-----------|------------|---------------|
| Botulinum Toxin | Inhibits release of acetylcholine at neuromuscular junction | Reversible, effective for focal spasticity, well-tolerated | Effect wears off within 3–6 mo, may cause weakness impairing function, potential to develop antibodies to toxin limiting effect, black box warning |
| Phenol/Alcohol | Destruction of myelin and disruption of muscle spindles | Permanent, phenol has immediate antinociceptive effect | Spasticity may return as a result of collateral sprouting; risk for chronic dysesthesia |
| Intrathecal Baclofen | GABA$_B$ receptor agonist | No need to cross BBB, allows lower doses, less side effects; may give additional oral doses as needed for spasm | Requires frequent follow-up and commitment to treatment course; risk of mechanical complications; abrupt withdrawal may cause seizure, coma, or death |

*Abbreviation:* BBB, blood-brain barrier.

level of the muscle to reduce spasticity by inhibiting release of acetylcholine at the neuromuscular junction.[38,39] Spasticity reduction generally begins within 1 to 2 days, peaks in 4 to 6 weeks, and wears off at 3 months.[40] Because of the reversibility, repeated treatments are required. Therapeutic effect may be limited by the development of antibodies to the toxin, although newer formulations are designed with less antigenic properties.[41] In addition, botulinum toxin carries a Food and Drug Administration (FDA) black box warning that warns that spread of the toxin far beyond the injection site is a rare but potentially life-threatening complication, including death.[42–47]

Neurolysis: focal nerve block can be accomplished with injection of either alcohol or phenol into muscles affected by spasticity.[48] Both agents work by denaturing proteins in neural tissue, resulting in demyelination and degeneration of muscle spindles. Care must be taken to identify motor branches of the nerves, because damage to sensory nerves may result in the development of dysesthesias.[49] Generally, because of its effects on muscle spindles and nervous tissue, treatment with phenol is considered irreversible, although reemergence of spasticity may occur secondary to partial nerve regeneration and sprouting.[50] In addition, phenol has anesthetic properties, so muscle relaxation may occur immediately, with neurolytic effects developing several hours after injection. Unintentional intravascular injection may result in cardiovascular and CNS effects, including hypotension, tremors, or convulsions.

### Nonpharmacologic treatments

**Noninvasive nonpharmacologic treatments** Nonpharmacologic therapies are the mainstay of spasticity management and should be included in every treatment plan.[17] Noninvasive therapeutic management strategies include physical and occupational therapy, passive stretching,[51,52] orthotics, splinting,[53] serial casting,[54–58] and taping[59,60] (**Table 6**). Specialized lycra garments may be used to maintain limb position, increase function, and prevent contracture without the need for serial casting.

| Table 6 Common nonpharmacologic treatments | |
|---|---|
| | **Treatment** |
| Low-load Passive Stretching | Physical therapy intervention uses positioning with equipment, casting, splints, orthoses, or taping to achieve sustained stretch |
| Low-load Active Stretching | Physical therapy intervention whereby patient actively engages antagonist muscles to achieve stretch in spastic muscles with goal of increasing and maintaining ROM |
| Serial Casting | Successive use of casts to achieve progressive sustained stretch of muscles, ligaments, and tendons to increase ROM |
| Splinting | Removable device used to support or immobilize limb, provide passive stretch, prevent contracture, and facilitate functional positioning |
| Orthosis | Device or appliance used to prevent or correct deformities, improve alignment, and augment musculoskeletal function |
| Taping | Use of adhesive strips to provide prolonged passive stretch to spastic muscles |
| Transcutaneous Electrical Nerve Stimulation (TENS) | TENS uses electrical current produced by a portable device to stimulate nerves; uses high-frequency stimulation below motor threshold to achieve effect |
| Functional Electrical Stimulation (FES) | FES uses low-energy-pulses to artificially generate muscle action in paralyzed limb; stimulation provided over muscles; may suppress motoneuronal excitability to reduce spasticity |

Transcutaneous electrical nerve stimulation or functional electrical stimulation may also be used to temporarily reduce spasticity.[61,62]

**Invasive nonpharmacologic management** Invasive nonpharmacologic therapies include a variety of orthopedic and neurosurgical techniques. Because the effects of these treatments are permanent, surgical interventions are often thought of as treatments of last resort, although they may be considered earlier if spasticity limits proper bone and muscle growth.[63] Common orthopedic interventions for spasticity include tendon lengthening procedures,[64] such as Achilles tendon lengthening, and tendon transfers, such as split anterior tibial tendon transfer.[65] Osteotomies may be performed to correct bony misalignment and to place muscles at more biomechanically favorable positions.[66] These interventions may be used to correct alignment, reduce deformity, manage contractures, and improve posture, but they do not directly address the mechanisms leading to the development of spasticity.

Neurosurgical options include ablative procedures, such as dorsal rhizotomy and selective neurotomy,[67–69] and nonablative interventions, such as spinal cord stimulation. Dorsal rhizotomy, or DREZ-otomy, is an ablative procedure in which the afferent fibers are divided at the dorsal root entry zone, resulting in destruction of nociceptive and myotactic fibers.[70] It is primarily indicated for severely affected patients with a significant pain component. Spinal cord stimulation involves the percutaneous placement of electrodes

---

**Box 1**
**Case 1**

A 66-year-old woman with primary progressive multiple sclerosis presents to her primary provider with complaint of a recent increase in her adductor spasticity that is interfering with hygiene tasks. She has been on oral baclofen 30 mg three times a day for more than 10 years but finds that it is no longer working. She has chronic bilateral flexion contractures of her wrists and fingers but is able to feed herself and operate her electric wheelchair. She has previously participated in physical therapy but is not currently enrolled in a program. She has not had injectable therapy or surgery in the past. Currently, she requires two caregivers overcome her spasticity to perform hygiene tasks. After evaluation by her physician, she was referred for further work-up and management.

In the emergency department, the patient was found to have a urinary tract infection, for which she was started on antibiotics. MRI head and spine showed no new lesions, but she was given a short course of oral steroids for possible multiple sclerosis exacerbation. She was then referred to Rehabilitation Medicine physician for further follow-up.

Factors to be taken into consideration, in discussion with the patient and her caregivers.

a. What is her baseline functional status? Has the recent decline been reversed or is this her new baseline after the urinary tract infection?

b. Should a different oral medication or injectable be tried? If so, what side effects may be anticipated and be tolerated?

c. Can reliable transportation be arranged for future clinic visits, given her impairment level?

Using the information ascertained by the physiatrist, an SMART goal was created by the provider, patient, and caregivers to increase hip abduction range of motion to 45° in each hip over the next 6 months. The patient underwent injection of botulinum toxin into both hip adductors with improvement in spasticity. Oral baclofen was reduced to 20 mg 3 times per day with a goal of being tapered off, if possible. An outpatient physical therapy program was initiated to improve the range of motion, transfers, and provide caregiver training. At her 6-month follow-up visit, she had met the set goal for her hip abduction, and new goal was set for improving self-care for toileting to maximum assist from total dependency in the next 6 months. New goals were also set for increasing use of wrist splints during sleeping hours.

---

**Box 2**
**Case 2**

A 54-year-old man presented to the emergency department for evaluation of acute onset of left-sided weakness (upper extremity > lower extremity) and left facial droop. Computed tomography angiography revealed flow void in left M1 segment and patient underwent thrombectomy with TICI 2a revascularization. Following thrombectomy, his left upper extremity weakness progressed to full paralysis. MRI showed diffuse chronic microischemic changes and evolution of stroke, but no hemorrhagic conversion. Once medically stable, the patient was transferred to an acute rehabilitation hospital for multidisciplinary rehabilitation. During his rehabilitation admission, the patient developed increasing tone in left upper extremity (LUE) wrist and finger flexors with spasticity. A resting hand splint was prescribed, and the patient was started on oral baclofen 5 mg three times per day. However, the patient was observed to be more lethargic and confused during therapy sessions, with worsening of his liver function.

What should be the rehabilitation team's approach?

The baclofen should be discontinued and a less hepatotoxic agent such as tizanidine should be used. Physical and occupational therapy options should be continued, including continuing use of resting hand splint, stretching, and use of modalities.

Following discharge to a subacute rehabilitation center, the patient was lost to follow-up. He reappeared at the outpatient rehabilitation clinic after 1 year. He had been transferred to a nursing home for the past 9 months during which time he received no formal rehabilitation therapy. However, he is now living at home with his wife and adult children who were willing to provide any necessary care.

On examination, he is awake, but only partially oriented with mild to moderate cognitive impairments. He has developed significant LUE spasticity and painful spasms. He has an internally rotated and adducted shoulder, flexed and pronated elbow, and flexed wrist with a clenched fist. In addition, he has hip adduction, flexed knee joint, and pronated foot.

What should be the rehabilitation team's approach?

1. Investigate what the underlying reasons for the patient's worsened condition are.

2. Establish what treatments the patient received in the interim and their effectiveness.

3. Using the Goal Attainment Scale methodology, SMART goals should be established in conjunction with the patient, family, and rehabilitation team.

The patient's oral tizanidine, which had been inadvertently discontinued, was restarted, with some improvement in range of motion. The initial SMART goal was to improve wrist and finger flexion to neutral to facilitate use of resting hand splint in the first 3 months using local injections of botox to the flexor carpi radialis, flexor carpi ulnaris, flexor digitorum superficialis, and flexor digitorum profundus. Therapy was also initiated to stretch and strengthen all the affected joints, improve transfers, and reduce caregiver burden. The rehabilitation team should continue setting new goals to further consider use of botox or other injectables to address the lower limb spasticity. Intrathecal baclofen pump implantation should also be considered. Finally, once all these options have been considered, surgical managements for any contractures or persistent, chronic pain should be considered.

---

over neural elements within the intrathecal space. This technique is primarily used for the management of chronic neuropathic pain, although recent literature suggests that this technique may be effective for the management of spasticity.[71]

### Treatment algorithm: summary

When determining a course of treatment, providers must consider several questions, including the following:

a. Establish cause of the spasticity.
b. Establish the physical and functional impairments as a result of the spasticity.

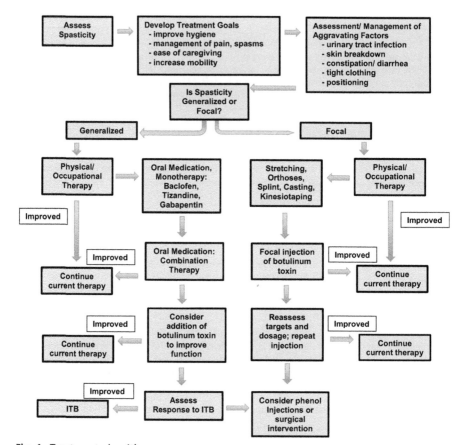

**Fig. 1.** Treatment algorithm.

c. Establish the role of other factors that can affect treatment options: for example, hematological and liver function, seizure, cognitive impairment, or mood disturbance

d. Identify all prior treatments and their results, benefits, and side effects.

e. Evaluate the logistical or financial limitations that may affect treatment options.

f. Create a priority list of functional goals that the patient and care team decides on together, using methodology such as Goal Attainment Scale to create a realistic and beneficial plan.

g. Determine the treatment options.

Traditionally a step-wise approach was used, using nonpharmacologic approaches first, progressing to oral medications, followed by injectables, and finally surgical options. However, more recently, practitioners advocate a parallel approach to management with a combination of both systemic and focal interventions to maximize functional outcome (**Boxes 1** and **2, Fig. 1**).

*Emerging therapies*
New modalities are emerging as potential options in the management of spasticity. These include both pharmacologic and nonpharmacologic treatments (**Table 7**).

| Table 7<br>Emerging noninvasive therapies | |
|---|---|
| | **Therapy** |
| Transcranial Direct Current Stimulation | Uses constant, low, direct current delivered via electrodes positioned on the scalp; direct refers to fact that current travels through the skull from one electrode to the other |
| Repetitive Transcranial Magnetic Stimulation | Uses creation of intracranial electrical field by application of extracranial magnetic field to modulate neuronal activity |
| Focal Vibration | Application of low-frequency vibration directly to focal area of spasticity |
| Whole Body Vibration | Application of low-frequency vibration to whole body via plate for treatment of more diffuse spasticity |
| Extracorporeal Shock Wave Therapy | Focal application of short-energy shock waves applied over spastic muscles |

Nonpharmacologic treatment options under investigation include acupuncture,[72] vibration,[73–76] extracorporeal shock wave therapy,[77,78] and noninvasive neural stimulation techniques, including transcranial direct current stimulation and repetitive transcranial magnetic stimulation.[79–82]

Emerging pharmacologic treatment options include the use of tetrahydrocannabinol (THC)/cannabidiol derivatives, such as Sativex, for the management of spasticity.[83] Widespread use of these medications is limited because of concern for cognitive side effects and risk of psychosis, but they are FDA-approved for use in the treatment of multiple sclerosis.[84,85] THC acts as a partial agonist to cannabinoid receptors, CB1 and CB2; it mimics the effects of endogenous endocannabinoids.[83] Although the mechanism of action for the reduction of spasticity has not been directly studied in humans, it is hypothesized that it may modulate excitatory signals through its presynaptic effects.

## REFERENCES

1. Lance J. What is spasticity? Lancet 1990;335:606.
2. Kheder A, Nair KP. Spasticity: pathophysiology, evaluation and management. Pract Neurol 2012;12:289–98.
3. Welmer AK, von Arbin M, Widén Holmqvist L, et al. Spasticity and its association with functioning and health-related quality of life 18 months after stroke. Cerebrovasc Dis 2006;21:247–53.
4. Lapeyre E, Kuks JBM, Meijler WJ. Spasticity: revisiting the role and the individual value of several pharmacological treatments. NeuroRehabilitation 2010;27:193–200.
5. National Collaborating Centre for Chronic Conditions (UK). Stroke: national clinical guideline for diagnosis and initial management of acute stroke and transient ischaemic attack (TIA). London: Royal College of Physicians (UK); 2008.
6. Sanger TD, Delgado MR, Gaebler-Spira D, et al. Classification and definitions of disorders caused by hypertonia in childhood. Pediatrics 2003;111:89–97.
7. Available at: http://www.neurorehabresource.org/Files/NRR_Differential_Diagnosis.pdf. Accessed October 21, 2017.

8. Bohannon RW, Smith MB. Interrater reliability of a modifilied Ashworth scale of muscle spasticity. Phys Ther 1987;67:206–7.

9. Boyd RN, Graham HK. Objective measurement of clinical findings in the use of botulinum toxin type A for the management of children with cerebral palsy. Eur J Neurol 1999;6:S23–35.

10. Kiresuk T, Sherman R. Goal attainment scaling: a general method of evaluating comprehensive mental health programmes. Community Ment Health J 1968;4: 443–53.

11. Stevenson VL, Playford D. Neurological rehabilitation and the management of spasticity. Neurol Rehabil 2016;44(9):530–6.

12. Elbasiouny SM, Moroz D, Bakr MM, et al. Management of spasticity after spinal cord injury: current techniques and future directions. Neurorehabil Neural Repair 2010;24(1):23–33.

13. Satkunam LE. Rehabilitation medicine: 3. Management of adult spasticity. CMAJ 2003;169(11):1173–9.

14. National Institute for Health and Care Excellence. Spasticity in Under 19s: Management. Clinical Guideline. 2012. Available at: http://www.nice.org.uk/guidance/cg145. Accessed October 20, 2017.

15. Balakrishnan S, Ward AB. Chapter 13: the diagnosis and management of adults with spasticity. Handb Clin Neurol 2013;110(3):145–60.

16. Francis HP, Wade DT, Turner-Stokes L, et al. Does reducing spasticity translate into functional benefit? An exploratory meta-analysis. J Neurol Neurosurg Psychiatry 2004;75:1547–51.

17. Naro A, Leo A, Russo M, et al. Breakthroughs in the spasticity management: are non-pharmacological treatments the future? J Clin Neurosci 2017;39:16–27.

18. Otero-Romero S, Sastre-Garriga J, Comi G, et al. Pharmacological management of spasticity in multiple sclerosis: systematic review and consensus paper. Mult Scler 2016;22(11):1386–96.

19. Chou R, Peterson K, Helfand M. Comparative efficacy and safety of skeletal muscle relaxants for spasticity and musculoskeletal conditions: a systematic review. J Pain Symptom Manage 2004;28(2):140–68.

20. Albright LA. Baclofen in the treatment of cerebral palsy. J Child Neurol 1996; 11(2):77–83.

21. Meythaler JM, Clayton W, Davis LK, et al. Orally delivered baclofen to control spastic hypertonia in acquired brain injury. J Head Trauma Rehabil 2004;19(2): 101–8.

22. Duncan GW, Shahani BT, Young RR. An evaluation of baclofen treatment for certain symptoms in patients with spinal cord lesions. Neurology 1976;26:441–6.

23. Bradley LJ, Kirker GB. Pregabalin in the treatment of spasticity: a retrospective case series. Disabil Rehabil 2008;30(16):1230–2.

24. Cutter NC, Scott DD, Johnson JC, et al. Gabapentin effect on spasticity in multiple sclerosis: a placebo-controlled, randomized trial. Arch Phys Med Rehabil 2000;81:164–9.

25. Kamen L, Henney HR, Runyan JD. A practical overview of tizanidine use for spasticity secondary to multiple sclerosis, stroke, and spinal cord injury. Curr Med Res Opin 2008;24(2):425–39.

26. Medici M, Pebet M, Ciblis D. A double-blind, long-term study of tizanidine ('sirdalud') in spasticity due to cerebrovascular lesions. Curr Med Res Opin 1989;11(6): 398–407.

27. Kim JY, Chun S, Bang MS, et al. Safety of low-dose oral dantrolene sodium on hepatic function. Arch Phys Med Rehabil 2011;92:1359–63.

28. Schmidt RT, Lee RH, Spehlmann R. Comparison of dantrolene sodium and diazepam in the treatment of spasticity. J Neurol Neurosurg Psychiatry 1976;39:350–6.

29. Dykes MHM. Evaluation of a muscle relaxant: dantrolene sodium (dantrium). JAMA 1975;231(8):862–4.

30. Ketel WB, Kolb ME. Long-term treatment with dantrolene sodium of stroke patients with spasticity limiting the return of function. Curr Med Res Opin 1984;9(3):161–9.

31. Meythaler JM, Guin-Renfroe S, Brunner RC, et al. Intrathecal baclofen for spastic hypertonia from stroke. Stroke 2001;32:2099–109.

32. Meythaler JM, Guin-Renfore S, Grabb P, et al. Long-term continuously infused intrathecal baclofen for spastic-dystonic hypertonia in traumatic brain injury: 1-year experience. Arch Phys Med Rehabil 1999;80:13–9.

33. Ertzgaard P, Campo C, Calabrese A. Efficacy and safety of oral baclofen in the management of spasticity: a rationale for intrathecal baclofen. J Rehabil Med 2017;49:193–203.

34. Saulino M, Ivanhoe CB, McGuire JR, et al. Best practices for intrathecal baclofen therapy: patient selection. Neuromodulation 2016;19:607–15.

35. Coffey RJ, Edgar TS, Francisco GE, et al. Abrupt withdrawal from intrathecal baclofen: recognition and management of a potentially life-threatening syndrome. Arch Phys Med Rehabil 2002;83:735–41.

36. Francois B, Vacher P, Roustan J, et al. Intrathecal baclofen after traumatic brain injury: early treatment using a new technique to prevent spasticity. J Trauma 2001;50(1):158–61.

37. Walker HW, Lee MY, Bahroo LB, et al. Botulinum toxin injection techniques for the management of adult spasticity. PM R 2015;7:417–27.

38. Fortuna R, Horisberger M, Vaz MA, et al. Do skeletal muscle properties recover following repeat onabotulinum toxin A injections? J Biomech 2013;46:2426–33.

39. Gracies JM, Lugassy M, Weisz DJ, et al. Botulinum toxin dilution and endplate targeting in spasticity: a double-blind controlled study. Arch Phys Med Rehabil 2009;90:9–16.

40. De Paiva A, Meuner FA, Molgo J, et al. Functional repair of motor endplates after botulinum neurotoxin type A poisoning: biphasic switch of synaptic activity between nerve sprouts and their parent terminals. Proc Natl Acad Sci U S A 1999;96:3200–5.

41. Zuber M, Sebald M, Bathien N, et al. Botulinum antibodies in dystonic patients treated with type A botulinum toxin: frequency and significance. Neurology 1993;43:1715–8.

42. Hyman N, Barnes M, Bhakta B, et al. Botulinum toxin (dysport) treatment of hip adductor spasticity in multiple sclerosis: a prospective, randomised, double blind, placebo controlled, dose ranging study. J Neurol Neurosurg Psychiatry 2000;68:707–12.

43. Bakheit AMO, Thilman AF, Ward AB. A randomized, double-blind, palcebo-controlled, dose-ranging study to compare the efficacy and safety of three doses of botulinum toxin type A (dysport) with placebo in upper limb spasticity after stroke. Stroke 2000;31:2402–6.

44. Bhakta BB, Cozens JA, Bamford JM, et al. Use of botulinum toxin in stroke patients with severe upper limb spasticity. J Neurol Neurosurg Psychiatry 1996;61:30–5.

45. Brashear A, Gordon MF, Elovic E, et al. Intramuscular injection of botulinum toxin for the treatment of wrist and finger spasticity after a stoke. N Engl J Med 2002; 347(6):395–400.
46. Caty GD, Detrembleur C, Bleyenheuft C, et al. Effect of upper limb botulinum toxin injections on impairment, activity, participation, and quality of life among stroke patients. Stroke 2009;40:2589–91.
47. Kirazli Y, On AY, Kismali B, et al. Comparison of phenol block and botulinum toxin type A in the treatment of spastic foot after stroke: a randomized, double-blind trial. Am J Phys Med Rehabil 1998;77(6):510–5.
48. Chau KSG, Kong KH. Alcohol neurolysis of the spastic nerve in the treatment of hemiplegic knee flexor spastcity: clinical outcomes. Arch Phys Med Rehabil 2000;81:1432–5.
49. Khalili AA, Betts HB. Peripheral nerve block with phenol in the management of spasticity. JAMA 1967;200(13):1155–7.
50. Wolf JH, English AW. Muscle spindle reinnervation following phenol block. Cells Tissues Organs 2000;166:325–9.
51. Bovend'Eerdt TJ, Newman M, Barker K, et al. The effects of stretching in spasticity: a systematic review. Arch Phys Med Rehabil 2008;89:1395–406.
52. Harvey LA, Katalinic OM, Herbert RD, et al. Stretch for the treatment and prevention of contractures [review]. Cochrane Database Syst Rev 2017;(1):CD007455.
53. Leung J, Harvey LA, Moseley AM, et al. Electrical stimulation and splinting were not clearly more effective than splinting alone for contracture management after acquired brain injury: a randomised trial. J Physiother 2012;58:231–40.
54. Dai AI, Demiryurek AT. Serial casting as an adjunct to botulinum toxin type A treatment in children with cerebral palsy and spastic paraparesis with scissoring of the lower extremities. J Child Neurol 2017;32(7):671–5.
55. Singer B, Singer KB, Allison G. Serial plaster casting to correct equino-varus deformity of the ankle following acquired brain injury in adults. Disabil Rehabil 2001;23(18):829–36.
56. Lannin NA, Novak I, Cusick A. A systematic review of upper extremity casting for children and adults with central nervous system motor disorders. Clin Rehabil 2007;21(11):963–76.
57. Mortenson PA, Eng JJ. The use of casts in the managament of joint mobility and hypertonia following brain injury in adults: a systematic review. Phys Ther 2003; 83(7):648–58.
58. Pohl M, Mehrholz J, Ruckriem S. The influence of illness duration and level of consciousness on the treatment effect and complication rate of serial casting in patients with severe cerebral palsy spasticity. Clin Rehabil 2003;17:373–9.
59. Karadag-Saygi E, Cubukcu-Aydoseli K, Kablan N, et al. The role of kinesiotaping combined with botulinum toxin to reduce plantar flexors spasticity after stroke. Top Stroke Rehabil 2010;14(4):318–22.
60. Santamato A, Micello MF, Panza F, et al. Adhesive taping vs. daily manual muscle stretching and splinting after botulinum toxin type A injection for wrist and fingers spastic overactivity in stroke patients: a randomized controlled trial. Clin Rehabil 2015;29(1):50–8.
61. Malhotra S, Rosewilliam S, Hermens H, et al. A randomized controlled trial of surface neuromuscular electrical stimulation applied early after acute stroke: effects on wrist pain, spasticity and contractures. Clin Rehabil 2012;27(7):579–90.
62. Oo WM. Efficacy of addition of transcutaneous electrical nerve stimulation to standardized physical therapy in subacute spinal spasticity: a randomized controlled trial. Arch Phys Med Rehabil 2014;95:2013–20.

63. Woo R. Spasticity: orthopedic perspective. J Child Neurol 2001;16(1):47–53.
64. Anakwenze OA, Namdari S, Hsu JE, et al. Myotendinous lengthening of the elbow flexor muscles to improve active motion in patients with elbow spasticity following brain injury. J Shoulder Elbow Surg 2013;22:318–22.
65. Limpaphayom N, Chantarasongsuk B, Osateerakun P, et al. The split anterior tibialis tendon transfer procedure for spastic equinovarus foot in children with cerebral palsy: results and factors associated with a failed outcome. Int Orthopaedics 2015;39:1593–8.
66. Aversano MW, Taha AMS, Mundluru S, et al. What's new in the orthopaedic treatment of cerebral palsy. J Pediatr Orthop 2017;37(3):210–6.
67. Buffenoir K, Decq P, Hamel O, et al. Long-term neuromechanical results of selective tibial neurotomy in patients with spastic equinus foot. Acta Neurochir 2013; 155:1731–43.
68. Deltombe T, Gustin T. Selective tibial neurotomy in the treatment of spastic equinovarus foot in hemiplegic patients: a 2-year longitudinal follow-up of 30 cases. Arch Phys Med Rehabil 2010;91:1025–30.
69. Deltombe T, Bleyenheuft C, Gustin T. Comparison between tibial nerve block with anaesthetics and neurotomy in hemiplegic adults with spastic equinovarus foot. Ann Phys Rehabil Med 2015;58:54–9.
70. Dudley RWR, Parolin M, Gagnon B, et al. Long-term functional benefits of selective dorsal rhizotomy for spastic cerebral palsy. J Neurosurg Pediatr 2013;12: 142–50.
71. Hofstoetter US, McKay WB, Tansey KE, et al. Modification of spasticity by transcutaneous spinal cord stimulation in individuals with incomplete spinal cord injury. J Spinal Cord Med 2014;37(2):202–11.
72. Lin SM, Yoo J, Lee E, et al. Acupuncture for spasticity after stroke: a systematic review and meta-analysis of randomized controlled trials. Evid Based Complement Alternat Med 2015;2015:870398.
73. Caliandro P, Celletti C, Padua L, et al. Focal muscle vibration in the treatment of upper limb spasticity: a pilot randomized controlled trial in patients with chronic stroke. Arch Phys Med Rehabil 2012;93:1656–61.
74. Seo HG, Oh BM, Leigh JH, et al. Effect of focal muscle vibration on calf muscle spasticity: a proof-of-concept study. PM R 2016;8:1083–9.
75. Sadeghi M, Sawatzky B. Effects of vibration on spasticity in individuals with spinal cord injury: a scoping systematic review. Am J Phys Med Rehabil 2014;93: 995–1007.
76. Miyara K, Matsumoto S, Uema T, et al. Feasibility of using whole body vibration as a means for controlling spasticity in post-stroke patients: a pilot study. Complement Ther Clin Pract 2014;20:70–3.
77. Santamato A, Notarnicola A, Panza F, et al. SBOTE study: extracorporeal shock wave therapy versus electrical stimulation after botulinum toxin type A injection for post-stroke spasticity-a prospective randomized trial. Ultrasound Med Biol 2013;39(2):283–91.
78. Moon SW, Kim JH, Jung MJ, et al. The effect of extracorporeal shock wave therapy on lower limb spasticity in subacute stroke patients. Ann Rehabil Med 2013; 37(4):461–70.
79. Leo A, Naro A, Molonia F, et al. Spasticity management: the current state of transcranial neuromodulation. PM R 2017;9:1020–9.
80. Gunduz A, Kumru H, Pacual-Leone A. Outcomes in spasticity after repetitive transcranial magnetic and transcranial direct current stimulations. Neural Regen Res 2014;9(7):712–8.

81. Glavao SCB, Costa dos Santos RB, Borba dos Santos P, et al. Efficacy of coupling repetitive transcranial magnetic stimulation and physical therapy to reduce upper-limb spasticity in patients with stroke: a randomized controlled trial. Arch Phys Med Rehabil 2014;95:222–9.

82. Wu D, Qian L, Zorowitz RD, et al. Effects on decreasing upper-limb poststroke muscle tone using transcranial direct current stimulation: a randomized sham-controlled study. Arch Phys Med Rehabil 2013;94:1–8.

83. Marinelli L, Balestrino M, Mori L, et al. A randomized controlled cross-over double-blind pilot study on THC: CBD oromucosal spray efficacy as an add-on therapy for post-stroke spasticity. BMJ Open 2017;7:1–6.

84. Syed YY, McKeage K, Scott LJ. Delta-9-tetrahydrocannabinol/cannabidiol (sativex): a review of its use in patients with moderate to severe spasticity due to multiple sclerosis. Drugs 2014;74:563–78.

85. Keating GM. Delta-9-tetrahydrocannabinol/cannsbidiol oromucosal spray (sativex): a review in multiple sclerosi-related spasticity. Drugs 2017;77:563–74.

# Pharmacologic Treatment Tools

## Systemic Medications and Toxins, Opportunities, and Pitfalls

Peter Riedel, DO[a], Michael H. Marino, MD[a,b],*

KEYWORDS

- Upper motor neuron syndrome • Spasticity • Muscle overactivity • Treatment
- Pharmacotherapy • Toxins

KEY POINTS

- Treatment of pathologic muscle overactivity associated with upper motor neuron syndrome can be multifaceted.
- One of the initial decisions to be made when formulating an overarching treatment plan is selecting a combination of strategies that is most applicable.
- Strategies may include physical interventions, such as stretching or splinting modalities, or surgery, whereas pharmacotherapeutic strategies encompass oral/systemic medications as well as agents, such as toxins and alcohols, used for focal chemodenervation.

## INTRODUCTION

Treatment of pathologic muscle overactivity associated with upper motor neuron (UMN) syndrome can be multifaceted. One of the initial decisions to be made when formulating an overarching treatment plan is selecting a combination of strategies that is most applicable. Strategies may include physical interventions such as stretching or splinting modalities or surgery, whereas pharmacotherapeutic strategies encompass oral/systemic medications as well as agents, such as toxins and alcohols used for focal chemodenervation. This article reviews the oral/systemic therapies as well as toxins that are used focally. Although medication can also be administered via intrathecal pumps, this treatment approach is discussed elsewhere.

Disclosure: The authors have nothing to disclose.
[a] Physical Medicine and Rehabilitation, Moss Rehab, 60 Township Line Road, Elkins Park, PA 19027, USA; [b] Physical Medicine and Rehabilitation, ReMed, 16 Industrial Boulevard, Paoli, PA 19301, USA
* Corresponding author. Physical Medicine and Rehabilitation, Moss Rehab, 60 Township Line Road, Elkins Park, PA 19027.
E-mail address: Marino01@einstein.edu

Phys Med Rehabil Clin N Am 29 (2018) 501–517
https://doi.org/10.1016/j.pmr.2018.04.008
1047-9651/18/© 2018 Elsevier Inc. All rights reserved.

## SYSTEMIC PHARMACOTHERAPY

Oral medications are frequently started as one of the initial treatments for muscle over-activity related to UMN syndrome. The use of these medications, as is discussed later, has significant associated risks. It must be emphasized that hypertonia not contributing to decreased function, pain, or increased burden of care need not be suppressed. Clinicians should always have a clear, goal-oriented approach for prescribing. Exacerbating factors such as visceral distension or other noxious stimuli should be identified and limited as much as possible before initiation of treatment. Most of the oral medications are likely to cause some degree of sedation so timing and environmental context of treatment are important considerations.

### Baclofen

Baclofen is the most commonly known and used oral medication to inhibit muscle overactivity. It binds to gamma-aminobutyric acid (GABA)-B receptors, inhibiting calcium influx that would otherwise allow release of excitatory neurotransmitters.[1] It is thought to have postsynaptic effects at the GABA-B receptor through multiple pathways and decreases activity of both the gamma motor neuron and intrafusal spindle muscles.[2–4] Both monosynaptic and polysynaptic reflexes are inhibited by baclofen.[5] Animal studies have also shown a possible mechanism for analgesic properties via reduction of substance P from nociceptive afferent nerve terminals.[6] Baclofen is mostly excreted through the kidneys (a small amount is metabolized by the liver) and has a short half-life of approximately 3.5 hours.

Baclofen has been studied most extensively in patients with spinal cord injury and those with multiple sclerosis and has been shown to reduce spasticity as well as painful flexor spasms in these populations.[7,8] There is less evidence supporting benefit in patients with spasticity of cerebral origin. Like many other oral medications for spasticity, there is no established evidence that baclofen alone can improve independence with mobility or activities of daily living. It has been used for more than 40 years and has a generally low incidence of drug tolerance and/or side effects.[9]

Side effects of baclofen include gastrointestinal upset, sedation, confusion, dizziness, insomnia, muscle weakness, euphoria, depression, and dyskinesia.[10] Baclofen can lower the seizure threshold in patients with epilepsy and decrease alertness in elderly patients with acquired brain injury.[11] Patients should be tapered appropriately off baclofen because of risk of seizures, temporarily increased spasticity, confusion, and hallucinations.[12]

### Diazepam

Like baclofen, benzodiazepines are a commonly known and used class of medications to treat spasticity. Benzodiazepines indirectly work through the GABA-A receptor by neuronal membrane hyperpolarization via increased chloride influx once GABA is already bound.[13] This presynaptic inhibition enhances the efficacy of GABA binding at spinal and supraspinal sites, which reduces both monosynaptic and polysynaptic reflexes at the spinal level.[14,15]

Diazepam, a long-acting benzodiazepine, has been used to treat spasticity in patients with spinal cord injury for more than 40 years and is the most commonly used drug for this purpose in its class.[16] However, because of its deleterious effects on attention and memory, it is not commonly used for spasticity in patients with acquired brain injury, although it has been shown to improve athetosis in addition to spasticity in patients with cerebral palsy.[17] Diazepam is metabolized by the liver and its half-life can be from 20 to 50 hours, with active metabolites lasting up to 100 hours.[18]

The most common side effects related to benzodiazepines are sedation, drowsiness, and ataxia. Sedation can worsen cognitive deficits caused by acquired brain injury or affect people with less cognitive reserve, such as the elderly, disproportionately. With increased dose, the sedative effect of the benzodiazepines can lead to physiologic dependence, coma, and/or death. If stopped abruptly or tapered incorrectly, withdrawal syndrome can occur with benzodiazepine, which includes anxiety, psychosis, seizures, and death.[18]

### Dantrolene

Dantrolene, compared with the previous 2 medications discussed, is a peripherally acting agent. By suppressing the release of calcium ions from the sarcoplasmic reticulum, excitation and contraction are decoupled, which diminishes the force of muscular contraction in spasticity.[19] This effect is more pronounced in fast-contracting fibers and affects both intrafusal and extrafusal fibers, indicating a component of muscle spindle sensitivity modulation.[20,21]

Because dantrolene works peripherally, it can be better tolerated in patients with spasticity of cerebral origin relative to baclofen and benzodiazepines. It has been shown to decrease spasticity in this population; however, it can still be associated with fatigue and muscle weakness, which limit functional improvement.[22,23] Patients with multiple sclerosis are most at risk for weakness caused by dantrolene.[24] Patients with spinal cord injury, stroke, and cerebral palsy have all been shown to tolerate dantrolene well.[25] Notably, dantrolene has been shown to be effective for treating clonus, although its overall effect of muscle weakness should be considered in functional terms. Dantrolene is primarily metabolized in the liver and has a half-life of approximately 15 hours.[19]

Dantrolene does have a US Food and Drug Administration (FDA) black box warning for hepatoxicity, with reactions occurring more frequently in higher doses and in women more than 35 year old on estrogen supplementation. The risk of fatality is 0.1% to 0.2% but hepatic injury is usually reversible if tests are being monitored and the medication is appropriately discontinued.[26] As previously mentioned, general weakness and malaise have been reported with dantrolene as well as gastrointestinal symptoms such as diarrhea. Dantrolene should be avoided in patients with multiple sclerosis, particularly with bulbar or respiratory muscle weakness.[25] The investigators recommend checking baseline liver function tests before starting dantrolene, then again at 1 month, and then every 3 months.

### Tizanidine

Tizanidine is a central alpha-2 adrenergic receptor agonist that is thought to act presynaptically to attenuate release of excitatory neurotransmitters at the spinal level and possibly through effects on interneurons and postsynaptic release of excitatory neurotransmitters.[27] The exact mechanism of action is incompletely understood, and it may also have supraspinal effects mediated though descending facilitatory coeruleospinal pathways.[28] Tizanidine is metabolized in the liver and has a half-life of approximately 3 hours.[29]

Tizanidine has been shown to improve spasticity in the spinal cord and in patients with multiple sclerosis but this was not correlated with functional improvement, similar to baclofen.[30–33] Tizanidine was also compared with diazepam and baclofen in patients with stroke and traumatic brain injury (TBI) and was found to have similar clinical efficacy; notably in 1 study it was associated with a superior walking distance compared with baclofen.[34,35]

Common side effects associated with tizanidine include xerostomia, sedation, muscle weakness, postural hypotension, and dizziness. From 5% to 7% of patients experience clinically significant increases in liver enzyme levels, particularly those on multiple medications metabolized by the liver.[36] Discontinuation of tizanidine is usually associated with improvement in transaminitis, but monitoring of liver function is recommended with this medication.

### Cyclobenzaprine

Cyclobenzaprine is a centrally acting muscle relaxant that is structurally similar to tricyclic antidepressants.[37] It has significant anticholinergic effects and is thought to have its primary effects through the brainstem, where it modulates the serotonergic system, reducing tonic somatic motor activity in both gamma and alpha motor systems.[38] Cyclobenzaprine is excreted by the kidneys with some minor metabolism by the liver and has a half-life of 8 hours.

Cyclobenzaprine has no recent or specific studies supporting its use in treatment of spasticity. A small study from 1972 did not find a clinically or electromyographically significant improvement with regular doses in patients with brain and spinal cord injury.[39] Cyclobenzaprine continues to be a commonly prescribed medication for a variety of conditions, including low back pain, neck pain, fibromyalgia, general pain, and sleep, and there is evidence showing moderate improvement in acute back pain and short-term fibromyalgia.[38]

The most common side effect of cyclobenzaprine is sedation, followed by lightheadedness, dizziness, and xerostomia. There is a potential risk of serotonin syndrome when prescribed alongside other serotonergic medications.

### Gabapentin

Gabapentin is an analogue of GABA that binds to intracellular sites that inhibit voltage-gated calcium channels and plasma membrane expression.[40] Its mechanism of action has been controversial; although it is not thought to bind directly to GABA receptors, it has been shown to increase GABA turnover.[41] Gabapentin is cleared by the kidneys and its half-life is approximately 6 hours.[42]

There are a few studies that show improvement in spasticity in patients with spinal cord injury and multiple sclerosis treated with gabapentin; however, there is little evidence of significant functional improvement.[43–45] Before the neuropathic and anticonvulsant indications were determined for gabapentin, it was originally designed as an antispasticity agent. Many patients who take gabapentin for neuropathic pain are likely to benefit from a minor adjuvant effect if they also have spasticity.

The most common side effect with gabapentin is sedation, followed by dizziness, ataxia, headache, tremor, and gastrointestinal upset.[46]

### Cannabis

Cannabis and its various herbal extracts represent some of the oldest medicine used by humans for many different conditions. It was first listed in the United States dispensatory in 1854 as a treatment of muscle spasms, neuralgia, tetanus, and pain and remained available for many other conditions effectively until 1937 with the Marihuana Tax Act.[47] The American Medical Association opposed the 1937 act because it limited doctors prescribing cannabis, unlike the similar Harrison Tax Act, which continued to allow prescription of opiates.[48] In 1970, the Controlled Substances Act was passed, which classified cannabis as having "no currently accepted medical use and a high potential for abuse."[49] Since then, many groups have lobbied for cannabis to return as a legally available medical treatment and, in 2018, 29 states in the United States, including Washington, DC, have laws supporting some form of medical marijuana with a recommendation from a doctor.[50]

The mechanism of action of the cannabinoids is not completely understood but they are known to interact with the cannabinoid receptors CB-1 and CB-2. CB-1 is the primary target with spasticity therapy and is found in the central nervous system, whereas CB-2 is distributed more broadly, including the immune system.[51] When CB-1 is activated by unopposed tetrahydrocannabinol (THC), anxiety and psychoses can occur more frequently. Coadministration of cannabidiol (CBD) can counter these effects, but it is not a CB-1 antagonist.[52] There is some thought that cannabinoid-based drugs could interrupt neurodegenerative processes, as in multiple sclerosis; however, this has not yet been proved in a large randomized placebo-controlled trial. The endocannabinoid system is also a target for spasticity therapy, and fatty acid amide hydrolase inhibitors have been successful in mouse multiple sclerosis models, which allow more anandamide (naturally occurring CB-1 ligand) to circulate and decrease spasticity.[53] Physical exercise has also been shown to increase endocannabinoid levels in the brain and sensitize CB-1 at central synapses, which indicates that epigenetics may play a part in CB-1 function and further research in this area could help tailor physical therapy as well as differentiate between appropriate individualize treatments.[51]

There are currently 2 synthetic preparations of the cannabinoid delta-9-THC, dronabinol (same structure as THC) and nabilone (synthetic derivative), which were developed to treat intractable nausea related to chemotherapy or acquired immunodeficiency syndrome. Cannabis is composed of at least 60 psychoactive cannabinoids, 2 of which, THC and CBD, compose in equal proportions the herbal extract nabiximols. Dronabinol is metabolized by the liver and has a half-life of up to 36 hours.[54] Nabilone is metabolized by the liver and has a half-life of 2 hours.[55] Nabiximols is metabolized in the liver and has a half-life of up to 5 hours. CBD is noted to be a cytochrome P450 inhibitor.[56]

There have not been large placebo-controlled studies with the synthetic cannabis medications in terms of spasticity treatment, only small blinded studies with electromyographic analysis or open-label subjective studies.[57,58] A large placebo-controlled trial with 630 patients with multiple sclerosis tested THC as well as oral cannabis extract but did not find improvement in Ashworth scores. The study did find objective improvement in mobility and subjective improvement in the patients' perception of pain.[59] The same patients who subjectively felt an improvement in symptoms with cannabis extract and THC were followed for another 12 months and did find a small improvement on Ashworth scores, but only in the THC group.[60] Two subsequent randomized placebo-controlled trials with nabiximols also showed significant subjective improvement of multiple sclerosis symptoms (and only within the group following the protocol in the second study) but not significant improvement on Ashworth scores.[61,62] In another 2 studies, 1 randomized and placebo controlled and the other noninterventional, about 20% to 25% of patients with multiple sclerosis had significantly increased subjective spasticity symptom scores with nabiximols.[63,64] Several of these nabiximols studies have had follow-up studies at 12 months showing maintained improvements and continued tolerance of treatment, and the relationship between Ashworth score and real functional improvement remains controversial for some. This body of research points toward a subset of patients with multiple sclerosis who would likely benefit from cannabis treatment of spasticity in lieu of combining some of the more traditional medications discussed previously and risking magnification of their associated side effects. There has yet to be much investigation of cannabis treatment of spasticity in patients with other spinal and cerebral neurologic disease, and further research into those populations and with multiple sclerosis are needed. In 2014, The American Academy of Neurology published a summary of evidence-based guidelines for complementary and alternative medicine in multiple sclerosis, which included level A and B recommendations respectively for oral cannabis extract and THC for spasticity symptoms and related pain.[65,66] In 2018, a systematic review found evidence supporting a trial of cannabinoids for spasticity or pain in patients with multiple sclerosis. This review included 11 systematic reviews considering 32 studies, 10 of which were moderate-quality to high-quality randomized controlled trials.[67] Nabiximols is approved in the United Kingdom for treatment of spasticity in multiple sclerosis and is in development for federal approval in the United States for symptom relief in patients with multiple sclerosis.

In the 2018 review, the following adverse effects of cannabis and cannabinoids were listed: dizziness, xerostomia, euphoria, diarrhea, and difficulty concentrating. There was no type of cannabinoid or route of administration that was specifically associated with any particular adverse effect.[67] Part of what has made cannabis difficult to standardize as a medication for more than a hundred years has been its heterogeneous effect, both in positive and negative effects. There is evidence for concern that smoking cannabis could be associated with negative cardiovascular effects, and health care practitioners should encourage their patients to use other forms of administration.[68] There is an approximately 1% chance of serious adverse mental disorders, so careful consideration should be given to patients with significant psychiatric histories and no children or adolescents with developing brains should be prescribed cannabis.[67]

## BOTULINUM TOXINS
### Mechanism of Action

Botulinum toxins (BoNT) are powerful neurotoxins produced by the gram-positive aerobic bacteria *Clostridium botulinum*.[69] There are several different serotypes produced, referred to as serotypes A through G, but only serotypes A and B are used in health care. All of the serotypes function at the presynaptic terminal by blocking release of acetylcholine into the synaptic cleft. A complex set of proteins called SNARE (soluble *N*-ethylmaleimide–sensitive factor attachment protein receptor) proteins are required for presynaptic vesicles containing acetylcholine to bind with the nerve terminal membrane and release their contents into the synaptic cleft. SNARE proteins include SNAP-25 (synaptosome-associated protein-25), synaptobrevin, and syntaxin.[1–4] Each neurotoxin molecule is composed of a heavy chain and a light chain. The heavy chain is responsible for presynaptic binding of the toxin to receptors. The light chain is responsible for inhibiting the action of a specific protein responsible for acetylcholine release.[1,3] Serotypes B, D, F, and G inhibit synaptobrevin. Serotypes A, C, and E inhibit SNAP-25. Serotype C also inhibits syntaxin.[1–4] By blocking acetylcholine release from the presynaptic membrane the muscle receives little to no stimulation from the nerve terminal and is functionally denervated.[70,71]

In 2009 the FDA suggested standardizations of the names of the available toxins to better identify and differentiate between the different formulations. BoNT type A, marketed as Botox and made by Allergan, is now referred to as onabotulinumtoxinA. BoNT type A, marketed as Dysport and manufactured by Ipsen, is now referred to as abobotulinumtoxinA. BoNT type A, marketed as Xeomin and manufactured by Merz, is now referred to as incobotulinumtoxinA. BoNT type B, marketed as Myobloc and manufactured by Solstice, is now referred to as rimabotulinumtoxinB[72] (**Table 1**).

**Table 1**
**Suggested standardizations**

| Name | Trade Name | Serotype | Mechanism of Action | Abbreviation |
|------|-----------|----------|--------------------|--------------|
| OnabotulinumtoxinA | Botox | A | Inhibits SNAP-25 | BoNT-ona |
| AbobotulinumtoxinA | Dysport | A | Inhibits SNAP-25 | BoNT-abo |
| IncobotulinumtoxinA | Xeomin | A | Inhibits SNAP-25 | BoNT-inc |
| RimabotulinumtoxinB | Myobloc | B | Inhibits synaptobrevin | BoNT-rim |

*Data from* Kedlaya D. Botulinum toxin 2016. Medscape: WebMD LLC. Available at: https://emedicine.medscape.com/article/325451-overview#showall. Accessed December 15, 2017; with permission.

## Opportunities

### Reviews

Most studies showing the efficacy of botulinum toxin for treating spasticity have been done in patients with stroke, with the minority of studies done in patients with brain injury and cerebral palsy. In 2009 a group of European clinicians published a consensus statement regarding the use of botulinum toxin type A in acquired brain injury (trauma, stroke, or hypoxia). The group had extensive experience in treating spasticity and represented 16 different European countries. They concluded that botulinum toxin type A was a valuable tool in treating upper limb and lower limb spasticity but still advised a multimodal approach.[73] Similarly, the American Academy of Neurology (AAN) also published an evidence-based review of botulinum toxin. The AAN group was also composed of a panel of experts with experience treating spasticity with botulinum toxin. This review included evaluations of spasticity in adults and children with several diagnoses including stroke, TBI, and cerebral palsy. The AAN group concluded that botulinum toxin types A and B are effective treatments for upper and lower limb spasticity in decreasing muscle tone and improving passive function.[74]

Note that these reviews, as well as several others, report findings primarily based on outcome measures of decreased muscle tone or passive function as measured by the Modified Ashworth Scale, Ashworth Scale, Tardieu Scale, passive range of motion, or spasm frequency. Reports of improved function after botulinum toxin injections have been more variable. Dong and colleagues[75] performed a systematic review with meta-analysis and trial sequential analysis on the efficacy and safety of botulinum toxin type A for upper limb spasticity after stroke or TBI. They reported on findings of both active and passive function. The review included studies evaluating all 3 available botulinum toxin type A preparations. They found firm evidence of a beneficial effect of botulinum toxin type A to decrease spasticity measured by Modified Ashworth Scale after stroke or TBI. There was also a statistically significant decrease in scores on the Disability Assessment Scale (DAS) at 4 weeks, 6 weeks, and 12 weeks postinjection, indicating improved report of function. The DAS addresses 4 domains: hygiene, dressing, limb position, and pain. Each domain is measured on a 4-point scale on which 0 indicates no disability and 3 indicates severe disability in which normal activities are limited.[76] The scale is subjectively reported and also contains measures of both active and passive function. In addition, the patients reported improved impression of functional disability at 4 weeks and 6 weeks postinjection as measured by the Global Assessment Scale. These impressions of self-improvement did not persist at 12 weeks postinjection. More rigorous measures of upper limb active function, including the Modified Frenchay Scale, Action Research Arm Test, and Motor Activity Log, did not show significant improvements with botulinum toxin injection at any time point after injection.

### Onabotulinum toxin A

Injection of BoNT-ona has shown positive effects on function in the lower limb in patients with TBI. Fock and colleagues[77] studied 7 patients with unilateral spastic equinus posture of the lower limb who were between 4 and 38 months postinjury, had failed other physical treatments, and were able to walk with or without aids independently for at least 50 m. They performed preinjection and postinjection tests of gait, including measuring walk speed, stride length, and cadence. A total of 300 units were injected per patient, with dosing distributed between both heads of the gastrocnemius, the soleus, and the tibialis posterior. Six subjects had improved walking speed at 2 weeks postinjection that continued at 12 weeks postinjection. Six subjects had a longer stride length at 12 weeks after the injection. Six subjects had increased cadence at 12 weeks postinjection; however, only 3 of those had shown improvement at 2 weeks postinjection. However, showing active functional improvements in the upper limbs of patients following botulinum toxin has proved more difficult. Childers and colleagues[78] studied 91 patients with upper limb spasticity from stroke. The patients were randomized into groups receiving placebo or 90 units, 180 units, or 360 units of botulinum toxin A (not specified but most likely BoNT-ona based on timing of article and dosing). Muscle groups injected included biceps brachii, flexor carpi radialis, flexor carpi ulnaris, flexor digitorum profundus, and flexor digitorum sublimis. The investigators found a dose-dependent improvement in muscle tone measured by Modified Ashworth Scale. They did not find any significant improvements in physician or patient global assessments, pain, FIM instrument, or Medical Outcomes Study 36-Item Short Form Health Survey (SF-36; a measurement of health-related quality of life).

### Abobotulinum toxin A

Treatment with BoNT-abo has also shown consistent improvement in measures of tone and passive function, with inconsistent improvements in active function. Dashtipour and colleagues[79,80] performed separate systematic reviews of BoNT-abo treatment of adults with lower limb spasticity and upper limb spasticity of multiple causes, including stroke, TBI, and multiple sclerosis. They found consistent improvements in measures of spasticity using the Modified Ashworth Scale for upper and lower limb muscles. Significant improvement in active movement was less consistently shown. Barbaud and colleagues[81] studied 23 hemiparetic patients with spasticity from stroke or TBI in a randomized, double-blind, placebo-controlled crossover study of BoNT-abo. Patients received placebo or 1000 units of BoNT-abo distributed into triceps surae, soleus, tibialis posterior, and flexor digitorum longus. The investigators found significant improvements in Modified Ashworth Scale values in the treatment group. They also found significant improvements in lower limb Fugl-Meyer assessment.

### Incobotulinum toxin A

Treatment with BoNT-inc has also shown consistent improvement in measures of tone and passive function in patients with stroke. In 2013, Santamato and colleagues[82] studied 71 patients with poststroke lower limb spasticity in an open-label trial using BoNT-inc. They Injected between 25 and 100 units into each of the medial and lateral gastrocnemius muscles and soleus muscles. They showed significant improvements in Modified Ashworth Scale score, in spasm frequency, and in ankle dorsiflexion range of motion. Improvements in passive and active function have been shown in the upper limb for patients with poststroke spasticity using BoNT-inc. In 2011, Kanovsky and colleagues[76] also used an open-label design to inject 145 patients with flexed elbow, pronated forearm, flexed wrist, thumb in palm, or clenched fist deformities. Muscle selection was based on clinical examination but included most major elbow flexors, wrist flexors, forearm pronators, and thumb and finger flexors. Up to 400 units of BoNT-inc was used at 12-week intervals. The investigators found significantly improved measures of muscle tone on the Modified Ashworth Scale and also showed significant improvement in DAS.

### Rimabotulinum toxin B

Similar findings regarding tone, passive function, and active function have been shown in BoNT-rim. Brashear and colleagues[83] evaluated 10 patients with stroke or TBI who had stable upper limb spasticity (6 months' duration or longer) in an open-label, single treatment session study. They injected a total dose of 10,000 units of BoNT-rim divided between biceps brachii, flexor carpi ulnaris, flexor carpi radialis, flexor digitorum sublimis, and flexor digitorum profundus. They found significant improvements in Ashworth Scale in elbow, wrist, and finger flexors across multiple intervals between injection and 12 weeks postinjection. They did not find any significant improvements on any functional measures, including the Nine Hole Peg Test and Jebsen Hand Function Test. More recently, in 2015, Gracies and colleagues[84] evaluated 24 patients who were at least 4 weeks poststroke or TBI and had disabling elbow flexor spasticity. They used a randomized, double-blind, placebo-controlled study design. They injected placebo, 10,000 units, or 15,000 units of BoNT-rim into overactive upper limb muscles per the investigator's discretion. They found that both doses significantly improved active elbow extension more than placebo. They did not find any significant improvement on the Modified Frenchay Scale, a measure of active function. However, the patients who were injected with 15,000 units of BoNT-rim showed significantly improved scores on the Global Self-assessment (GSA). The GSA is a patient-rated tool that is a subjective measure of function based on pain, stiffness-induced discomfort, and active function. This study represents one of the few to show improvement in active function as measured by an objective scale (in this case the patient's ability to actively extend the elbow) and on a subjective scale (the GSA).

### Pitfalls

### Dosing issues

Although injection of botulinum toxin represents a valuable clinical tool for physicians treating patients with spasticity, there is also a variety of potential pitfalls that physicians must be aware of. In 2009, the FDA announced black-box warnings on labeling for botulinum toxin products because of the risk of systemic spread of the toxin resulting in botulismlike symptoms. Symptoms of systemic spread of toxin include weakness, voice hoarseness, dysarthria, bladder incontinence, respiratory distress, dysphagia, vision changes, and eyelid drooping. Most of these events occur in children with cerebral palsy who received high doses of botulinum toxin to treat muscle spasticity. Severe cases resulted in hospitalizations and some deaths.[85] Cases of botulinum toxin–related death caused by anaphylaxis have also been reported.[86] Between December 1989 and May 2003, there were 28 reported deaths related to therapeutic botulinum toxin use.[87] In order to decrease the chances of adverse reactions, careful dosing strategy should be used by the injector. It is imperative that injectors have comfort and familiarity with the formulation of botulinum toxin that they are injecting. Dosing guides are available from the products' manufacturers. Extreme caution should be taken when converting between different formulations of botulinum toxin. Units of one formulation are not equivalent to units of another formulation. For example, a typical dose of BoNT-ona is 100 to 300 units, whereas a typical dose for BoNT-rim is 5000 to 15,000 units. No universally accepted conversion system has been developed, and dosing should be determined on a patient-by-patient basis.[88] Although distal spread can cause systemic effects such as a botulismlike syndrome, local spread of medication to adjacent muscles is also of concern.[89,90] The desired clinical effect of treating spastic muscle with botulinum toxin is to produce weakness. Complications arise when too much weakness is produced either systemically or locally. Using a careful case-by-case approach helps to mitigate this risk.

### Localization issues

One of the biggest challenges in injection of botulinum toxin is ensuring that the medication is delivered within the correct muscle. There are several techniques used to localize muscles for injection. Anatomic localization involves the use of anatomic landmarks to identify the target muscles. Injectors often use electromyography (EMG) texts as guides, which is the simplest and quickest technique for injection and does not require additional equipment. The primary disadvantage is the potential to inadvertently inject a nontarget muscle. EMG guidance is another technique used to identify target muscles. Advantages include a wide availability of EMG equipment and familiarity of physicians with EMG techniques. Using EMG also allows the injector to select the most electrically active muscles or regions of muscles to inject. In addition, EMG equipment is relatively inexpensive. Potential disadvantages include prolonged procedure time, increased pain because of prolonged time of the needle in the muscle, cost of insulated EMG needles, and the cost of the EMG machines. In addition, although using EMG guidance aids in the identification of target muscles, it does not guarantee that the needle is in the target muscle. Electrical stimulation (e-stim) is another technique used to aid identification of target muscles. Injectors can use e-stim to stimulate a target muscle and then use direct visual correlation of muscle contraction to determine that they are indeed in the target muscle. The amplitude of stimulation can then be slowly decreased while still observing muscle contraction. In this way precise localization is enhanced, allowing lower doses of botulinum toxin to be used more effectively. Disadvantages include prolonged time to perform the injection, more training required for injectors, increased discomfort/pain for the patient, the cost of the needle electrode, and the cost of the e-stim device. Ultrasonography is another technique to aid identification of target muscles. Advantages include real-time visualization of needle advancement into target muscles, the ability to avoid penetrating neurovascular structures, and more precise identification of target muscles. In skilled hands this technique can be quick; however, significant training and experience are required. In addition, simultaneous operation of the ultrasonography transducer and advancement of the needle may necessitate an assistant during the injection. The cost of an ultrasonography machine may be too great for some practices.[91]

The use of EMG guidance, e-stim guidance, and ultrasonography guidance have all been shown to be more effective clinically than using anatomic localization alone.[92–94] Mayer and colleagues[95] evaluated the clinical effectiveness of botulinum toxin injection using EMG versus e-stim guidance in a parallel-group, randomized controlled trial of patients with acquired brain injury and elbow flexor spasticity. They evaluated efficacy based on Ashworth Scale, Tardieu catch angle, and surface EMG activity of the elbow flexor muscles. The investigators concluded that EMG guidance and e-stim guidance produce similar clinical results. Picelli and colleagues[96] evaluated the clinical effectiveness of botulinum toxin injection using anatomic localization versus e-stim guidance versus ultrasonography guidance in a single-blinded, randomized controlled trial of 60 patients with chronic stroke with clenched fist or flexed wrist deformity. Primary outcome measures were Modified Ashworth Scale scores, Tardieu angle, and passive range of motion, and e-stim was superior to anatomic localization in all measures. Similarly, ultrasonography guidance was superior to anatomic localization in all measures. However, there was no difference in clinical outcome between the e-stim and ultrasonography guidance groups.

*Immunogenicity*
Another pitfall in the effective use of botulinum toxin is the development of neutralizing antibodies. As a result of the protein content in botulinum toxins (particularly the heavy chains), the body's immune system can form antibodies against the toxin, which may block its effect. Early studies of BoNT-ona used for cervical dystonia revealed rates of neutralizing antibodies as high as 17%. However, BoNT-ona was reformulated in 1998 with a 5-fold reduction in protein load, which has led to reduced incidence of neutralizing antibodies. Current estimates of the incidence of blocking antibodies range between 0.5% and up to 6.6% of patients treated with botulinum toxin.[97,98] The presence of neutralizing antibody should be considered in any patient who initially responded to treatment with botulinum toxin but later developed treatment failure. A variety of laboratory assays are available to test for neutralizing antibodies, including enzyme-linked immunosorbent assay and Western blot. There are also several clinical techniques to diagnose neutralizing antibodies that involve injecting a small dose of botulinum toxin into small muscles and observing the clinical response using the naked eye or motor nerve conduction study measurements.[88] Current recommendations to minimize the potential for development of neutralizing antibodies include using an injection schedule that separates injections at a minimum of 3 months, using the lowest effective dosage, and avoiding booster injections, which are injections given in the interval between the every-3-months injection schedule.[99]

*Bleeding complications*
Botulinum toxin injectors often experience trepidation regarding performing injections on patients who are on antiplatelet agents or anticoagulants because of concern for major bleeding events. Several reviews have examined this issue. Phadke and colleagues[100] retrospectively reviewed the charts of 110 patients with stroke treated for spasticity with BoNT-ona or BoNT-inc and who were on warfarin, a new oral anticoagulant agent, an antiplatelet agent, or no anticoagulant. These 110 patients underwent a total of 674 injection cycles and there were no incidences of compartment syndrome or major bleeding events. Lavallee and colleagues[101] retrospectively reviewed the charts of 15 patients who underwent a total of 328 ultrasonography-guided injections of botulinum toxin for spasticity. Eight patients were on anticoagulants (warfarin, dabigatran, enoxaparin, rivaroxaban) and 7 were on antiplatelet agents (aspirin, clopidogrel). Only 8% of the patients on warfarin had a supratherapeutic International Normalized Ratio. The investigators found only 2 incidences of bleeding complications (1 subcutaneous hematoma and 1 intermuscular hematoma). They concluded that the risk of significant bleeding complications is small but still advised collaboration between the injector and the physician managing the anticoagulation medication to determine whether it should be discontinued before the procedure.

## REFERENCES

1. Curtis DR, Gynther BD, Lacey G, et al. Baclofen: reduction of presynaptic calcium influx in the cat spinal cord in vivo. Exp Brain Res 1997;113(3):520–33.
2. Misgeld U, Bijak M, Jarolimek W. A physiological role for GABAB receptors and the effects of baclofen in the mammalian central nervous system. Prog Neurobiol 1995;46(4):423–62.

3. Lev-Tov A, Meyers DE, Burke RE. Activation of type B gamma-aminobutyric acid receptors in the intact mammalian spinal cord mimics the effects of reduced presynaptic Ca2+ influx. Proc Natl Acad Sci U S A 1988;85(14):5330–4.

4. Harrison FG. The effects of baclofen on gamma motoneurones supplying gastrocnemius muscle in the rabbit. Neuropharmacology 1982;21(10):973–9.

5. Ito T, Furukawa K, Karasawa T, et al. Effects of chlorpromazine, imipramine and baclofen on the spinal polysynaptic reflex in acute, chronic and 6-hydroxydopamine-treated spinal rats. Jpn J Pharmacol 1982;32(6):1125–33.

6. Henry JL. Pharmacological studies on the prolonged depressant effects of baclofen on lumbar dorsal horn units in the cat. Neuropharmacology 1982;21(11):1085–93.

7. Duncan GW, Shahani BT, Young RR. An evaluation of baclofen treatment for certain symptoms in patients with spinal cord lesions. A double-blind, crossover study. Neurology 1976;26(5):441–6.

8. Feldman RG, Kelly Hayes M, Conomy JP, et al. Baclofen for spasticity in multiple sclerosis. Double-blind crossover and three-year study. Neurology 1978;28(11):1094–8.

9. Roussan M, Terrence C, Fromm G. Baclofen versus diazepam for the treatment of spasticity and long-term follow-up of baclofen therapy. Pharmatherapeutica 1985;4(5):278–84.

10. Dario A, Tomei G. A benefit-risk assessment of baclofen in severe spinal spasticity. Drug Saf 2004;27(11):799–818.

11. Hulme A, MacLennan WJ, Ritchie RT, et al. Baclofen in the elderly stroke patient its side-effects and pharmacokinetics. Eur J Clin Pharmacol 1985;29(4):467–9.

12. Terrence CF, Fromm GH. Complications of baclofen withdrawal. Arch Neurol 1981;38(9):588–9.

13. Olsen RW. GABA-benzodiazepine-barbiturate receptor interactions. J Neurochem 1981;37(1):1–13.

14. Skerritt JH, Willow M, Johnston GA. Diazepam enhancement of low affinity GABA binding to rat brain membranes. Neurosci Lett 1982;29(1):63–6.

15. Polc P, Möhler H, Haefely W. The effect of diazepam on spinal cord activities: possible sites and mechanisms of action. Naunyn Schmiedebergs Arch Pharmacol 1974;284(4):319–37.

16. Corbett M, Frankel HL, Michaelis L. A double blind, cross-over trial of Valium in the treatment of spasticity. Paraplegia 1972;10(1):19–22.

17. Marsh HO. Diazepam in incapacitated cerebral-palsied children. JAMA 1965;191:797–800.

18. Riss J, Cloyd J, Gates J, et al. Benzodiazepines in epilepsy: pharmacology and pharmacokinetics. Acta Neurol Scand 2008;118(2):69–86.

19. Ward A, Chaffman MO, Sorkin EM. Dantrolene. A review of its pharmacodynamic and pharmacokinetic properties and therapeutic use in malignant hyperthermia, the neuroleptic malignant syndrome and an update of its use in muscle spasticity. Drugs 1986;32(2):130–68.

20. Jami L, Murthy KS, Petit J, et al. Action of dantrolene sodium on single motor units of cat muscle in vivo. Brain Res 1983;261(2):285–94.

21. Leslie GC, Part NJ. The effect of dantrolene sodium on intrafusal muscle fibres in the rat soleus muscle. J Physiol 1981;318:73–83.

22. Ketel WB, Kolb ME. Long-term treatment with dantrolene sodium of stroke patients with spasticity limiting the return of function. Curr Med Res Opin 1984;9(3):161–9.

23. Chyatte SB, Birdsong JH, Bergman BA. The effects of dantrolene sodium on spasticity and motor performance in hemiplegia. South Med J 1971;64(2): 180–5.
24. Gelenberg AJ, Poskanzer DC. The effect of dantrolene sodium on spasticity in multiple sclerosis. Neurology 1973;23(12):1313–5.
25. Pinder RM, Brogden RN, Speight TM, et al. Dantrolene sodium: a review of its pharmacological properties and therapeutic efficacy in spasticity. Drugs 1977; 13(1):3–23.
26. Utili R, Boitnott JK, Zimmerman HJ. Dantrolene-associated hepatic injury. Incidence and character. Gastroenterology 1977;72(4 Pt 1):610–6.
27. Davies J. Selective depression of synaptic transmission of spinal neurones in the cat by a new centrally acting muscle relaxant, 5-chloro-4-(2-imidazolin-2-yl-amino)-2, 1, 3-benzothiodazole (DS103–282). Br J Pharmacol 1982;76(3): 473–81.
28. Coward DM. Tizanidine: neuropharmacology and mechanism of action. Neurology 1994;44(11 Suppl 9):S6–10 [discussion: S10–1].
29. Granfors MT, Backman JT, Laitila J, et al. Tizanidine is mainly metabolized by cytochrome p450 1A2 in vitro. Br J Clin Pharmacol 2004;57(3):349–53.
30. Nance PW, Bugaresti J, Shellenberger K, et al. Efficacy and safety of tizanidine in the treatment of spasticity in patients with spinal cord injury. North American Tizanidine Study Group. Neurology 1994;44(11 Suppl 9):S44–51 [discussion: S51–2].
31. United Kingdom Tizanidine Trial Group. A double-blind, placebo-controlled trial of tizanidine in the treatment of spasticity caused by multiple sclerosis. Neurology 1994;44(11 Suppl 9):S70–8.
32. Newman PM, Nogues M, Newman PK, et al. Tizanidine in the treatment of spasticity. Eur J Clin Pharmacol 1982;23(1):31–5.
33. Hassan N, McLellan DL. Double-blind comparison of single doses of DS103-282, baclofen and placebo for suppression of spasticity. J Neurol Neurosurg Psychiatry 1980;43(12):1132–6.
34. Bes A, Eyssette M, Pierrot-Deseilligny E, et al. A multi-centre, double-blind trial of tizanidine, a new antispastic agent, in spasticity associated with hemiplegia. Curr Med Res Opin 1988;10(10):709–18.
35. Medici M, Pebet M, Ciblis D. A double-blind, long-term study of tizanidine ('Sirdalud') in spasticity due to cerebrovascular lesions. Curr Med Res Opin 1989; 11(6):398–407.
36. Wagstaff AJ, Bryson HM. Tizanidine. A review of its pharmacology, clinical efficacy and tolerability in the management of spasticity associated with cerebral and spinal disorders. Drugs 1997;53(3):435–52.
37. Spiller HA, Winter ML, Mann KV, et al. Five-year multicenter retrospective review of cyclobenzaprine toxicity. J Emerg Med 1995;13(6):781–5.
38. Cimolai N. Cyclobenzaprine: a new look at an old pharmacological agent. Expert Rev Clin Pharmacol 2009;2(3):255–63.
39. Ashby P, Burke D, Rao S, et al. Assessment of cyclobenzaprine in the treatment of spasticity. J Neurol Neurosurg Psychiatry 1972;35(5):599–605.
40. Hendrich J, Van Minh AT, Heblich F, et al. Pharmacological disruption of calcium channel trafficking by the $\alpha2\delta$ ligand gabapentin. Proc Natl Acad Sci U S A 2008;105(9):3628–33.
41. Welty DF, Schielke GP, Vartanian MG, et al. Gabapentin anticonvulsant action in rats: disequilibrium with peak drug concentrations in plasma and brain microdialysate. Epilepsy Res 1993;16(3):175–81.

42. McLean MJ. Clinical pharmacokinetics of gabapentin. Neurology 1994;44(6 Suppl 5):S17–22 [discussion: S31–2].

43. Rabchevsky AG, Patel SP, Duale H, et al. Gabapentin for spasticity and autonomic dysreflexia after severe spinal cord injury. Spinal Cord 2011;49(1): 99–105.

44. Cutter NC, Scott DD, Johnson JC, et al. Gabapentin effect on spasticity in multiple sclerosis: a placebo-controlled, randomized trial. Arch Phys Med Rehabil 2000;81(2):164–9.

45. Gruenthal M, Mueller M, Olson WL, et al. Gabapentin for the treatment of spasticity in patients with spinal cord injury. Spinal Cord 1997;35(10):686–9.

46. Shorvon S, Stefan H. Overview of the safety of newer antiepileptic drugs. Epilepsia 1997;38(Suppl 1):S45–51.

47. Abel E. Marihuana: the first twelve thousand years. Boston (MA): Springer; 1980. p. 182, 247.

48. Statement of Dr. William C. Woodward, legislative council, American Medical Association; 2017. Available at: http://www.druglibrary.org/Schaffer/hemp/taxact/woodward.htm. Accessed March 11, 2018.

49. DEA/Drug Scheduling 2018. Available at: https://www.dea.gov/druginfo/ds.shtml. Accessed March 11, 2018.

50. State Medical Marijuana Laws. National Conference of State Legislatures. Available at: http://www.ncsl.org/research/health/state-medical-marijuana-laws.aspx. Accessed November 3, 2017.

51. Chiurchiù V, van der Stelt M, Centonze D, et al. The endocannabinoid system and its therapeutic exploitation in multiple sclerosis: Clues for other neuroinflammatory diseases. Prog Neurobiol 2018;160:82–100.

52. McPartland JM, Duncan M, Di Marzo V, et al. Are cannabidiol and Δ(9)-tetrahydrocannabivarin negative modulators of the endocannabinoid system? A systematic review. Br J Pharmacol 2015;172(3):737–53.

53. Pryce G, Cabranes A, Fernández-Ruiz J, et al. Control of experimental spasticity by targeting the degradation of endocannabinoids using selective fatty acid amide hydrolase inhibitors. Mult Scler 2013;19(14):1896–904.

54. Solvay Pharmaceuticals. Product information: Marinol®, dronabinol oral capsules. Marietta (GA): Solvay Pharmaceuticals; 2006.

55. Valeant Pharmaceuticals. Product information: Cesamet™, nabilone oral capsules. Costa Mesa (CA): Valeant Pharmaceuticals; 2006.

56. GW Pharma. Product information: Sativex® oromucosal spray summary of product characteristics, 2014. Available at: http://www.medicines.org.uk/emc/medicine/23262. Accessed March 11, 2018.

57. Petro DJ, Ellenberger C Jr. Treatment of human spasticity with delta 9-tetrahydrocannabinol. J Clin Pharmacol 1981;21(8–9 Suppl):413S–6S.

58. Consroe P, Sandyk R, Snider SR. Open label evaluation of cannabidiol in dystonic movement disorders. Int J Neurosci 1986;30(4):277–82.

59. Zajicek J, Fox P, Sanders H, et al, UK MS Research Group. Cannabinoids for treatment of spasticity and other symptoms related to multiple sclerosis (CAMS study): multicentre randomised placebo-controlled trial. Lancet 2003; 362(9395):1517–26.

60. Zajicek JP, Sanders HP, Wright DE, et al. Cannabinoids in multiple sclerosis (CAMS) study: safety and efficacy data for 12 months follow up. J Neurol Neurosurg Psychiatry 2005;76(12):1664–9.

61. Collin C, Davies P, Mutiboko IK, et al, Sativex Spasticity in MS Study Group. Randomized controlled trial of cannabis-based medicine in spasticity caused by multiple sclerosis. Eur J Neurol 2007;14(3):290–6.
62. Collin C, Ehler E, Waberzinek G, et al. A double-blind, randomized, placebo-controlled, parallel-group study of Sativex, in subjects with symptoms of spasticity due to multiple sclerosis. Neurol Res 2010;32(5):451–9.
63. Novotna A, Mares J, Ratcliffe S, et al, Sativex Spasticity Study Group. A randomized, double-blind, placebo-controlled, parallel-group, enriched-design study of nabiximols* (Sativex(®)), as add-on therapy, in subjects with refractory spasticity caused by multiple sclerosis. Eur J Neurol 2011;18(9): 1122–31.
64. Flachenecker P, Henze T, Zettl UK. Nabiximols (THC/CBD oromucosal spray, Sativex®) in clinical practice–results of a multicenter, non-interventional study (MOVE 2) in patients with multiple sclerosis spasticity. Eur Neurol 2014; 71(5–6):271–9.
65. Yadav V, Bever C Jr, Bowen J, et al. Summary of evidence-based guideline: complementary and alternative medicine in multiple sclerosis: report of the guideline development subcommittee of the American Academy of Neurology. Neurology 2014;82(12):1083–92.
66. Koppel BS, Brust JC, Fife T, et al. Systematic review: efficacy and safety of medical marijuana in selected neurologic disorders: report of the Guideline Development Subcommittee of the American Academy of Neurology. Neurology 2014; 82(17):1556–63.
67. Nielsen S, Germanos R, Weier M, et al. The use of cannabis and cannabinoids in treating symptoms of multiple sclerosis: a systematic review of reviews. Curr Neurol Neurosci Rep 2018;18(2):8.
68. Piano MR. Cannabis smoking and cardiovascular health: it's complicated. Clin Pharmacol Ther 2017;102(2):191–3.
69. Simpson LL. The origin, structure, and pharmacological activity of botulinum toxin. Pharmacol Rev 1981;33(3):155–88.
70. Brashear A. Botulinum toxin in the treatment of upper limb spasticity. In: Brashear A, Ellovic E, editors. Spasticity diagnosis and management, vol. 11. New York: Demos Medical; 2011. p. 131–40.
71. Blasi J, Chapman ER, Link E, et al. Botulinum neurotoxin A selectively cleaves the synaptic protein SNAP-25. Nature 1993;365(6442):160–3.
72. Botulinum toxin safety warnings updated and name changes issued. Available at: https://www.medscape.com/viewarticle/706934. Accessed December 16, 2017.
73. Wissel J, Ward AB, Erztgaard P, et al. European consensus table on the use of botulinum toxin type A and adult spasticity. J Rehabil Med 2009;41(1):13–25.
74. Simpson DM, Gracies JM, Graham HK, et al. Assessment: botulinum neurotoxin for the treatment of spasticity (and evidence-based review): report of the therapeutics and technology assessment subcommittee of the American Academy of Neurology. Neurology 2008;70(19):1691–8.
75. Dong Y, Wu T, Hu X, et al. Efficacy and safety of botulinum toxin type A for upper limb spasticity after stroke or traumatic brain injury: systematic review with meta-analysis and trial sequential analysis. Eur J Phys Rehabil Med 2017;53(2): 256–67.
76. Kanovsky P, Slawek J, Denes Z, et al. Efficacy and safety of treatment with incobotulinum toxin A (botulinum neurotoxin type a free from complexing proteins; NT 201) in poststroke upper limb spasticity. J Rehabil Med 2011;43:486–92.

77. Fock J, Galea M, Stillman B, et al. Functional outcome following botulinum toxin A injection to reduce spastic equinus in adults with traumatic brain injury. Brain Inj 2004;18(1):57–63.

78. Childers MK, Brashear A, Jozefczyk P, et al. Dose-dependent response to intra-muscular botulinum toxin type a for upper-limb spasticity in patients after a stroke. Arch Phys Med Rehabil 2004;85:1063–9.

79. Dashtipour K, Chen JJ, Walker HW, et al. Systematic literature review of abobo-tulinumtoxinA in clinical trials for adult upper limb spasticity. Am J Phys Med Rehabil 2015;94(3):229–38.

80. Dashtipour K, Chen JJ, Walker HW, et al. Systematic literature review of abobo-tulinumtoxinA in clinical trials for lower limb spasticity. Medicine 2016;95(2):1–13.

81. Barbaud P, Wiart L, Dubos JL, et al. A randomized, double blind, placebo-controlled trial of botulinum toxin in the treatment of spastic foot in hemiparetic patients. J Neurol Neurosurg Psychiatry 1996;61:265–9.

82. Santomato A, Micello MF, Panza F. Safety and efficacy of incobotulinum toxini type A (NT 201-Xeomin) for the treatment of post-stroke lower limb spasticity: a prospective open-label study. Eur J Phys Rehabil Med 2013;49:483–9.

83. Brashear A, McAfee AL, Kuhn ER, et al. treatment with botulinum toxin type B for upper limb spasticity. Arch Phys Med Rehabil 2003;84:103–7.

84. Gracies MJ, Bayle N, Goldberg S, et al. Botulinum toxin type B in the spastic arm: a randomized, double-blind, placebo-controlled, preliminary study. Arch Phys Med Rehabil 2014;95:1303–11.

85. Kuehn B. FDA requires black box warnings on labeling for botulinum toxin products. JAMA 2009;301(22):2316.

86. Li M, Goldberger BA, Hopkins C. Fatal case of BOTOX-related anaphylaxis? J Forensic Sci 2005;50(1):169–72.

87. Cote TR, Mohan AK, Polder JA, et al. Botulinum toxin type A injections: adverse events reported to the US Food and Drug Administration in therapeutic and cosmetic cases. J Am Acad Dermatol 2005;53(3):407–15.

88. Smith AG. Pearls and pitfalls in the therapeutic use of botulinum toxin. Semin Neurol 2004;24(2):165–74.

89. Yaraskavitch M, Leonard T, Herzog W. Botox produces functional weakness in non-injected muscles adjacent to the target muscle. J Biomech 2008;41(4):897–902.

90. Eleopra R, Tugnoli V, Caniatti L, et al. Botulinum toxin treatment in the facial muscles of humans: evidence of an action in untreated near muscles by peripheral local diffusion. Neurology 1996;46(4):1158–60.

91. Walker HW, Lee MY, Bahroo LB, et al. Botulinum toxin injection techniques for the management of adult spasticity. PMR 2015;7:417–27.

92. Ploumis A, Varvarousis D, Kotsiotis S, et al. Effectiveness of botulinum toxin injection with and without needle electromyographic guidance for the treatment of spasticity and hemiplegic patients: a randomized control trial. Disabil Rehabil 2014;36:313–8.

93. Xu K. A randomized controlled trial to compare to botulinum toxin injection techniques on the functional improvement of the leg of children with cerebral palsy. Clin Rehabil 2009;2009:800–11.

94. Py AG, Zein AG, Perrier Y, et al. evaluation of the effectiveness of botulinum toxin injections in the lower limb muscles of children with cerebral palsy. Preliminary prospective study of the advantages of ultrasound guidance. Ann Phys Med Rehabil Med 2009;52:215–23.

95. Mayer NH, Whyte J, Wannstedt G, et al. Comparative impact of 2 botulinum toxin injection techniques for elbow flexor hypertonia. Arch Phys Med Rehabil 2008;89:982–7.

96. Picelli A, Lobba D, Midiri A, et al. Botulinum toxin injection into the forearm muscles for wrist and fingers spastic overactivity in adults with chronic stroke: a randomized controlled trial comparing 3 injection techniques. Clin Rehabil 2014;28: 232–42.

97. Naumann M, Boo LM, Ackerman AH, et al. Immunogenicity of botulinum toxins. J Neural Transm 2013;120:275–90.

98. Benecke R. Clinical relevance of botulinum toxin immunogenicity. BioDrugs 2012;26(2):e1–9.

99. Francisco GE. Botulinum toxin: dosing and dilution. Am J Phys Med Rehabil 2004;83(suppl):S30–7.

100. Phadke CP, Thanikachalam V, Ismail F, et al. Patterns of botulinum toxin treatment for spasticity and bleeding complications in patients with thrombotic risk. Toxicon 2017;138:188–90.

101. Lavallee J, Royer R, Smith G. Prevalence of bleeding complication following ultrasound guided botulinum toxin injection in patients on anticoagulation of antiplatelet therapy. PMR 2017;9:1217–24.

# Neurolysis
## A Brief Review for a Fading Art

Steven Escaldi, DO[a,b],*

## KEYWORDS

- Spasticity management • Neurolysis • Hypertonia

## KEY POINTS

- For the clinician attempting to address the focal manifestations of hypertonia without surgical intervention, there have been 2 primary options: neurolysis or chemodenervation.
- Before the introduction of the botulinum toxins, neurolysis was the only focal spasticity treatment option available to the previous generation of physical medicine and rehabilitation practitioners.
- The goal of this chapter is to present the historical events and describe the treatment approaches that were common prior to the use of botulinum toxin. Case studies will be presented to provide support for the importance for the continued use and training in this technique.

 Video content accompanies this article at http://www.pmr.theclinics.com/.

The key to the successful treatment of patients with spasticity is contingent upon choosing appropriate interventions tailored to meet the needs, goals, and specific presentation of each patient. The physician's toolbox to address spasticity has remained relatively unchanged over the past 25 years. Specifically, for the clinician attempting to address the focal manifestations of hypertonia without surgical intervention, there have been 2 primary options: neurolysis or chemodenervation. Chemodenervation using botulinum toxin has become the primary treatment choice to address focal hypertonia across all diagnostic classes. The past decade alone has seen nearly monthly journal articles exploring the different formulations, dosing, and refinements of technique and localization. Although the attention and accolades for chemodenervation using botulinum toxin are warranted, this article focuses on the procedure whose role over the past decade has diminished. Before the introduction of the botulinum toxins, neurolysis was the only focal spasticity treatment option available to the previous generation of physical medicine and rehabilitation (PMR) practitioners.

Disclosure Statement: The author has nothing to disclose.
[a] Spasticity Management Program, Department of Rehabilitation Medicine, JFK-Johnson Rehabilitation Institute, Edison, NJ 08818, USA; [b] Rutgers Robert Wood Johnson Medical School, Piscataway, NJ 08854, USA
* Spasticity Management Program, Department of Rehabilitation Medicine, JFK-Johnson Rehabilitation Institute, Edison, NJ 08818.
E-mail address: sescaldi@jfkhealth.org

Phys Med Rehabil Clin N Am 29 (2018) 519–527
https://doi.org/10.1016/j.pmr.2018.03.005
1047-9651/18/© 2018 Elsevier Inc. All rights reserved.

pmr.theclinics.com

The term "nerve block" refers to the process of applying chemical agents to various nerve structures to intentionally interfere with nerve conduction. Nerve blocks were initially performed to address painful conditions such as cancer-related pain. Nerve blocks to manage spasticity typically focus on the intramuscular nerve (motor point), motor branches of nerves, or peripheral nerves. The blocks can be further subdivided based on the intended duration and mechanism of action.

Diagnostic nerve blocks (anesthetic nerve block)

- Term used when a short-acting anesthetic is placed over the nerve
- Typical agents used include lidocaine (0.5%–2.0% concentration) and bupivacaine (0.25%–0.75% concentration)
- Mechanism of action: works by interfering with the ion channels on the axon by decreasing membrane permeability to sodium ions. This prevents depolarization of the membrane, which interrupts signal transmission. Block occurs without residual damage to the nerve.
- Onset of action: within 5 minutes (lidocaine) to 15 minutes (bupivacaine)
- Duration of effect: approximately 1 to 3 hours for lidocaine, 4 to 6 hours for bupivacaine
- Common uses:
  - Evaluation of the functional benefit from spasticity
  - Improve comfort and ease of serial casting
  - Investigate extent of soft tissue contracture
  - Assist in planning for more permanent procedures

Therapeutic nerve blocks (neurolysis):

- Term used when applying longer-acting agents.
- Agents and the most commonly used concentrations include phenol 3% to 6% and ethyl alcohol 10% to 50%.
- Mechanism of action: destruction of nerve tissue via protein necrosis, the higher the concentration the more tissue damage noted.
- Onset of action: anesthetic effect occurs immediately, maximal neurolytic effect 24 to 48 hours.
- Duration of action: Variable based on type of block and amount placed. Generally, 2 to 6 months expected.
- Common uses: In conjunction with botulinum toxin or alone to address significant postures, such as the equinovarus foot, adducted hips, internally rotated shoulder, flexed elbow and wrist.

## HISTORIC MILESTONES IN MEDICINE RELATED TO SPASTICITY AND NEUROLYSIS

- 1860s: Sir Joseph Lister began using phenol as an antiseptic agent during surgery.
- 1903: Schlosser reports injection of alcohol into nerves for the treatment of neuralgia and other painful conditions.
- 1912: May publishes results of functional and histologic effects of intraneural and intraganglionic injections of alcohol of various concentrations in cats. Concludes that the alcohol causes local necrosis and fibrosis when placed over a peripheral nerve. Partial regeneration of the nerve was noted.[1]
- 1919: Liljestrand and Magnus report reduction of triceps rigidity in a decerebrate cat after an intramuscular injection of procaine.
- 1959: Nathan and Kelly separately described techniques for Intrathecal phenol injections to treat spasticity.[2,3]

- 1964: Tardieu and Hariga report results performing motor point injections using dilute alcohol and electrical stimulation.[4]
- 1964: Khalili and associates publish findings and present injection technique of 39 peripheral nerve blocks using 2% to 3% phenol solution.[5]
- 1965: Halpern and Meelhuysen publish findings and present injection technique for motor point blocks using small doses of 3% to 7% phenol solution.[6]

## Technique

### External and internal stimulation technique

The injection technique and materials required for motor point and peripheral nerve injection are similar. Motor points typically require multiple injection sites and less volume injected per site. The use of external stimulation to localize motor points and nerve branches before injection may improve patient comfort by decreasing the duration of needle stimulation and localization (**Fig. 1**, Video 1). The use of ultrasound combined with internal stimulation has become a more common technique for neurolysis. It offers the benefit of direct visualization of the nerve and identification of vascular structures. Ideally, the combination of ultrasound and electrical stimulator guidance should provide maximal safety with decreased medication volume required due to the increased ability to localize the target nerve. This will also minimize the time required for needle localization and stimulation-based discomfort. However, this technique requires additional equipment and skill in ultrasound technique.

### Materials and equipment

- Teflon-coated injection needle 22 to 28 gauge, length based on site and procedure ranging (1.2–3.0 inches) (**Fig. 2**)
- 1-mL to 5-mL syringe with extension port connector to needle hub; the extension port provides improved stabilization of needle during aspiration and medication injection
- Nerve stimulator capable of delivering an electrical impulse once or twice per second
- Gel electrodes
- Gauze, betadine, and alcohol
- Medication for injection

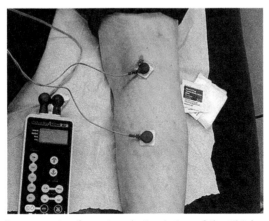

**Fig. 1.** Technique demonstration for external stimulation of the tibial nerve.

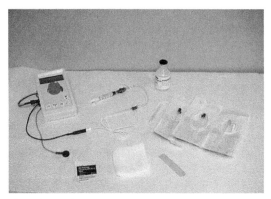

**Fig. 2.** Materials and equipment.

*Procedure*

- Clean site with alcohol and betadine (**Fig. 3**, Video 2).
- Draw up injectant.
- Attach syringe to needle and port.
- Connect internal stimulator to reference electrode.
- Insert needle into site advancing and adjusting output of stimulator with the goal of attaining a maximum contraction of the target muscle with only a minimal current; goal is to reduce the current below 1.0 milliamp.
- Withdraw plunger to ensure no intravascular administration.
- Inject 0.5 to 3.0 mL as needed, monitoring for extinction of contraction.
- Phenol has the potential to cause serious systemic side effects including seizures, central nervous system (CNS) depression, and cardiovascular collapse; 8.5 g of phenol is considered as a potential lethal dose.[7] Ten milliliters of a 5% phenol solution contains 0.5 g of phenol. Safe practice suggests using less than 1 g per treatment session.[8,9] Typical volumes used per motor point 0.5 to 1.0 mL, peripheral nerve 0.5 to 3.0 mL. There is no such concern regarding maximal dose per treatment session with ethanol (ETOH).
- ETOH has a benefit of simple storage and handling requirements. It can be diluted to the desired concentration by the physician at the time of the procedure.

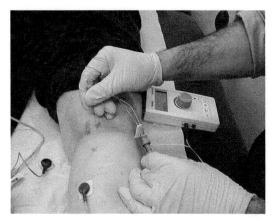

**Fig. 3.** Procedure.

Phenol solutions have to be produced by the pharmacist using strict storage and handling guidelines.

The advantages of nerve blocks:

- Low cost
- Rapid onset of action
- Able to treat large muscle groups to address specific limb postures (**Table 1**).
- Effect and dosing can be titrated to need (eg, multiple vs single motor point injections to a target muscle)
- Can be performed in a series over days to weeks, can reinject same nerve or area more frequently (booster effect)

Disadvantages of nerve blocks:

- Potential for trauma to injection site: tissue swelling, muscle necrosis, fibrosis, granuloma formation, muscle atrophy, scarring, skin slough
- Risk of dysesthesias; reported incidence varies 10% to 30%[6]; most common when injecting mixed motor and sensory nerves
- Increased procedure time and resources needed compared with botulinum toxin

**Table 1**
**Examples of common sites for peripheral nerve blocks**

| Problem | Nerve | Ideal Patient Position | Needle Position | Precautions |
|---|---|---|---|---|
| Flexed elbow | Musculocutaneous | Supine, arm abducted, and shoulder externally rotated | Proximal arm, medial aspect, between the tendons of the coracobrachialis and short head of the biceps | If needle is too posterior, it will encounter the axillary artery, too medial will encounter the median nerve |
| Adducted thigh | Obturator | Supine, hip abducted and externally rotated | Anterior approach in triangle made by add long tendon, femoral group, and inguinal ligament. (alternative approach, in between the add longus and gracilis tendons) | If needle placed too laterally risk injecting femoral nerve, artery or vein. |
| Extended knee | Femoral | Supine, knee extended | Distal to the inguinal ligament, lateral to the femoral artery | If needle placed too medially, risk injecting obturator nerve |
| Equinovarus foot | Tibial | Prone, knee extended to 30° of flexion, foot off edge of table | Popliteal fossa below the apex formed by the tendons of the biceps femoris and semimembranosus | If needle placed too lateral or proximal to branch off sciatic will affect common peroneal nerve |

- Potential for more discomfort for patient during procedure
- Increased requirement to remain immobilized during procedure
- Inadvertent systemic absorption or intravascular injection can result in cardio-vascular or CNS effects
- Permanent weakness due to nerve damage.

### Discussion

Despite the long history and safety profile performing neurolysis for spasticity, the frequency of its use in clinical practice has declined. Anecdotal evidence through discussion among PMR colleagues typically reveals that the procedure is being less frequently performed or completely abandoned. Insight gained from my personal experience training brain injury fellows over the past 10 years reveals that none reported feeling confident in performing nerve blocks and most recently some reported never performing one during their residency.

The following cases serve as my primary justification for the importance of the continued need to practice and promote the use of nerve blocks for spasticity management.

### CASE EXAMPLE 1: RATIONALE FOR DIAGNOSTIC NERVE BLOCK

This case is presented as a clinical situation in which a diagnostic block is useful in the evaluation and formulation of a treatment plan.

### History

The patient is a 58-year-old man with a history of hemorrhagic cerebrovascular accident (CVA) with left-sided weakness occurring 6 months ago. He is currently receiving outpatient therapies 3 times a week and performing a self-directed home exercise and stretching program daily. He presents with a chief complaint of increased difficulty with walking and tightness in the left inner thigh muscles. He and his therapist report increased left hip "scissoring," which is limiting his ability to advance the leg and also causes him to lose his balance. He is not walking at home due to fear of falls, but he is able to take a few steps to perform transfers with assistance. He denies any other areas of spasms or tightness. He reports taking multiple medications for other medical conditions, including seizures. He notes significant sleepiness and fatigue from the seizure medications.

### Evaluation

Focused examination reveals left leg weakness grading 3/5 for the knee extensors, 2-/5 for hip flexors, 0/5 for knee flexion and dorsiflexion of the ankle. Tone at rest reveals a 2 modified ashworth scale for the hip adductors, 1+ for the knee extensors and plantar flexors of the foot. Sensation is intact to light touch and pinprick. Functional evaluation reveals that he uses a left ankle foot orthosis and hemi-walker. He requires minimal assist to perform a sit to stand transfer. Gait examination reveals a right trunk lean to advance the left leg with hip external rotation and adduction of the left leg. With successive steps, the adduction of the hip increases and crosses midline, which results in loss of balance to the left.

### Treatment Premise

Focal reduction of the left leg adductor spasticity will improve leg position, base of support, and gait ability.

### Treatment Concern

Because of the left hip flexor weakness, the hip adductor spasticity could be functionally assisting the leg advancement during swing. Removal of the tone may result in loss of the ability to advance the left leg. This effect would limit his transfer ability and function at home.

### Treatment Decision

A diagnostic nerve block was performed targeting the anterior branch of the obturator nerve. A total of 2.0 mL 0.5% bupivacaine was injected.

### Treatment outcome and plan

**Positive functional result** The patient was noted with reduced hip adductor tone. There was improved left leg position and base of support on standing. His gait pattern was noted with decreased trunk lean to the right, increased left leg step length, and better foot placement during stance. He was able to increase his walking distance. With fatigue, there was noted return of the hip adduction but it did not cross midline. There was no loss of balance. This result proves the premise and demonstrated that the hip adduction is not functionally benefiting the patient. This allows confidence that a "longer- term" procedure, such as neurolysis or chemodenervation, can be performed.

**Negative functional result** Patient was noted with resolution of the hip adductor tone. There was improved left leg position and base of support on standing. With attempted walking, he was unable to advance the left leg without significant right trunk lean and pelvic rotation. This result confirms the treatment concern and demonstrated that the hip adduction was functionally benefiting the patient. A longer-term treatment option would have resulted in decreased transfer ability and safety. An appropriate treatment decision would be an increased focus in therapy on hip adductor stretching and strengthening of the left hip flexors and core. A reevaluation of his status after 4 weeks would be appropriate.

## CASE PRESENTATION 2: NEUROLYSIS
### History

The patient is a 65-year-old man with a history of atrial fibrillation and traumatic spinal cord injury secondary to a motor vehicle accident 2 years ago. He was diagnosed with a T9 AIS A paraplegia. During the course of his hospitalization, he was taken off oral anticoagulation to perform a procedure. During this time period off the anticoagulation therapy, he unfortunately sustained an embolic CVA, which resulted in deficits including decreased cognition and mild left arm weakness. Because of his impairments, he is dependent in self-care and transfers. His wife and daughter perform transfers using a mechanical lift. He is able to independently manage his power wheelchair once transferred. He presents with the chief complaint of painful and frequent lower extremity spasms. The family explains these symptoms occur randomly throughout the day, numerous times per hour. They also report significant increase in symptoms with any tactile stimulation of the legs. As a result, there is significant difficulty when performing dressing, toileting, and hygiene of the legs. They are also reporting decreased safety when transferring to the wheelchair due to the leg extension while in the mechanical lift. His feet do not remain on the wheelchair foot rest despite using Velcro straps. He was trialed on several oral antispasticity agents but did not receive any significant benefit due to severe negative effects on his cognition and arousal.

### Examination

Pertinent focal examination reveals complete motor and sensory paraplegia. While in the wheelchair, the knees would remain extended if they were not strapped to the footplate. Visible extensor spasms were witnessed at rest and they significantly increased in intensity with any tactile stimulation or attempted passive range of motion (PROM). While supine, the resting position of the hips were fully adducted with inability to attain any passive abduction from this resting position. The knees were only able to obtain 30° of flexion with significant effort.

### Treatment

All available treatment options were discussed (other oral medications, Intrathecal Baclofen Therapy, chemodenervation, and neurolysis). Although the patient appeared an ideal intrathecal baclofen candidate, the family was unwilling to discontinue anticoagulation to allow procedure or trial. We proceeded with botulinum toxin injection to address the bilateral hip adductors and knee extensors. The procedure was performed twice in a 6-month period (400 units initially, 600 units the second time). Results of both injections provided benefit with decreased tone and improved ease of dressing and activities of daily living. There was prolonged tone reduction with the higher dosing and decreased frequency and intensity of the spasms. There was, however, never complete resolution of the knee extensor spasms. While preparing for the third course of injections, the family reported that because of a change in insurance their out-of-pocket cost for the injection would not allow them to proceed. Rather than discontinuing treatment, we decided to proceed with the neurolysis. Because the primary concern at the time was the knee extensor spasms, bilateral femoral nerve blocks were performed. A total dose of 3.0 mL 50% ETOH was performed in 2 sites per leg. The patient tolerated the procedure without complication. Three months post injection there was no extensor tone noted on PROM. The family and patient reported resolution of the knee extensor spasms and that dressing and transfers were significantly easier and safer.

This case, although not complex, represents an ideal situation in which neurolysis became the most appropriate (and only) option for this patient. It meets the criteria for a successful treatment plan from both a symptom improvement and cost-efficient perspective. The complete nature of his injury allows injection to the larger peripheral nerves of the legs due to removed concerns regarding sensory or functional loss.

### SUMMARY

- Although there has been a decline in their use over the past decade, nerve blocks continue to offer an important treatment approach for spasticity management.
- The safety and side-effect profile of the procedure significantly improves with a skilled injector using a refined technique.
- Despite its well-established history of use and technique, more research is needed to evaluate the ideal medication and concentration choice, as well as the long-term effects on tissues and function.
- Consider as an early treatment option in cases with poor potential for functional recovery in which avoidance of contracture, pain, and ease of hygiene are primary goals (ie, patients with complete spinal cord injury, patients with severe traumatic brain or stroke patients with severe lower extremity spasticity and sensory loss).

### SUPPLEMENTARY DATA

Supplementary data related to this article can be found online at https://doi.org/10.1016/j.pmr.2018.03.005.

## REFERENCES

1. May O. The functional and histological effects of intraneural and intraganglionic injections of alcohol. Br Med J 1912;31:465.
2. Nathan PW. Intrathecal phenol to relieve spasticity in paraplegia. Lancet 1959;2: 1099–102.
3. Kelly RE, Gauthier-Smith PC. Intrathecal phenol in the treatment of reflex spasms and spasticity. Lancet 1959;ii:1102–5.
4. Tardieu G, Hariga J. Traitment des raideurs musculaires d'origine cerebrale par infiltration d'alchol dilue. Arch Franc Pedia 1964;21:25–41.
5. Khalili AA, Harmel MH, Forster S, et al. Management of spasticity by selective peripheral nerve block with dilute phenol solutions in clinical rehabilitation. Arch Phys Med Rehabil 1964;45:513–9.
6. Halpern D, Meelhuysen FE. Phenol motor point block in the management of muscular hypertonia. Arch Phys Med Rehabil 1966;47:659–64.
7. Wood KE. The use of phenol as a neurolytic agent: a review. Pain 1978;42(5): 726–32.
8. Glenn MB. Nerve blocks. In: Glenn MB, Whyte J, editors. The practical management of spasticity in children and adults. Philadelphia: Lea & Febiger; 1990. p. 227–58.
9. Khalili AA, Betts HB. Peripheral nerve block with phenol in the management of spasticity: indications and complications. JAMA 1967;200:1155–7.

## FURTHER READINGS

Cuccurullo S, Lee J. Physical Medicine and Rehabilitation Board Review. Demos Medical 2015;868–9.
Gracies J-M, Elovic E, McGuire J, et al. Traditional Pharmacological Treatments for Spasticity Part 1: Local Treatments. Muscle Nerve Suppl 1997;6:S61–91.
Zafonte RD, Munin MC. Phenol and alcohol blocks for the treatment of spasticity. Phys Med Rehabil Clin N Am 2001;12(4):817–832, vii.

# Muscle Overactivity in the Upper Motor Neuron Syndrome

## Assessment and Problem Solving for Complex Cases: the Role of Physical and Occupational Therapy

Kimberly Miczak, PT, NCS[a],*, Joseph Padova, OTR/L[b]

**KEYWORDS**

- Spasticity • Upper motor neuron syndrome • Physical • Occupational • Therapy

**KEY POINTS**

- Assessment of abnormal tone includes evaluation of neural and nonneural features of musculature, with emphasis on functional implications.
- Treatment interventions should consider severity and chronicity of impairments, in addition to the client's goals, resources, and support.
- Often, optimal outcomes are achieved via a multidisciplinary approach using a blend of compensation and remediation techniques.

## INTRODUCTION

The presence of muscle overactivity may have undesirable implications for an individual that includes decreased range of motion, abnormal posture, abnormal movement patterns, and limited movement capabilities.[1] The functional impact of such deficits may lead to pain, skin breakdown, decreased movement repertoire, inefficiency of movements (leading to fatigue), and limited ability to interact in meaningful ways in a variety of environments.[2] The role of the physical or occupational therapist is to determine the implication of muscle overactivity, via an evaluation that includes a comprehensive assessment of active and passive movements, neural and nonneural

---

Disclosure Statement: The authors have nothing to disclose.
[a] Drucker Brain Injury Center, MossRehab Hospital, 60 Township Line Road, Elkins Park, PA 19027, USA; [b] MossRehab Outpatient Center, 60 Township Line Road, Elkins Park, PA 19027, USA
* Corresponding author.
*E-mail address:* miczakk@einstein.edu

Phys Med Rehabil Clin N Am 29 (2018) 529–536
https://doi.org/10.1016/j.pmr.2018.03.006
1047-9651/18/© 2018 Elsevier Inc. All rights reserved.

structures, cognition, social support system, and patient goals. Collectively, this information assists the clinician in determining the optimal plan of care for the individual. This article discusses examination and intervention techniques that the physical or occupational therapist may use as a framework for managing muscle overactivity in the presence of upper motor neuron syndrome (UMNS) in complex cases.

The initial examination of an individual with muscle overactivity in the presence of UMNS should include assessment of[3]

- Passive range of motion (PROM)
- Active motion, including
  ○ Force production: grading of force, timing, presence of cocontraction
  ○ Ability to isolate movements in single joints (segments) and with multiple joints
  ○ Movement analysis (initial conditions, initiation, execution, termination)
- Standardized assessment tools, including but not limited to
  ○ Modified Ashworth Scale, Tardieu scale
  ○ Outcome tools, such as Barthel Index, Rivermead Mobility Index, Gait Speed

When performing the evaluation and treatment of individuals who have hemiparesis following lesions to the corticospinal system it is important for the clinician to be able to have a working understanding of the terminology of UMNS and how the terminology is applied during the rehabilitation process of the affected body parts. For example, when working with individuals who have hemiparesis following a stroke, it is not appropriate for therapists to describe the abnormal volitional movement patterns of the upper limb as spastic movement. Spasticity only describes one sign of UMNS.[4] When using the term spasticity in conjunction with a volitional movement, it is not being used correctly and does not provide a clear clinical picture of either the movements available to the patient or the anomalies of the intended motion that need to be more completely analyzed for effective therapeutic interventions. For therapeutic analysis, a clinician needs to understand the positive and negative signs of UMNS.[4] Combinations of positive and negative signs produce imbalances of muscle force across a joint of a limb creating maladaptive postural influences of the limb and abnormalities in movement patterns.[4] Negative signs include a lack of muscle activity. For example, weakness, lack of volitional recruitment of muscle groups, and a lack of reflexive activity are considered negative signs of UMNS.[4] Positive signs include spasticity, associated reactions, clonus, cocontraction, and spastic dystonia.[4] Included with the impaired movement patterns associated with the positive and negative signs of UMNS are also the consequences of the UMNS in regards to shortening of soft tissues of the muscles, joints, structures, and osteoporotic considerations of the bones and the skin.

Spasticity is defined as resistance of the antagonistic muscle group in reaction to a passive stretch. The strength of the resistance is velocity driven. When using this definition in the clinical picture of therapy, the effects of spasticity is seen during PROM of the joint (not active volitional movements).[4]

## PASSIVE RANGE OF MOTION ASSESSMENT

Because the effects of spasticity are velocity driven, the faster the joint is stretched the greater the antagonistic muscle groups of the joint resist the stretch. The effects of spasticity may also be a contributing factor to shortening of the muscle and soft tissues of the joints and weakness of the bones because of osteoporosis related to muscular imbalances and long periods of immobilization caused by lack of ability of the limb to change positions.[4] Therapists need to take these effects of spasticity into account when performing PROM of the affected limb. If moving the limb too quickly the effects of spasticity can limit how far the limb is ranged. A slow prolonged stretch using inhibitory positioning and placement of the patient supine to limit trunk overcompensatory motions is more advantageous than attempting faster PROM of the limb while the patient is seated.

## ACTIVE MOVEMENT ASSESSMENT

When assessing active movements of a limb with muscle overactivity, the clinician should use careful observational skills to analyze movement patterns. There may be a variety of deficits noted including associated reactions, clonus, or dystonia. These deficits may contribute to decreased active range of motion (AROM), force production deficits, and limit isolation of single joint movements. Activation in various postures and with different demands may result in variability of performance skills (discussed later).

An associated reaction is an involuntary reaction of a limb that is associated with a voluntary or involuntary effort made in another limb.[4] An example is that of a weight-lifter when flexing his or her elbow while curling a heavy load in one hand, and because of the effort, the opposite limb performs portions of the same curling motion. For an individual who has associated reaction of the affected upper extremity (UE) the limb may move from a more relaxed extended position when the patient is seated relaxed; however, the limb may move to a synergistic posture when the patient puts forth the effort to move to stand. This can also be seen when the patient is standing, and the therapist works on the patient to relax the affected UE, but the relaxed position is lost and moves to a synergistic pattern once a weight shift occurs that challenges the postural system, or during the effort of ambulation.[4] It can also be seen when the patient attempts to perform activities of daily living and the effort to reach with the intact limb, or performance of fast postural shifts increases the tightness, or synergistic posturing of the affected UE. In this case it becomes important to find postures and effort levels that limit the impact of associated reactions during activities of daily living and during therapeutic interventions.

Clonus is a phasic, or time-varying phenomenon, consisting of low-frequency rhythmic oscillation observed in one or more limb segments.[4] It occurs when there is an involuntary or voluntary movement of the affected limb and the antagonistic muscle groups stretch receptors are activated by the quick stretch and fight the movement. Conversely, the agonistic muscle groups that initiated the motion also react to the fast stretch from the antagonists and also fight to move in the opposite direction and the resulting activation of the agonistic and antagonistic muscle groups reaction becomes self-sustaining. This result is the limb moving in a shaking fashion. This clonus reaction is seen during passive repositioning of the affected limb when the movement to the new position is too fast. It can also be seen when the effort to produce volitional motions of the upper limb, such as when reaching for targets, objects, or specific ranges during an intervention, requires an effort level that triggers the clonus reaction. The clonus is controlled when careful attention is given to slowly reposition the shaking limb, keep the effort of the targeted AROM within parameter of the available active range, and slowly advance the parameters of the range as the patient's muscle strength and volitional movement improves within carefully designed work space.

Cocontraction is described as the activation of antagonistic muscle groups when attempting to perform motions.[4] For example, when an individual with UMNS attempts to extend the affected elbow and the elbow extensors begin to fire and the elbow flexors also activate blocking the motion. This results in rigidity of the limb and increased effort during volitional movement. When the cocontraction also has super-imposed stretch reflex generated by stretching the antagonist the combined phenom-ena is described as spastic cocontraction.[4] This is related to the amount of effort required to perform the volitional effort, the speed of the motion, and inability to isolate antagonistic muscle groups.

Dystonia occurs when a muscle is continually firing in the absence of an obvious stretch, or voluntary effort.[4] This is best observed during electromyographic (EMG) studies. In the therapy setting the phenomenon is likely to be evident in situations when a patient is able to perform a complete motion, such as fully extending the digits for release once, but on repeated attempts the digits have progressively less active extension, cramping, or impaired skilled fine motor dexterity. It may also be suspect in individuals who have posturing of the affected UE even when at rest. However, because of influences of other positive signs of UMNS and soft tissue shortening, dys-tonia without EMG studies is difficult to confirm.

The use of standardized assessment tools that quantify the abnormal tone, such as the Modified Ashworth Scale or the Tardieu scale, allows succinct description of the quantity and quality of abnormal tone. Use of activity- and participation-based tools allows the clinician to objectively identify functional skills, which may be influenced by the presence of UMNS. Once deficits have been identified, the clinician must deter-mine which deficits are most functionally limiting, which deficits may become detri-mental if not addressed (ie, tissue shortening, contracture), and which deficits are amenable to therapeutic intervention.

It is imperative for the clinician to collaborate with the patient, the caregivers, and the therapy team, including physicians regarding the functional implications of UMNS, including hygiene, positioning, presence of pain, and ability to actively use the involved limbs. Even if deficits are not functionally limiting, the clinician may choose to provide interventions as a means of preventing detrimental sequelae in the future, such as tissue shortening or contracture. The clinician need not use signif-icant time or resources for preventative measures and may opt for education and/or home management program as a means of preventing negative consequences in the affected limb.

When considering amenability to therapeutic intervention, the clinician must consider the following:

- Severity of deficits: More complex or severe deficits are less amenable to quick changes and may not be as responsive to conservative interventions.
- Chronicity of condition: Presence of overactivity has neural and nonneural impli-cations at a joint, with potential implications at proximal and distal joints. Chronic posturing often leads to joint contracture, which is less amenable to conservative interventions.
- Response to previous interventions: Knowing which interventions have been tried, their success, and the client's feelings toward those interventions may in-fluence the selection of interventions for the current episode of care.
- Cognitive status, compliance, and social support: Many persons with chronic neurologic conditions may also have concurrent cognitive dysfunction. This dysfunction has potential to influence comprehension of treatment interven-tions, tolerance to uncomfortable or challenging interventions, and thus compli-ance with therapeutic interventions. Hence, the role of caregivers or other support systems should be considered when determining feasibility of particular interventions.

Therapeutic interventions are targeted at the negative consequences of the effects of UMNS, not at altering the UMNS itself. Although there are a small number of studies that indicate that therapeutic interventions may have positive effect on abnormal tone, most studies demonstrate that therapeutic interventions do not decrease the overactivity of the musculature.[5] Rather, the interventions address secondary consequences because of the presence of abnormal excitability.

To address deficits, the clinician may choose (a hierarchal) approach when considering interventions with goals that address maintaining or improving PROM, facilitating active movement of antagonist or agonist musculature, and working toward multijoint movements in functional contexts.[6]

The use of low load, long duration stretching is the most widely used intervention to maintain or increase range of motion in joints affected by muscle overactivity. There is limited literature to support use of stretching to influence muscle overactivity, range of motion, pain, or participation.[5,7] Caution is advised in concluding therefore that stretching is not effective in preventing contractures or increasing range of motion in the presence of hyperexcitable musculature. Rather, consideration of potential risks/adverse effects (skin breakdown, discomfort, wound infection, costs of supplies and time) should be carefully weighed against potential gains and clinical experience should be included in this clinical decision-making process. Use of serial casts, dynamic splints, resting splints, weight-bearing postures, and manual stretching interventions are all viable options. Serial casts offer the ability to achieve low load, long duration stretch while concurrently limiting inputs that trigger the stretch reflex, therefore having the ability to impact neurophysiologic and morphologic components of overactive muscles. They have demonstrated most effectiveness when used in conjunction with chemodenervation interventions.[8] However, in situations when positive signs of UMNS are present it is important to consider referral to a motor control laboratory for EMG studies to see if there is a need for chemodenervation of the overactive muscle groups. If needed, chemodenervation is used to decrease the influence of overactive muscular forces that may be a contributing factor to the contracture and allow for improved result from the serial casting.[9] Similar to serial casts, splints offer long-duration stretch in a fashion that is easily removed and reapplied for situations in which casting is not an option, such as in the instance of fluctuating edema, or integumentary concerns. Mechanical stretching via sustained postures, such as use of tilt tables, may elicit a positive impact on range of motion while concurrently addressing other realms of dysfunction that are common in the presence of neurologic insults, such as endurance, alertness, and active motor contractions in a low-cost, time-efficient manner.

To facilitate active movement of antagonist or agonist musculature in a limb with overactivity, a variety of options exist. Active movement patterns that include elements of force production, muscular endurance, muscle timing of activation, and coordination of multiple segments in the effected limb can all lead to improved function of the effected limb.[10] The experienced clinician analyzes movement patterns to determine prioritization of treatment interventions related to strengthening, while concurrently considering such variables as postural demands, positioning, external cues, and level of muscular fatigue when progressing the interventions. Consideration of agonist and antagonistic musculature in the involved limb should be analyzed. The presence of abnormal tone in a particular muscle group has been shown to demonstrate underlying deficits in regards to volitional force production.[11,12] Concurrently, the antagonistic muscle group may also exhibit weakness caused by limited opportunities to engage in volitional activation patterns, especially in the presence of restricted range of motion.

Supplemental modalities that may assist the client's success with active movement training include use orthotics, electrical stimulation,[3,13] augmented feedback (EMG or biofeedback), and robotic devices. When applying supplemental modalities with individuals who have the positive and negative signs of UMNS it is important to take into consideration the specific deficits that the therapist is trying to address. For example, an individual who when attempting arm flexion at the shoulder complex cocontracts the arm extensors may find it beneficial to work on graded reaching tasks with a dual channel biofeedback to learn to activate the flexors in isolation of the extensors. Following chemodenervation with Botox of the wrist and finger flexors, functional electrical stimulation (FES) or EMG biofeedback, or EMG-triggered FES is a rehabilitation option to increase the strength of the extensors.

The use of therapeutic robotics interventions has shown to be valuable in improving components of proximal upper limb control.[14,15] The use of therapeutic robotics allows for increased repetition/practice or higher intensity of practice with increased consistency of performance, which align with current science.[14,15] When using therapeutic robotics it is important for the therapist to consider the client presentation in terms of the positive and negative signs of UMNS in addition to cognitive and perceptual skills. The therapist uses this information to design the number of repetitions, the size of the work space in which the patient will move the affected UE, speed of the movement, and the effort level and resistance level required to move the affected UE. If these are not taken into account, there is a risk that the interventions chosen could require abnormal movement patterns. If the intervention is graded too low, there may not be enough repetitions to allow for learning the intended motions. If the effort level is too low, the targeted muscle groups may not become strong enough to move the affected UE when no longer supported by the robotic upper limb support system.

It is important for the treating therapist to recognize that the incorporation of technologies, such as those mentioned previously, are tools that are used as a part of the rehabilitation process to improve movement patterns, strength, and range of motion. Evidence suggests that high repetitive practice with carefully graded task-specific training using activities that are relevant to the patients real life situation is integral for learning how to integrate the affected upper extremity.[16,17] If the patient is to learn the timing, strength, AROM requirements, and bilateral integration to use the affected upper limb to hold a container while the unaffected upper limb opens it, or to reach for, pick up, and place a cup, then it is important to practice that task.[16,17]

Lastly, the direct relationship between muscle overactivity and function is not well established.[18,19] Therefore, the clinician should be mindful of the resources allocated to normalizing impairments in lieu of addressing functional skills. A delicate balance of remediation and compensatory interventions may allow the client the opportunity to address impairments while concurrently improving functional capacity in the home and/or community. In terms of promoting functional integration of the affected UE it is important for the therapist to be able to not only consider the application of interventions that are designed to promote restorative function, but also to consider compensatory integrative interventions. Compensatory integration of the affected upper extremity takes into account that despite significant restorative efforts there still remains residual signs of UMNS that limit functional use of the upper limb. For example, an individual who has been living with the effects of a stroke for several years, had many courses of outpatient therapy, and still presents with synergistic patterns, can move the affected hand to touch the unaffected hand at midline, can volitionally create adequate flexor recruitment of the digits of the affected hand to generate a 4/5 gripping force (using manual muscle test), is able to stop the gripping force when cued, and is only able to passively extend the digits. In this scenario, therapeutic problem-solving needs to consider different ways that the patient may be able to integrate the affected UE. For example, the patient may be trained to use the upper limb to stabilize objects between the trunk and the affected UE. This hypothetical patient could be trained to use the hand as a holder. For example, the patient could be trained to place objects, such as a wallet or envelope, into the affected hand while the unaffected hand opens them and removes or replaces the contents. Some individuals can learn to use tenodesis to open the affected hand and use active grip force to hold objects while the uninvolved UE is used to manipulate them. For individuals who cannot relax the wrist to use tenodesis, functional hand splints are designed to extend the digits. Splinting options are static, dynamic, or a combination of the two. The therapist can adjust the extension force to allow the person to actively close the hand and hold objects. The patient can be trained to relax the hand to allow the splint to help release the object. When functional splinting is being considered the treating therapist needs to consider the multiple effects that signs of UMNS can have with regards to functional splinting options. Resistance and speed of the orthotic system being used to open the hand must be considered. If the patient has flexor spasticity, the tension used to extend the digits should be graded to not open the hand too quickly, or flexor spasticity may fight the extension force and limit the ability of the outrigger to open the hand for pregrasp. Individuals with spasticity may have weakness in the affected muscle groups. If the attempt to allow full extension of the hand requires too strong of an opening force, the patient may not have enough strength to close the affected hand and hold the desired object. If the flexion force is weak, it may be important to fabricate a splint to support the wrist in addition to the dynamic hand component. In this case, stabilizing the wrist in various degrees of extension and preventing flexion may improve grip force by biomechanically increasing tension on the extrinsic digit flexors that cross the wrist. In cases when the extrinsic finger flexors have shortened over time, opening of the hand is improved by fabrication of a splint that positions the wrist in varying degrees of flexion. In some cases, the wrist may hyperextend, which combined with tightness of the digit flexors that cross the wrist can also limit opening of the affected hand. A splint that blocks the hyperextension or flexes the wrist can promote opening of the digits using a modified tenodesis.

Careful dosing of chemodenervations that decreases the effects of associated reactions or spasticity in select muscle groups can be used in conjunction with functional splinting. Collaboration should be taken between the injecting physician and the therapist to help identify the muscle groups targeted for the chemodenervation and not overweaken them if active flexion is needed for function.

## SUMMARY

The physical or occupational therapist's role in persons with muscle overactivity caused by a UMNS is to evaluate the implications of the abnormal muscle activity on function. A thorough assessment that considers the consequences on movement patterns and the longer-term consequences on soft tissue allows for a thoughtful plan of care that incorporates a variety of factors and leads to patient-centered optimization of functional outcomes.

## REFERENCES

1. Fheodoroff K, Jacinto J, Geurts A, et al. How can we improve current practice in spastic paresis? Eur Neurol Rev 2016;11(2):79–86.
2. Zorowitz RD, Gillard PJ, Brainin M. Poststroke spasticity. Sequelae and burden on stroke survivors and caregivers. Neurology 2013;80:S45–52.

3. Gracies JM. Physical modalities other than stretch in spastic hypertonia. Phys Med Rehabil Clin N Am 2001;12:769–92.

4. Mayer NH, Herman RM. Positive signs and consequences of upper motor neuron syndrome. In: Brashear A, Mayer N, editors. Spasticity and other forms of muscle overactivity in upper motor neuron syndrome etiology, evaluation, management, and the role of Botulinum Toxin. WeMove. 2008. p. 11–26.

5. Bovend'Eerdt TJ, Newman M, Barker K, et al. The effects of stretching in spasticity: a systematic review. Arch Phys Med Rehabil 2008;89:1395–406.

6. Yelnik AP, Simon O, Parratte B, et al. How to clinically assess and treat muscle overactivity in spastic paresis. J Rehabil Med 2010;42:801–7.

7. Harvey LA, Katalinic OM, Herbert RD, et al. Stretch for the treatment and prevention of contractures. Cochrane Database Syst Rev 2017;(1):CD007455.

8. Farina S, Migliorini C, Gandolfi M, et al. Combined effects of botulinium toxin and casting treatments on lower limb spasticity after stroke. Funct Neurol 2008;23: 87–91.

9. Albany K, Myers R, Hunt D. Physical and occupational therapy considerations in adult patients receiving botulin toxin injections for muscle overactivity. In: Brashear A, Mayer N, editors. Spasticity and other forms of muscle overactivity in upper motor neuron syndrome etiology, evaluation, management, and the role of Botulinum Toxin. WeMove. 2008. p. 219–30.

10. Smania N, Picelli A, Munari D, et al. Rehabilitation procedures in the management of spasticity. Eur J Phys Rehabil Med 2010;46:423–38.

11. Sommerfeld DK, Gripenstedt U, Welmer A-K. Spasticity after stroke: an overview of prevalence, test instruments, and treatments. Am J Phys Med Rehabil 2012;91: 814–20.

12. Sunnerhagen KS, Olver J, Francisco GE. Assessing and treating functional impairment in poststroke spasticity. Neurology 2013;80(Suppl 2):S35–44.

13. Watanabe T. The role of therapy in spasticity management. Am J Phys Med Rehabil 2004;83:S45–9.

14. Chang WH, Kim YH. Robot-assisted therapy in stroke rehabilitation. J Stroke 2013;15(3):174–81. Available at: http://j-stroke.org/upload/pdf/jos-15-174.pdf. Accessed December 27, 2017.

15. Prange GB, Jannink MJ, Groothuis-Oudshoorn CG, et al. Systematic review of the effect of robot-aided therapy on recovery of the Hemiparetic arm after stroke. J Rehabil Res Dev 2006;43(2):171–84. Available at: https://www.rehab.research. va.gov/jour/06/43/2/pdf/prange.pdf. Accessed December 27, 2017.

16. Lum PS, Mulroy S, Amdur RL, et al. Gains in upper extremity function after stroke via recovery or compensation: potential differential effects on amount of real-world limb use. Top Stroke Rehabil 2009;16(4):237–53.

17. Hayner K, Gibson G, Giles GM. Comparison of constraint-induced movement therapy and bilateral treatment of equal intensity in people with chronic upper-extremity dysfunction after cerebrovascular accident. Am J Occup Ther 2010; 64(4):528–39. Available at: https://ajot.aota.org/article.aspx?articleid=1854540. Accessed December 27, 2017.

18. Malhotra S, Pandyan AD, Rosewilliam S, et al. Spasticity and contractures at the wrist after stroke: time course of development and their association with functional recovery of the upper limb. Clin Rehabil 2011;25(2):184–91.

19. Ng SSM, Hui-Chan CWY. Ankle dorsiflexion, not plantarflexion strength, predicts the functional mobility of people with spastic hemiplegia. J Rehabil Med 2013;45: 541–5.

# Intrathecal Therapies

Michael Saulino, MD, PhD[a,b,*]

## KEYWORDS

- Intrathecal therapy • Intrathecal baclofen • Spasticity • Intraventricular baclofen

## KEY POINTS

- Intrathecal baclofen therapy is an effective therapy for multifocal and global presentation of spasticity.
- Positive results have been seen in several diagnoses, including multiple sclerosis, spinal cord injury, brain injury, stroke, and cerebral palsy.
- The classic algorithm for intrathecal baclofen therapy is a sequence of patient selection, trialing, implantation of a permanent system, and chronic maintenance therapy.
- At times, derivation from the traditional treatment for intrathecal baclofen therapy is appropriate to achieve reasonable outcomes in selected patient populations.

## INTRODUCTION

Intrathecal baclofen therapy (IBT) is a form of targeted drug delivery that has been used for three decades in the management of spastic hypertonia associated with the upper motor neuron syndrome.[1] This condition includes pathology affecting the spinal cord as well as the brain. Intrathecal baclofen infusion exerts its therapeutic effect by delivering liquid baclofen directly into the cerebrospinal fluid (CSF), thus affording enhanced access of this agent to target neurons in the spinal cord. This article provides a brief review of IBT because it is currently used in routine clinical practice as well as a series of hypothetical cases that will explore unusual techniques and strategies for targeted drug delivery in the management of the hypertonic condition. It is pertinent to recognize that the cases will explore treatment approaches that are not approved by Food and Drug Administration (FDA). Although clinicians are allowed to explore these "off-label" methodologies, they should fully acknowledge the risks and benefits of these procedures and apprize their patients accordingly.[2]

Disclosure Statement: Speakers bureau, fellowship support and research grant: Medtronic (19107). Speakers bureau, and research grant: Jazz Pharmaceuticals (19107). Speakers bureau: Ipsen. Patent compensation: Saol Therapeutics.
[a] MossRehab, 60 Township Line Road, Elkins Park, PA 19027, USA; [b] Department of Rehabilitation Medicine, Thomas Jefferson University, Philadelphia, PA, USA
* 60 Township Line Road, Elkins Park, PA 19027.
*E-mail address:* Docsaulino@msn.com

## PHARMACOLOGY OF INTRATHECAL BACLOFEN

Baclofen exerts its therapeutic effect by binding to gamma-aminobutyric acid (GABA) B receptors located in the laminae I–IV of the spinal cord, where primary sensory fibers end. After binding with the presynaptic terminal of GABAergic interneurons, membrane hyperpolarization arises, leading to a restriction of the influx of calcium into the presynaptic terminal. This leads to a reduction of endogenous transmitter release, which leads to inhibition of monosynaptic and polysynaptic spinal reflexes. Baclofen is rapidly absorbed after oral administration, partially metabolized by the liver, and mainly excreted by kidneys in unchanged form. Oral baclofen has several significant pharmacokinetic limitations, including restricted absorption in the upper small intestine by saturable active transport mechanism, a short half-life of 3 to 4 hours, partial hepatic metabolization, rapid renal clearance, and poor passage through the blood brain barrier.[3,4] There is also the possibility of pharmacogenomic variability with regard to baclofen metabolism.[5] Relatively common side effects of oral baclofen are sedation, respiratory depression, confusion, dizziness, headache, insomnia, depression, tremor, ataxia, paresthesia, hallucinations, orthostatic hypotension, dry mouth, visual accommodation troubles, nausea, vomiting, constipation, diarrhea, hyperhidrosis, rashes, and aggravation of a preexistent dysuria.[5] Significant adverse effects have been demonstrated with oral baclofen in both elderly stroke population and a mixed population with acquired brain injury.[6] Adherence to prescribed oral baclofen is often limited.[7] The rationale for intrathecal administration has been the delivery of the drug directly into the spinal fluid in order to allow higher concentrations in the spinal cord using lower doses than the oral route,[8] thus optimizing the benefit/risk ratio. This method of administration allows for GABA-mediated inhibition of spasticity while minimizing side effects secondary to high levels of baclofen in the brain. Although IBT can be tremendously beneficial for the management of spasticity related to central nervous system pathology, there is the potential for serious adverse effects related to this therapy. The improved potency of IBT compared with oral baclofen particularly predisposes patient to the possibilities of withdrawal and overdose syndromes.[9]

## TRADITIONAL UTILIZATION OF INTRATHECAL BACLOFEN THERAPY

IBT is formally indicated for the management of severe spasticity of spinal and cerebral origins.[10] Despite its ubiquity, spasticity is a challenging entity to delineate with an evolving definition. Perhaps the best description that captures the depth and breath of this phenomenon is "a disordered sensorimotor control, resulting from an upper motor neuron lesion, presenting as intermittent or sustained involuntary activation of muscles."[11] The next level of medical decision making for spasticity management is to determine the gravity of the condition. Colloquial definitions of "severe" include terminology such as "causing discomfort or hardship" as well as "very painful or harmful." It is certainly reasonable to consider spasticity as severe when it is problematic, interfering with comfort, function, or caregiving. Spasticity intensity should include both the clinician's impression as well as the patient's perception. Clinicians should consider how problematic the spasticity is to the patient/caregiver, than solely relying on a numerical rating of a particular spasticity assessment measure. For example, modest resistance to passive motion, which could be evaluated as mild to the physician, may have a significant functional impact on the patient, who could describe the same phenomenon as severe. Given the diversity of spasticity presentations and the variety of diseases that create spasticity, it is not unexpected there are a multiplicity of treatment options. These therapeutic modalities can be divided into nonpharmacologic, oral agents, chemodenervation techniques, IT therapy, orthopedic surgical techniques, and neurosurgical interventions.[12–15] **Table 1** summarizes the nature of each intervention with their associated advantages and disadvantages. How each of these techniques is applied to each patient population is an evolving art and science. The role of IBT, within the armamentarium of spasticity modification, continues to evolve and define itself. It is also relevant to mention that each of these techniques can be applied in monotherapy or in combination. It is possible that there could be a synergistic benefit when multiple approaches are used simultaneously.[16]

Once a decision to proceed with IBT is made, the patient will undergo a trial or test dose.[17] The typical method for intrathecal baclofen trialing is to perform a lumbar puncture and inject a bolus of a baclofen solution into the CSF. Fifty micrograms of baclofen is the most commonly used initial screening dose.[18] The onset of clinical effects from a screening bolus occurs within 1 to 3 hours postinjection, and peak effects are typically observed 4 to 6 hours postinjection. The effects of the screening bolus are always temporary with the effects routinely lasting 6 to 8 hours.[19] Prolonged effects of single test bolus have been reported.[7] Screening boluses can be repeated if the initial injection is unsuccessful. It is a commonly accepted practice to wait at least 24 hours before repeating a trial in order to insure that the patient's neuromuscular status has completely returned to baseline. "Positive" responses are reported in 80% to 90% of bolus trials.[18] Generally, antibiotic prophylaxis is not needed for a bolus trial.[20] For patients on antiplatelet or anticoagulant therapy, recommendations from the American Society of Regional Anesthesia are followed.[21]

Once a patient has had a positive test intrathecal baclofen dose, the patient can then proceed to implantation of the intrathecal delivery system. Some centers proceed immediately to implantation following the trial dose, whereas others have patient undergo a more extensive preadmission testing for permanent implantation compared with the initial trial. Although the implantation procedure might be considered a relatively minor surgery, the patient population served by intrathecal baclofen therapy can be somewhat fragile. Patients should be clinically stable before surgery to minimize perioperative complications. The risks of the permanent pump implantation and infusion are same as the screening trial, with the additional risks of drug overdose, drug withdrawal, and device complications.

Dose adjustments can commence immediately after system implantation. In general, 24 hours is a reasonable time to wait between each dosing adjustment to allow for the full effects of the IBT to be observed. Dose modifications are performed by "interrogating" the system with a handheld programmer, programming the needed adjustments, and then updating the dosing schedule. Various modes of administration include simple continuous (dose delivered continuously throughout a 24h cycle), complex continuous (variable dose delivered continuously during 24h cycle), and periodic bolus (regularly scheduled boluses of ITB within 24h cycle). These various modes of delivery are represented diagrammatically in **Fig. 1**. In this example, the total, daily dosing for the three modes of delivery is the same but the dose, at any particular time, is variable. The complex, continuous, dosing mode allows for differential effects throughout the course of the day. For example, a patient may find it beneficial to be on a lower dose during the day (in order to minimize weakness and maximize functional mobility) and a higher dose during the night (in order to minimize nocturnal, spontaneous spasms). Periodic, bolus dosing delivers several boluses rapidly over a few minutes with relatively low delivery between the boluses. This mode of delivery may allow for greater distribution of drug with enhanced access to more cephalad, spinal levels. This mode of delivery may be particularly beneficial for addressing upper, extremity hypertonia. The periodic bolus delivery mode potentially places a patient at a higher

**Table 1**
Various options for spasticity management

| Category | Intervention | Description/Example | Advantages | Disadvantage |
|---|---|---|---|---|
| Nonpharmacologic | Removal/avoidance of noxious stimuli | • Treatment of neurogenic bladder<br>• Treatment of neurogenic bowel<br>• Pressure sore management | • Returns patient to baseline hypertonia<br>• May eliminate ongoing stimuli<br>• Low cost<br>• Minimal adverse events | • May not easily be reversible<br>• Modulation may not be predictable |
| | Manual stretching | Physical movement of limbs | • Low cost<br>• Minimal risk | • Short duration of action |
| | Passive stretching | • Bracing<br>• Splinting<br>• Serial casting | • Low cost<br>• Minimal risk | • Potential for skin breakdown<br>• Restricts patient movement<br>• Requires some expertise in prescribing |
| Oral Medications | GABAergic agents<br><br>α-adrenergic agonists<br><br>Serotonin antagonists<br>Peripheral acting agents<br>GABA analogues | Benzodiazepines<br>Baclofen<br>Clonidine<br>Tizanidine<br>Cyproheptadine<br>Dantrolene<br>Pregabalin<br>Gabapentin | • Noninvasive<br>• Low cost<br>• Allows patient control<br>• Global effectiveness<br>• Secondary indications (eg, sleep aide, pain, etc.) | • Poor patient tolerability<br>• Weakness<br>• Sedation<br>• Hepatotoxicity |

| Category | Treatments | Mechanism/Target | Advantages | Disadvantages |
|---|---|---|---|---|
| Chemodenervation | Motor point or nerve blocks<br><br>Botulinum toxins | Local anesthetics<br>Alcohol<br>Phenol<br>Botox<br>Dysport<br>Xeomin<br>Myobloc | Excellent effect for focal hypertonia | • Multiple injections needed for global tone<br>• Technical skill for localization<br>• Difficulty with procurement (phenol)<br>• Cost (toxins)<br>• Need to repeat injections |
| IT Therapy | GABAergic agents | Baclofen | • Highly potent<br>• Affords precise delivery | • Surgical procedure<br>• Risk of overdose and withdrawal<br>• Need for constant maintenance |
| Orthopedic Surgery | Tendon lengthening<br>Tendon transfers | • Alters length-tension relationship<br>• Reduces efferent signaling from muscles | • Corrects underlying deformity<br>• Long duration of action | • Invasive<br>• Destructive<br>• May require extensive gait/motor control analysis |
| Neurosurgical | Rhizotomy<br>Myelotomy | Ablation of spinal nerve roots (rhizotomy) or spinal cord (myelotomy) | • Long duration of action | • Invasive<br>• Destructive<br>• Neuropathic pain |

*From* Saulino M. Intrathecal baclofen therapy for the control of spasticity. In: Krames E, Peckham PH, Rezai AR, editors. Neuromodulation: comprehensive textbook of principles, technologies, and therapies, vol. 2. 2nd edition. London (United Kingdom): Elsevier; 2018. p. 892; with permission.

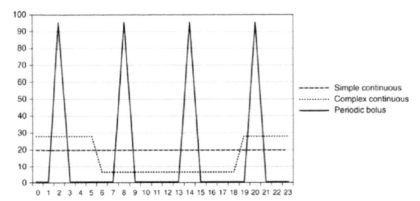

**Fig. 1.** Various modes of intrathecal delivery. (*From* Saulino M. Baclofen pump management. In: Buvanendran A, Diwan S, Deer T, editors. Intrathecal drug delivery for pain and spasticity, vol. 2. 71646th edition. Philadelphia: Elsevier; 2011. p. 167; with permission.)

risk of overdose, although this has not been observed clinically.[22] Both the complex continuous and periodic bolus modes of delivery are purported to be beneficial for the management of pharmacologic tolerance.[23,24] If a clinician is unsure if a dosing adjustment is warranted, a single bolus (at a given dose per day) can be programmed for several days followed by an automatic return to the baseline delivery. This mode of delivery is called single bolus/simple continuous delivery and allows a patient to be exposed to two different dosing levels automatically without the need for a physician visit. This mode of delivery can also be used for stepwise titration of IT delivery.

During the titration phase of IBT, patients are usually weaned from oral, antispasticity medications. The amount of each IT adjustment varies depending on patient tolerability. Nonambulatory patients may tolerate dose adjustments of 20% of total daily dose, whereas others, especially ambulatory patients, will require lower titration increments (5%–10%). Adverse effects that may be seen during this phase of therapy include excessive hypotonia, changes in bowel[25,26] and bladder status,[27] and increased thromboembolic risk.[28,29] The frequency and size of dosing adjustments should be individualized, based on the response to prior changes. Some patients tolerate rapid titration with daily, dosing adjustments, whereas others may require longer periods of observation and accommodation before undertaking further adjustments. Although there is no evidence-based ideal titration frequency, dose adjustments 1–2 times weekly until optimal dosing is achieved is reasonable and practical. Some patients may also benefit from some residual use of oral medications to address variable breakthrough spasms or to address upper extremity spasticity that is not addressed by IBT. The titration phase of IBT could last 6 to 9 months after implantation.

Because IBT has the capacity to affect a patient's active functional status, a rehabilitation program after implantation is appropriate. Postimplant rehabilitation may also be needed for caregiver training. The setting, scope, and complexity of this program will vary depending on the patient's individual goals as well as the availability of these services, in a given region. The timing of rehabilitation is also subject to some debate. Some centers defer therapies for few weeks after the implant because of concerns of catheter fracture or incisional dehiscence, whereas others favor immediate postimplant rehabilitation. Some implanters limit thoracolumbar flexion or twisting for a few weeks to minimize any potential issues relative to catheter migration or incisional dehiscence. However, there are no reports of incisional or catheter difficulties specifically related to a specific activity. Potential disciplines involved in the rehabilitation process include physiatry/neurorehabilitation, physical therapy, occupational therapy, and rehabilitation nursing. Issues that potentially require attention during this phase of therapy include incisional care, medical management (spinal headache, pain assessment, medication adjustment, dosing changes), mobility, self-care ability, and bowel/bladder function. Patients, especially ambulatory individuals, should be thoroughly counseled on the need for postimplant rehabilitation in order to maximize the benefits of IBT.[30]

## CASE 1
### Presentation

A 35-year-old woman with spastic paraparesis due to primary progressive multiple sclerosis presents in outpatient clinic. She is alert and cognitively intact, with a primary complaint of poorly controlled spasticity. She requires assistance for transfers, but once out of bed she is reasonably mobile at household distances with a manual wheelchair. During most nights, she awakes 3–4 times from uncomfortable leg spasms. The spasms also occur intermittently during the day. Her past medical history is significant for pulmonary embolism 1 year ago (currently on anticoagulation), placement of a suprapubic catheter 6 months ago, and two incidences of stage 2 sacral decubitus over the past 18 months, both now well-healed. As part of the workup for multiple sclerosis, she received a lumbar puncture after which she experienced a significant spinal headache. Her past treatments for tone included oral baclofen, which was discontinued at a dose due to sedation, and injection of botulinum toxin into key leg muscle with little noticeable improvement. She is currently on 24 mg/d of tizanidine and 6 mg/d diazepam, which she tolerates but does not adequately control her symptoms. On inspection, she demonstrates a "wind-swept" appearance of legs, with flexion at the bilateral hips and knees and equinovarus at both ankles. Although the patient herself has little ability to actively move her lower extremity muscles, surprisingly the legs can be somewhat straightened passively with effort. All lower extremity muscles consistently demonstrated Modified Ashworth scores of 3 on examination. The patient is willing to proceed with IBT. The clinical question is whether a bolus trial is absolutely necessary before implantation.

### Discussion

The patient already has demonstrated a pharmacologic responsiveness to baclofen. The patient's suboptimal response to baclofen to date likely represents the limitations of the drug when administered orally. The application of baclofen by intrathecal delivery is likely to bypass oral pharmacologic shortcomings.

The rate of success of intrathecal baclofen trialing is quite high, with levels of 85% to 90% being reported. The medical literature does not provide significant insight into what constitutes a "failed trial." A significant percentage of patients who do not respond to a single test dose level will respond to higher test dose amount. Thus, a "failure" of a specific test dose amount does not represent a failure of the therapy rather a case of relative underdosing. A failed trial could represent difficulty in accessing the lumber cistern.[31] In this instance, it is not a failure of the intervention but technical difficulty that could potentially be overcome with better localization techniques, such as fluoroscopy,[32] ultrasound,[32] or computed tomography.[33]

Conceivably, fixed contracture (which is not responsive to intrathecal baclofen) could be perceived as severe spasticity. In this scenario, it is not the intervention that has failed but a case of misdiagnosis. This possibility is not in play with the described case because the passive range of motion can be accomplished in the lower extremities. This observation eliminates the possibility of erroneously attributing fixed contracture from dynamic hypertonia. A failed trial could also represent an individual who demonstrated an excess reduction in spasticity where problematic hypotonia was observed. Excessive hypotonia resulting in cardiovascular collapse is extraordinarily rare with a single bolus trial. In summary, the 10% to 15% "failure" rate of intrathecal baclofen test dose administration may actually represent an artificially inflated percentage. Given these reflections, it is quite reasonable to assume that the described patient would have a positive response to a trial. From the perspective of both the patient and the clinician, an intrathecal baclofen trial may just be "proving the obvious."

Although intrathecal baclofen trialing is considered a relatively safe procedure, it is not completely risk-free undertaking. The rate of complications during intrathecal baclofen trialing has been reported to be as high as 30% to 40%.[34,35] Adverse events include spinal headaches, hypotonia, dizziness, paresthesia, hypotension, respiratory depression, infection, nausea/vomiting, urinary retention, seizures, drowsiness/sedation, and coma. Spinal headaches occur in up to 30% of patients undergoing a lumbar puncture and can vary in severity from mild to incapacitating.[36] The patient's history of spinal headache might place her at a higher risk for developing a second spinal headache.[37] There is also some evidence to suggest that patients with multiple sclerosis who are on disease modifying therapy are at higher risk for infectious complications.[38] An added difficulty in this is patient in his anticoagulation status. As noted, the patient is on anitcoagulation for pulmonary embolism. Recent guidelines suggest that a lumbar puncture is an intermediate risk procedure with regard to potential risk for a serious bleeding event.[21] Removal of anticoagulant therapy places the patient at risk for a recurrent thromboembolic event. The patient would then need to be restarted on anticoagulation after the trial only to again be discontinued before the implant procedure. The requirement for two anticoagulation holidays can be excessively burdensome for the patient. In total, this patient has the potential to experience several negative effects with an intrathecal test dose.

Conversely, the managing clinicians in this case should consider what disadvantages the direct-to-implant approach would bestow on the patient. Some might argue that the trial offers some degree of insight into the patient's future sensitivity to chronic intrathecal baclofen infusion. Admittedly, patients with multiple sclerosis may represent a patient group that demonstrates a higher level of susceptibility to adverse events with dosing adjustments. Recognizing this possibility, the concern could be alleviated by initiating a chronic infusion at a very low dose, such as 25 mcg/d or even lower. It is increasingly recognized that the pharmacodynamic responses to bolus administration of intrathecal medications is substantial different compared with long-term infusion.[39,40] There is minimal evidence to suggest that the patient's response to single bolus test dose is predictive of the patient's long-term dosing levels or other outcomes.[41] Thus the disadvantages of a direct-to-implant strategy do not appear insurmountable.

Lastly, a prompt implant and subsequent commencement with long-term intrathecal baclofen infusion can be significantly advantageous to this patient. The patient can experience a rapid decrement of hypertonia in short order. His dose can be titrated early in the postoperative period in an effort to obtain optimal spasticity reduction. A direct-to-implant approach without trial has been described by Borowski and colleagues.[42] In this study, 26 pediatric patients were directly implanted with an intrathecal delivery system followed by immediate commencement of intrathecal baclofen therapy. These patients had an inaccessible intrathecal space. The patients underwent simultaneous system implant and posterior spinal fusion for scoliosis. The positive outcomes of this cohort are identical to patients who underwent a trial without a concomitant increase in complications.

In summary, the calculus of decision making in this case results in a positive trend toward applications of intrathecal baclofen therapy without a trial. The risks associated with this strategy do not seem to be overwhelming and are outweighed by the benefits of prompt initiation of chronic intrathecal baclofen infusion. This option is entirely reasonable and should be presented to the patient as a potential approach.[43]

## CASE 2
### Presentation

A 28-year-old white man with C5 ASIA A spastic quadriplegia due to a traumatic spinal cord injury presents to clinic for spasticity management. He resides in a long-term care facility. He has used IBT for 3 years with overall good results. He does not use his spasticity for functional mobility. Spasticity reduction results in improved wheelchair tolerance and socialization. He reports erratic episodes of increased spasms. There is no obvious predisposing trigger or temporal pattern for these occurrences. These spasms are global in presentation, involving all four extremities. This irregularity is confirmed by the staff at the patient's facility. Transportation from the patient's facility to the clinic is adequate but somewhat challenging to attain urgent appointments. The patient has been seen monthly for the last 18 months in an effort to improve spasticity control. Several intrathecal dosing strategies have attempted without dramatic improvement because of the irregularity of the spasticity pattern. Physical examination result is negative for any obvious source of increased spasticity. Routine laboratory inquiry was similarly unrewarding. Investigation of the intrathecal system via radiotelemetry did not demonstrate any electronic abnormalities. Residual volume during pump refills was equal to the expected volume. The patient has undergone a computed tomographic myelogram with dye injection through the side port of the system, which demonstrated good subarachnoid flow and no abnormalities of the catheter portion of the system. The clinical question is whether the patient can achieve better control of spasticity reduction.

### Discussion

An irregular pattern of increased spasticity is not an unusual presentation. Many individuals, especially those with spinal cord injury, report variations in spasm frequency and intensity.[44] Spasticity levels can be affected by many factors, including temperature, emotional status, time of day, level of pain, body position, and the amount of prior stretching. Given this potential variability, interpretation of serial measurements can be problematic.[45] The first step in management of this presentation is to explore potential noxious stimuli that could be artificially elevating the hypertonicity.[46] In the described case, this strategy would seem to be reasonably well examined. The next step would be to inquire as to any potential abnormalities with regard to intrathecal drug delivery.[47] This possibility also seems to be fully investigated in this case.

One option for management is the additional of oral medications to the patient's approach to spasticity management. Indeed, it is the only on-label method of spasticity management that allows for patient control of a variable spasticity pattern. There is no contraindication for the combined use of oral medications with intrathecal drug delivery. Given the relative rapid onset of the patient's symptoms, short-acting oral medications would be preferable. Perhaps the best medication class that fits the description of having both a short half-life and spasticity reduction potential would be the benzodiazepines.[48] Certainly, practitioners must proceed with caution with this approach because both intrathecal baclofen and oral benzodiazepines have the potential to result in central nervous system depression. In addition, benzodiazepines have the potential for dependence, tolerance, and withdrawal, which would be undesirable in any patient population.[49]

A handheld accessory for implanted intrathecal delivery systems has become available that allows for patient-controlled, preprogrammed boluses. The amount, frequency, and lockout period for these boluses are set by the physician. At present, this device is only FDA-approved for intrathecal delivery for pain control.[50] Although this device allows the patient to vary their intrathecal dosing to address the variability of the spastic condition, it does have the theoretic risk of masking ongoing or progressive noxious stimuli that may be driving the increased tone. In the neurologic patient, increased spasticity may be the only sign of a potentially serious medical condition, such as urolithiasis or appendicitis. Thus, use of the handheld, patient activation device could potentially delay the patient's need to seek medical attention. The combination of programming options described earlier allows for extraordinarily wide variety of options for IT delivery.

There are no published manuscripts on the use of this strategy for spasticity management although abstracts from medical conference are available.[44,51] These reports, as well as the author's clinical experience suggest that boluses of 5% to 10% of the total daily dose are a safe maneuver. Caution must be used with regard to the lockout interval in an effort to prevent undue dose stacking.

## CASE 3
### Presentation

A 40-year-old man with spastic right hemiparesis due to a traumatic brain injury presents to clinic for spasticity management. He has severe spasticity involving most muscle groups on the right side and also has involvement of the right paraspinal muscles resulting in scoliosis. He has a well-documented allergy to oral baclofen—diffuse itching and a rash within an hour after oral administration. This was observed in two separate occasions and confirmed by the patient's family. He has tried oral dantrolene without a significant response. He has received botulinum toxin injections in the past, with some degree of positive benefit. However, his insurance carrier limits the amount of toxin that can be administered in any one injection session, thus limiting the overall success of this therapy. He has no obvious contraindication for intrathecal delivery. The clinical question is whether other intrathecal agents could be beneficial to this patient.

### Discussion

Intrathecal agents other than baclofen currently play a small role in the management of the hypertonic patient. Given the effects that intrathecal baclofen has on the GABAergic system, the use of other GABA agonists would seem to be sound strategy for long-term intrathecal delivery. Benzodiazepines suppress GABA-mediated activity in the spinal reflex pathways and have the potential to modulate spasticity. The two oral agents that have the most clinic exposure in this agent are diazepam and clonazepam, which have been used orally for many years.[13] There are no recent reports that explore the use of benzodiazepines via intrathecal delivery. Another potential GABAergic agent is gabapentin. This agent is structurally similar to the GABA, but it does not bind to GABA receptors and its exact mechanism of action is unknown. There is preclinical and early clinical exploration of gabapentin as an intrathecal analgesic agent[52,53] but minimal investigation into its potential therapeutic benefit for spasticity. Another neurotransmitter that is involved in spasticity modulation is the adrenergic system. Tizanidine and, to a lesser extent, clonidine are adrenergic agonists that have been used orally (and in the case of clonidine, transdermally) to modulate spasticity. Intrathecal clonidine is well recognized as adjuvant therapy in the algorithm for intrathecal analgesic therapy.[54] There is limited discussion in the utility of this approach for spasticity.[55] IT tizanidine presents an intriguing possibility as an alternative agent for spasticity management. Oral tizanidine, in both monotherapy and in combination therapy with baclofen, has been used for many years for spasticity management. Although there has been some preclinical investigation into intrathecal tizanidine,[56,57] there is minimal reported human experience with this approach. Lastly, it is well recognized that noxious stimuli can drive increased spasticity; it is reasonable to extrapolate the possibilities that intrathecal agents for chronic pain might be useful in this patient population. There are rare reports of IT opiates, particularly morphine, being undertaken for this patient population.[58–60] Continued investigatory efforts would be worthwhile to further elucidate the potential utility of other agents for chronic IT infusion.

## CASE 4
### Presentation

A 22-year-old white man with spastic quadriparesis present with his parents to spasticity clinic for a second opinion. The patient has diffuse hypertonia with a combination of spasticity and dystonia that involve all four extremities. He has used IBT for many years with erratic and inconsistent results. His first system was placed when he was 12 years old. He has undergone multiple revisions for catheter disruptions and loculations. The catheter tip has been in multiple locations within the spinal canal over the last decade without a clear advantage of one site over another. Multiple dosing regimens have also been attempted with similarly inconsistent results. His most recent system became infected 18 months ago subsequently requiring explantation. Several oral medication trials have been undertaken without significant benefit. He has taken botulinum toxin injections in the past, but the benefits were short-lived. His past medical history is notable for a complete spinal fusion (occiput to sacrum), multiple tendon releases/lengthenings, spastic dysarthria, well-controlled seizure disorder, neurogenic bowel, and neurogenic bladder. The clinical question is whether targeted drug delivery is of any further utility in this patient.

### Discussion

This presentation has a similar approach to the second clinician discussion. The initial steps in management would of suboptimal spasticity control involve a thorough search for noxious stimuli that could be driving increased hypertonicity should be undertaken. It is conceivable that there is an underlying trigger that is falsely elevating the increased tone. Particular attention should be paid to neurogenic bladder investigation.[46] Assuming this workup result is negative, it is possible that the patient has developed arachnoiditis. There are animal models that suggest intrathecal catheters can develop scarring in the subarachnoid space.[61,62] The incidence of arachnoiditis with human long-term spinal intrathecal delivery is unknown. It is similarly uncertain as to whether arachnoiditis develops in a similar mechanism to catheter tip granuloma.[63] Baclofen is unlikely to cause neurologic inflammation is isolation.[64]

One potential option for this patient would be intraventricular delivery of baclofen. This strategy involves the same device construct as intrathecal baclofen therapy with the catheter positioned within the third ventricle.[65] This approach has been described most commonly with children with cerebral palsy.[66] It is a reason to cautiously approach the family with this treatment approach. Similar to IBT, complication of this strategy can occur. Perhaps most concerning is the potential for severe hypotonia with the most rostral presentation of the liquid baclofen. This method of targeted drug delivery should only be undertaken with an experienced multidisciplinary team that is well versed in device management.

## SUMMARY

Targeted drug delivery for spasticity management is a mature therapy with more than a three decade experience of clinical success. Despite its long history, IBT is probably underused.[67,68] Most of the patients can be managed with the traditional approaches to IBT. This article reviews the classical methodologies of this modality as well as novel strategies that may be worth of consideration in selected patients. Further investigations are warranted into the utility of targeted drug delivery in the modulation of muscle overactivity associated with central nervous system pathology.

## REFERENCES

1. Francisco GE, Saulino MF, Yablon SA, et al. Intrathecal baclofen therapy: an update. PM R 2009;1(9):852–8.
2. McCarthy M. Off-label drug use is associated with raised risk of adverse events, study finds. BMJ 2015;351:h5861. British Medical Journal Publishing Group;351.
3. Wuis EW, Dirks MJ, Vree TB, et al. Pharmacokinetics of baclofen in spastic patients receiving multiple oral doses. Pharm Weekbl Sci 1990;12(2):71–4.
4. Lapeyre E, Kuks JB, Meijler WJ. Spasticity: revisiting the role and the individual value of several pharmacological treatments. NeuroRehabilitation 2010;27(2):193–200.
5. Kita M, Goodkin DE. Drugs used to treat spasticity. Drugs 2000;59(3):487–95.
6. Hulme A, MacLennan WJ, Ritchie RT, et al. Baclofen in the elderly stroke patient its side-effects and pharmacokinetics. Eur J Clin Pharmacol 1985;29(4):467–9.
7. Halpern R, Gillard P, Graham GD, et al. Adherence associated with oral medications in the treatment of spasticity. PM R 2013;5(9):747–56.
8. Albright AL, Thompson K, Carlos S, et al. Cerebrospinal fluid baclofen concentrations in patients undergoing continuous intrathecal baclofen therapy. Dev Med Child Neurol 2007;49(6):423–5.
9. Shirley KW, Kothare S, Piatt JH Jr, et al. Intrathecal baclofen overdose and withdrawal. Pediatr Emerg Care 2006;22(4):258–61.
10. Saulino M, Ivanhoe CB, McGuire JR, et al. Best practices for intrathecal baclofen therapy: patient selection. Neuromodulation 2016;19(6):607–15.
11. Pandyan AD, Gregoric M, Barnes MP, et al. Spasticity: clinical perceptions, neurological realities and meaningful measurement. Disabil Rehabil 2005;27(1–2):2–6.
12. Watanabe T. The role of therapy in spasticity management. Am J Phys Med Rehabil 2004;83(10 Suppl):S45–9.
13. Watanabe TK. Role of oral medications in spasticity management. PM R 2009;1(9):839–41.
14. Elovic EP, Esquenazi A, Alter KE, et al. Chemodenervation and nerve blocks in the diagnosis and management of spasticity and muscle overactivity. PM R 2009;1(9):842–51.

15. Lynn AK, Turner M, Chambers HG. Surgical management of spasticity in persons with cerebral palsy. PM R 2009;1(9):834–8.

16. Kunz KD, Ames SL, Saulino MF. Multimodality approach to spasticity management - how patients treated with intrathecal baclofen also utilize other spasticity interventions. Am J Phys Med Rehabil 2009;88(3):S57.

17. Boster AL, Bennett SE, Bilsky GS, et al. Best practices for intrathecal baclofen therapy: screening test. Neuromodulation 2016;19(6):616–22.

18. Stempien L, Tsai T. Intrathecal baclofen pump use for spasticity: a clinical survey. Am J Phys Med Rehabil 2000;79(6):536–41.

19. Horn TS, Yablon SA, Stokic DS. Effect of intrathecal baclofen bolus injection on temporospatial gait characteristics in patients with acquired brain injury. Arch Phys Med Rehabil 2005;86(6):1127–33.

20. Deer TR, Provenzano DA, Hanes M, et al. The Neurostimulation Appropriateness Consensus Committee (NACC) recommendations for infection prevention and management. Neuromodulation 2017;20(1):31–50.

21. Narouze S, Benzon HT, Provenzano DA, et al. Interventional spine and pain procedures in patients on antiplatelet and anticoagulant medications: guidelines from the American Society of Regional Anesthesia and Pain Medicine, the European Society of Regional Anaesthesia and Pain Therapy, the American Academy of Pain Medicine, the International Neuromodulation Society, the North American Neuromodulation Society, and the World Institute of Pain. Reg Anesth Pain Med 2015;40(3):182–212.

22. Skalsky AJ, Fournier CM. Intrathecal baclofen bolus dosing and catheter tip placement in pediatric tone management. Phys Med Rehabil Clin N Am 2015; 26(1):89–93.

23. Heetla HW, Staal MJ, van Laar T. Tolerance to continuous intrathecal baclofen infusion can be reversed by pulsatile bolus infusion. Spinal Cord 2010;48(6): 483–6.

24. Heetla HW, Staal MJ, Kliphuis C, et al. The incidence and management of tolerance in intrathecal baclofen therapy. Spinal Cord 2009;47(10):751–6.

25. Kofler M, Matzak H, Saltuari L. The impact of intrathecal baclofen on gastrointestinal function. Brain Inj 2002;16(9):825–36.

26. Morant A, Noe E, Boyer J, et al. Paralytic ileus: a complication after intrathecal baclofen therapy. Brain Inj 2006;20(13–14):1451–4.

27. Vaidyanathan S, Soni BM, Oo T, et al. Bladder stones - red herring for resurgence of spasticity in a spinal cord injury patient with implantation of Medtronic Synchromed pump for intrathecal delivery of baclofen - a case report. BMC Urol 2003;3:3.

28. Carda S, Cazzaniga M, Taiana C, et al. Intrathecal baclofen bolus complicated by deep vein thrombosis and pulmonary embolism. A case report. Eur J Phys Rehabil Med 2008;44(1):87–8.

29. Murphy NA. Deep venous thrombosis as a result of hypotonia secondary to intrathecal baclofen therapy: a case report. Arch Phys Med Rehabil 2002;83(9): 1311–2.

30. Boster AL, Adair RL, Gooch JL, et al. Best practices for intrathecal baclofen therapy: dosing and long-term management. Neuromodulation 2016;19(6):623–31.

31. Fettes PD, Jansson JR, Wildsmith JA. Failed spinal anaesthesia: mechanisms, management, and prevention. Br J Anaesth 2009;102(6):739–48.

32. Eskey CJ, Ogilvy CS. Fluoroscopy-guided lumbar puncture: decreased frequency of traumatic tap and implications for the assessment of CT-negative acute subarachnoid hemorrhage. AJNR Am J Neuroradiol 2001;22(3):571–6.

33. Brook AD, Burns J, Dauer E, et al. Comparison of CT and fluoroscopic guidance for lumbar puncture in an obese population with prior failed unguided attempt. J Neurointerv Surg 2014;6(4):324–8.

34. Sayer C, Lumsden DE, Perides S, et al. Intrathecal baclofen trials: complications and positive yield in a pediatric cohort. J Neurosurg Pediatr 2015;1–6 [Epub ahead of print].

35. Phillips MM, Miljkovic N, Ramos-Lamboy M, et al. Clinical experience with continuous intrathecal baclofen trials prior to pump implantation. PM R 2015;7(10):1052–8.

36. Ahmed SV, Jayawarna C, Jude E. Post lumbar puncture headache: diagnosis and management. Postgrad Med J 2006;82(973):713–6.

37. Amorim JA, Valenca MM. Postdural puncture headache is a risk factor for new postdural puncture headache. Cephalalgia 2008;28(1):5–8.

38. Williamson EM, Berger JR. Infection risk in patients on multiple sclerosis therapeutics. CNS Drugs 2015;29(3):229–44.

39. Heetla HW, Staal MJ, Proost JH, et al. Clinical relevance of pharmacological and physiological data in intrathecal baclofen therapy. Arch Phys Med Rehabil 2014;95(11):2199–206.

40. Flack SH, Bernards CM. Cerebrospinal fluid and spinal cord distribution of hyperbaric bupivacaine and baclofen during slow intrathecal infusion in pigs. Anesthesiology 2010;112(1):165–73.

41. Clearfield JS, Nelson ME, McGuire J, et al. Intrathecal baclofen dosing regimens: a retrospective chart review. Neuromodulation 2015;19(6):642–9.

42. Borowski A, Shah SA, Littleton AG, et al. Baclofen pump implantation and spinal fusion in children: techniques and complications. Spine (Phila Pa 1976) 2008;33(18):1995–2000.

43. Bilsky GS, Saulino M, O'Dell MW. Does every patient require an intrathecal baclofen trial before pump placement? PM R 2016;8(8):802–7.

44. Delhaas EM. Posters. Pain Pract 2007;7:23–102.

45. Sheean G, McGuire JR. Spastic hypertonia and movement disorders: pathophysiology, clinical presentation, and quantification. PM R 2009;1(9):827–33.

46. Phadke CP, Balasubramanian CK, Ismail F, et al. Revisiting physiologic and psychologic triggers that increase spasticity. Am J Phys Med Rehabil 2013;92(4):357–69.

47. Saulino M, Anderson DJ, Doble J, et al. Best practices for intrathecal baclofen therapy: troubleshooting. Neuromodulation 2016;19(6):632–41.

48. Vinkers CH, Tijdink JK, Luykx JJ, et al. Choosing the correct benzodiazepine: mechanism of action and pharmacokinetics. Ned Tijdschr Geneeskd 2012;155(35):A4900.

49. Reeve E, Ong M, Wu A, et al. A systematic review of interventions to deprescribe benzodiazepines and other hypnotics among older people. Eur J Clin Pharmacol 2017;73(8):927–35.

50. Ilias W, le Polain B, Buchser E, et al, oPTiMa study group. Patient-controlled analgesia in chronic pain patients: experience with a new device designed to be used with implanted programmable pumps. Pain Pract 2008;8(3):164–70.

51. Derian A, Khurana S, Hoffmann BL, et al. Poster 248 a novel infusion method of intrathecal baclofen using personal therapy manager: a case series. PM R 2018;8(9):S241.

52. Takasusuki T, Yaksh TL. The effects of intrathecal and systemic gabapentin on spinal substance P release. Anesth Analg 2011;112(4):971–6.

53. Rauck R, Coffey RJ, Schultz DM, et al. Intrathecal gabapentin to treat chronic intractable noncancer pain. Anesthesiology 2013;119(3):675–86.
54. Deer TR, Pope JE, Hayek SM, et al. The Polyanalgesic Consensus Conference (PACC): recommendations on intrathecal drug infusion systems best practices and guidelines. Neuromodulation 2017;20(2):96–132.
55. Prudhomme M, Cottin S, Roy J, et al. Intrathecal clondine pump as a treatment for spasticity and walking: a multiple case study. Neuromodulation 2014;17(2): e1–14.
56. Ochs G, Loew M, Tonn J, et al. Distribution, tolerability and tissue compatibility of intrathecal tizanidine in the sheep. Acta Anaesthesiol Scand 1998;42(7):786–93.
57. Leiphart JW, Dills CV, Levy RM. Alpha2-adrenergic receptor subtype specificity of intrathecally administered tizanidine used for analgesia for neuropathic pain. J Neurosurg 2004;101(4):641–7.
58. Rogano LA, Greve JM, Teixeira MJ. Use of intrathecal morphine infusion for spasticity. Arq Neuropsiquiatr 2004;62(2B):403–5.
59. Erickson DL, Lo J, Michaelson M. Control of intractable spasticity with intrathecal morphine sulfate. Neurosurgery 1989;24(2):236–8.
60. Vidal J, Gregori P, Guevara D, et al. Efficacy of intrathecal morphine in the treatment of baclofen tolerance in a patient on intrathecal baclofen therapy (ITB). Spinal Cord 2004;42(1):50–1.
61. Jones LL, Tuszynski MH. Chronic intrathecal infusions after spinal cord injury cause scarring and compression. Microsc Res Tech 2001;54(5):317–24.
62. Zhang SX, Huang F, Gates M, et al. Extensive scarring induced by chronic intrathecal tubing augmented cord tissue damage and worsened functional recovery after rat spinal cord injury. J Neurosci Methods 2010;191(2):201–7.
63. Coffey RJ, Burchiel K. Inflammatory mass lesions associated with intrathecal drug infusion catheters: report and observations on 41 patients. Neurosurgery 2002;50(1):78–86 [discussion: 86–7].
64. Deer TR, Raso LJ, Coffey RJ, et al. Intrathecal baclofen and catheter tip inflammatory mass lesions (granulomas): a reevaluation of case reports and imaging findings in light of experimental, clinicopathological, and radiological evidence. Pain Med 2008;9(4):391–5.
65. Albright AL. Technique for insertion of intraventricular baclofen catheters. J Neurosurg Pediatr 2011;8(4):394–5.
66. Turner M, Nguyen HS, Cohen-Gadol AA. Intraventricular baclofen as an alternative to intrathecal baclofen for intractable spasticity or dystonia: outcomes and technical considerations. J Neurosurg Pediatr 2012;10(4):315–9.
67. Dvorak EM, Ketchum NC, McGuire JR. The underutilization of intrathecal baclofen in poststroke spasticity. Top Stroke Rehabil 2011;18(3):195–202.
68. Erwin A, Gudesblatt M, Bethoux F, et al. Intrathecal baclofen in multiple sclerosis: too little, too late? Mult Scler 2011;17(5):623–9.

# Neurosurgical Approaches

Peter J. Madsen, MD[a], Han-Chiao Isaac Chen, MD[a],
Shih-Shan Lang, MD[a,b],*

## KEYWORDS

- Neurosurgery • Spasticity • Dystonia • Rhizotomy • Deep brain stimulation

## KEY POINTS

- Neurosurgeons play an important role in the treatment of muscle hyperactivity, and should be included in multidisciplinary efforts to treat these patients.
- Focal spasticity can be treated through identification and lesioning of a nerve target.
- Patients with generalized spasticity, especially ambulatory children with spastic diplegia, should be considered for selective dorsal rhizotomy.
- Dorsal root entry zone lesioning is an option for severe cases of spasticity in a nonfunctioning limb.
- Deep brain stimulation has demonstrated efficacy in the treatment of primary dystonias, especially those caused by DYT-1 gene mutation.

## INTRODUCTION

Neurosurgeons have historically played a significant role in the management of patients with upper motor neuron conditions that result in muscle hyperactivity, such as spasticity or dystonia. Nerve lesioning procedures for the treatment of spasticity were first proposed in the early twentieth century and have since undergone considerable surgical refinement and study.[1] The introduction of intrathecal infusion devices and the advent of deep brain stimulation have also expanded the neurosurgeon's role in this field. The aim of this article is to describe these techniques and the anatomy and pathophysiology involved, as well as delineate the indications for each procedure and associated data on efficacy and complications. Surgical techniques discussed in this article include the broad class of nerve lesioning procedures for spasticity (selective peripheral neurotomy, selective dorsal rhizotomy, and dorsal root entry zone lesioning) and deep brain stimulation for dystonia. Intrathecal baclofen delivery, an

---

Disclosure Statement: The authors have no relevant financial conflicts of interest.
[a] Department of Neurosurgery, Hospital of the University of Pennsylvania, Perelman School of Medicine, University of Pennsylvania, Silverstein 3rd Floor, 3400 Spruce Street, Philadelphia, PA 19104, USA; [b] Division of Neurosurgery, Children's Hospital of Philadelphia, Wood Center, 6th Floor, 3401 Civic Center Boulevard, Philadelphia, PA 19104-399, USA
* Corresponding author.
E-mail address: chens4@email.chop.edu

area where neurosurgeons are also involved, will only be examined in its relationship to selective dorsal rhizotomy. General knowledge regarding these surgical interventions is essential for those clinicians treating patients with conditions of muscle hyperactivity, as proper referral and patient selection can provide meaningful symptom relief and improve the quality of life for patients. For this reason, it is also important to include the field of neurosurgery within the comprehensive multidisciplinary team that is often required to adequately care for these complex patients.

## NERVE LESIONING

Since early work by Lorenz and Stoffel in the peripheral nervous system and Foerester in the central nervous system in the late nineteenth and early twentieth centuries, multiple sites and techniques for nerve lesioning have been proposed and include lesion to the peripheral nerve, spinal roots, dorsal root entry zone, and spinal cord.[2] The physiologic principles behind nerve lesioning depend upon which level of the nerve is being targeted, and each technique comes with its own set of indications, preoperative work-up, efficacy data, and set of complications. These factors will be discussed for each of the nerve lesioning procedures.

### Selective Peripheral Neurotomy

First introduced by Lorenz in 1887 for hip adduction spasticity[3] and Stoffel in 1912 for control of spastic foot,[4] selective peripheral neurotomy (SPN) involves the identification and surgical lesioning of pathologic peripheral nerves or nerve fascicles that contribute to spasticity. The disruption of the nerve supplying motor innervation to a spastic muscle or muscle group abolishes the motor reflex arc and limits the spastic potential of the muscle, theoretically resetting the balance between agonist and antagonist muscle groups.[2,5] Lesioning should be performed on at least 50% to 80% of the fibers innervating the muscle to expect a positive outcome.[2] Because the lesion disrupts only a population of efferent ($\alpha$-motor) and afferent (Ib proprioceptive spindle fibers) neurons, some of the remaining efferent inputs are capable of some muscle reinnervation. The afferent fibers are unable to reconnect in a cohesive manner, therefore allowing for the return of some motor function with continued loss of the afferent limb of the reflex arc that contributes to muscle hyperactivity.[6] The technique has been refined to include the use of identification of individual nerve fascicles within the nerve that contribute to the motor reflex arc by means of intraoperative electrophysiology. This process also allows for the identification and avoidance of sensory fibers, which if found and avoided, can help to prevent the development of painful postoperative allodynia or neuralgia.[5]

SPN is indicated for cases of focal or multifocal spasticity for which a clear muscular culprit can be identified preoperatively and for which repeated injection of botulinum toxin has become ineffective. Underlying causes of the focal spasticity can be numerous, but include cerebral palsy (CP), stroke, traumatic brain injury (TBI), or spinal cord injury (SCI). Examples of relevant nerve targets for SPN and the spastic conditions they are intended to ameliorate are summarized in **Table 1**.[2,6] Preoperative assessment of patients being considered for SPN is critical for proper target identification. In addition to a complete neurologic examination to determine the muscular groups(s) involved, peripheral nerve blocks using long-acting local anesthetics (eg, bupivacaine) or botulinum toxin should be performed.[5,7] Use of these agents allows for the simulation of the expected effects of SPN, and, following their administration, assessments of both symptom relief (ie, effect on spasticity) and adverse effects (ie, effect on ambulation or other

**Table 1**
Common targets for selective peripheral neurotomy in the treatment of focal spastic conditions and their common surgical sites

| Nerve(s) Targeted | Muscle(s) Affected | Disorder Treated | Surgical Site |
|---|---|---|---|
| **Upper limb** | | | |
| Ansa of the medial and lateral pectoral n. | Pectoralis major and | Spastic shoulder (internal rotation, adduction) | Deltopectoral sulcus |
| Lower subscapular n. | Teres major | | Between teres major and minor |
| Musculocutaneous n. | Biceps brachii and brachialis | Elbow flexion spasticity | Medial bicipital groove |
| Median n. | Pronator teres, quadratus | Pronation spasticity | Cubital fossa |
| | Flexor carpi radialis, palmaris longus | Spastic wrist flexion with radial deviation | |
| | Flexor digitorum superficialis/ profundus | Finger flexion spasticity | |
| Ulnar n. | Flexor carpi ulnaris | Spastic wrist flexion with ulnar deviation | Medial elbow (cubital tunnel) |
| | Flexor digitorum profundus | Spastic lateral finger flexion | |
| | Adductor pollicis | Spastic thumb adduction-flexion | Guyon canal at the wrist |
| **Lower limb** | | | |
| Obturator n. | Adductor muscles | Hip adduction spasticity ("scissoring" gait) | Hip flexion fold |
| Sciatic n. | Semitendinosus (and other hamstring muscles) | Knee flexion deformity | Between ischial tuberosity and greater trochanter |
| Tibial n. | Soleus | Equinovarus spastic foot | Popliteal fossa |
| Femoral n. | Quadriceps (rectus femoris and vastus intermedius) | Spastic knee extension | Hip flexion fold |

Data from Refs.[2,5,6]

function) should be performed. If the patient experiences the desired effects from these interventions with a tolerable level of adverse effect, then the definitive SPN procedure should be considered and performed on the location of the nerve block that gave the best results. Efficacy data of SPN have been mostly limited to case series, but these studies have shown promise in the procedure's ability to enhance function and limit symptomatic focal spasticity.[8–11] A randomized trial performed by Bollens and colleagues[12] comparing SPN with botulinum toxin injection for equinovarus spastic foot showed a greater level of spasticity reduction with SPN, with equivalent function outcomes between the groups. Long-term complications of the procedure are mostly limited to symptomatic allodynia or neurogenic pain if sensory fibers are lesioned, but this adverse effect is often temporary and can be treated with medication if sustained and severe.[6,8]

### Selective Dorsal Rhizotomy

Lesioning of the central nervous system for treatment of spasticity was first proposed and studied by Otfrid Foerester in 1908, who described a selective dorsal rhizotomy (SDR) technique for treatment of lower limb spasticity in CP.[13] SDR has since become one of the most widely utilized surgical interventions for spasticity. Its effect is thought to be mediated by a reduction in Ia afferent input from the spastic muscle, which allows for enhanced function of the inhibitor spinal interneurons, providing more inhibitory input on the hyperactive alpha motor neuron, diminishing the hyperactive tone.[5] It is most commonly performed in the lumbosacral region for the treatment of spastic diplegia in children with CP, but can also be used in the cervical spine for patients with severe upper extremity spasticity. Typically, the procedure is performed on dorsal roots from the L1 to S2 level, but can be tailored depending on the myotomes most effected. SDR is performed in a variety of technically different ways, but in general requires exposure of the lumbosacral nerve roots in the thecal sac (either at the level of the conus medullaris for a limited-exposure approach, or at multiple levels in lumbar spine for a wider exposure), identification of pathologic dorsal rootlets within the dorsal, and sectioning of these rootlets.[2] (**Fig. 1**). The exposure of the nerve roots can be accomplished by laminectomy (removal of the lamina covering the thecal sac) or laminoplasty (removal of a contiguous segment of the lamina or hemilamina so that it can be secured back in place at the completion of the procedure to recreate the spinal architecture). After opening the thecal sac and exposing the nerve roots, intraoperative electrical

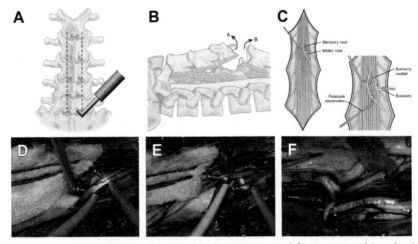

Fig. 1. (*A*) Illustration of bilateral cuts in the lamina required for its removal in a laminoplasty technique. Longitudinal cuts at these locations allow for reattachment of the bone back to the spine at the conclusion of the procedure. (*B*) Illustration of the elevation and removal of the cut lamina to expose the thecal sac. (*C*) Illustration of cauda equina after opening of the thecal sac and steps involved in the dissection, identification, and sectioning of selected roots. (*D*) Ventral nerve roots are identified by their larger caliber and significant vascularity. (*E*) Sensory rootlets can be isolated out from motor roots with the help of electrical stimulation. (*F*) Following identification of proper nerve rootlets for lesioning, the root is sharply sectioned. (*Adapted from* Drazin D, Auguste K, Danielpour M. Contemporary dorsal rhizotomy surgery for the treatment of spasticity in childhood. In: Quiñones-Hinojosa A, editor. Schmidek and Sweet's operative neurosurgical techniques. 6th edition. Philadelphia: Elsevier; 2012. p. 755–7; with permission.)

stimulation is used to identify the dorsal rootlets that contribute to spasticity. To accomplish this, rootlets are separated in each dorsal root and are stimulated to identify those that cause sustained, exaggerated muscle activation or spread to other myotomes.[2,5] This allows for the selective lesioning of only a subset of rootlets that contribute the most to spasticity in hopes of preserving sensory function with the remaining rootlets.[14] Once the desired roots have been lesioned, the dura is closed as tightly as possible in an attempt to prevent cerebrospinal fluid leak. Following surgery, physical rehabilitation is especially important, but protocols for implementation vary widely, with some institutions recommending as much as 3 months of inpatient rehabilitation.[15] Rehabilitation plans should be tailored to each patient, but in all cases their implementation is crucial to promote maximal functional improvement following SDR.

The efficacy of SDR, particularly for spastic diplegia in children with CP, has been studied extensively. In a meta-analysis of 3 randomized trials, SDR with physical therapy in this population was shown to be superior to physical therapy alone in terms of both spasticity and functional outcome scores.[16] Outcomes were also shown to be correlated with the number or rootlets transected, suggesting a dose-response relationship for the therapy. Most studies have focused on short-term outcomes, leading some to question the long-term effects of the surgery,[17,18] but sustained, positive outcomes for the procedure have been demonstrated out as far as 28 years, especially in those with less severe levels of spasticity.[19–23] Improvements have also been shown in gait parameters for ambulatory patients and in activities of daily living for patients with varied levels of spasticity.[24–26] Interestingly, lumbosacral SDR has also been shown to lead to a significant reduction in upper extremity spasticity in many patients, and has even been suggested to lead to improvements in cognitive performance indirectly (ie, through improvement in mode or decreased physical discomfort) and possibly even direct mechanisms.[27,28] With regard to the use of SDR in conditions other than spastic CP, limited reports of positive outcomes have been reported in children with SCI[29] and spasticity related to multiple sclerosis, TBI, and stroke, but lack of standardization of outcomes in these groups makes generalization of their results difficult.[30]

As with other lesioning surgeries, SDR is irreversible; therefore, much effort and thought should go into the patient selection process surrounding the surgery. Unfortunately, no agreed-upon selection criteria exist to assist clinicians in this endeavor.[14] In general, SDR should be considered for patients with diffuse spasticity of a limb or limbs rather than focal or multifocal types better treated by botulinum toxin injection or SPN. Patients who fit these criteria are most often children with CP, especially those with spastic diplegia. Because SDR has been studied the most in this group, predictive factors for success following SDR in this population have been identified and include age between 4 to 7 and a gross motor function measure test between 65% and 85%.[31] These patients are also thought to receive the most benefit form SDR, because they have not yet reached a plateau for gross motor development and with surgery can continue to develop rather than decline during adolescence.[20] Outside of this patient population, there has been little reported on outcomes, but small studies have shown some benefit of SDR in ambulatory adults with spastic diplegia.[32]

Common complications of SDR include postoperative sensory disturbances, cerebrospinal fluid leak, neurogenic bladder, bowel incontinence, chronic back pain, and spinal deformity.[5] Transient urinary retention is common following surgery, as high as 24%, but chronic changes to bladder function are uncommon.[24] Back pain can occur in 4% to 7% of patients but rarely interferes with function.[24] Spinal deformity following SDR has been a contentious issue in the literature, and its occurrence has led to the suggestion that limited laminectomies or laminoplasty should be performed over more extensive laminectomies in hopes of avoiding the complication.[5,24]

Although elaborated upon elsewhere in this text, the use of intrathecal baclofen pumps (ITBPs) should be discussed in the context of SDR. General thinking has held that SDR should be reserved for ambulatory patients with CP whereas ITBP should be used in those who are nonambulatory,[33] but this has recently been challenged in the literature. Two series in nonambulatory patients showed a benefit of SDR in terms of spasticity and ease of nursing care over their prior long-term ITBP use.[34,35] Randomized control trials have yet to be performed comparing the 2 interventions, but a study of matched cohorts compared SDR with ITBP and showed greater improvement in spasticity measures and functional outcomes, and less need for subsequent orthopedic interventions in the SDR group.[33] The decision between SDR and ITBP in these patients is complex, and should involve multidisciplinary discussions that take into account numerous factors such as the irreversible nature of SDR, the need for multiple interventions and titrations related to ITBP, the presence of dystonia (treatable by ITBP but not SDR), and the desired effect of the therapy chosen (improved motor function versus improved spasticity).[36]

### Dorsal Root Entry Zone Lesioning

Dorsal root entry zone lesioning (DREZL) was originally developed as a treatment for chronic severe pain, but was found by Sindou in the 1970s to provide relief of spasticity in addition to pain.[37] The procedure is similar to SDR, but instead of lesioning the dorsal roots, a lesion is created in the DREZ of the spinal cord.[2] The spinal cord is exposed by means of a laminectomy or laminoplasty and opening of the dura. The DREZ is identified where the dorsal roots enter the spinal cord, and a lesion is created starting at the level of the dorsolateral sulcus and extended deep into the dorsal horn of the spinal cord.[2] (**Fig. 2**) The lesion is created in an attempt to disrupt the

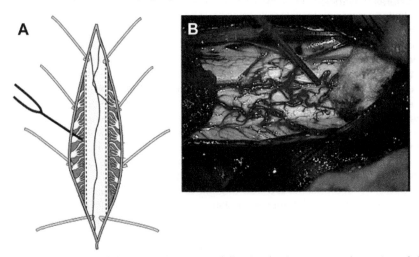

**Fig. 2.** (*A*) Illustration of the surgical exposure following laminectomy and opening of the dura. The site for DREZL is shown as a dotted line. This point marks the dorsolateral sulcus of the spinal cord. (*B*) Intraoperative photograph showing the spinal cord with patient's head to the left of the image. Intact left dorsal nerve rootlets can be seen entering the spinal cord at the bottom of the image. The right dorsal nerve rootlets had been previously injured. DREZL is being performed on the right side using a radiofrequency probe. (*From* Cahill K, Belzberg AJ, Anderson WS. Dorsal root entry zone lesions. In: Quiñones-Hinojosa A, editor. Schmidek and sweet's operative neurosurgical techniques. 6th edition. Philadelphia: Elsevier; 2012. p. 1484; with permission.)

large Ia afferent centrally located tonigenic fibers of the dorsal roots and related cir-cuitry of the ventral horn contributing to spasticity.[2,38] Focal dystonia can also be affected if the lesion is carried deep enough into the ventral horn.[2] It can be performed in the cervical spine (C5-C8 cord segments) or lumbar spine (L1-S1 cord segments) for upper and lower limb pathology, respectively.[39] The procedure is generally reserved for patients with severe, painful spasticity of an entire nonfunctioning limb given its considerably more destructive nature than other options.[5,39] The cause for the spas-ticity can be from stroke, TBI, SCI, or CP. Small studies have shown that DREZL is effective at decreasing severe spasticity and associated pain, and is typically better at controlling proximal versus distal spasticity.[39,40] The most significant complication of the procedure is the damaging of the corticospinal tracts and subsequent weakness if the lesion is performed too laterally.[41] Although performed much less frequently for the treatment of spasticity than SDR, DREZL should be considered in patients with se-vere, painful spasticity of a nonfunctional limb for whom conservative measures have failed.

## DEEP BRAIN STIMULATION

Deep brain stimulation (DBS) has achieved extensive use and acceptance in the neurosurgical field, especially in the relief of tremor related to adult movement disor-ders. Its role in the treatment of disorders of muscle hyperactivity, especially dystonia, has also been born out in numerous studies and will be further discussed in this section.

Dystonia is a heterogeneous category of movement disorders that result in sus-tained, intermittent muscle hyperactivity, which often causes repetitive motions and/or postures.[42] Traditionally classified as either primary or secondary dystonia, new ter-minology is emerging to better describe this complex set of disorders,[42] but for the purposes of this text, these terms will still be used. Primary dystonia is considered to be those disorders that consist of solely dystonic symptoms not caused by another underlying etiology. The dystonic symptoms of secondary dystonias are caused by another underlying disease and often coexist with other neurologic symptoms. Dysto-nias are often further classified by the distribution of the body that is effected, such as generalized, segmental, or cervical. Importantly, some primary dystonias have recently been characterized by several underlying genetic mutations.[43] Multiple med-ical interventions exist for the treatment of dystonia, but many are ineffective and come with multiple adverse effects. Historically, surgical lesions to the thalamus or basal ganglia have been performed for dystonia, but the irreversible, destructive na-ture of the procedures and their inconsistent results led to the study of DBS for dystonia.[44]

In general, DBS systems consists of 1 unilateral or 2 bilateral electrodes that have been precisely inserted into a subcortical brain structure using image-guided stereo-taxis. The electrodes are connected to leads that are tunneled posteriorly behind the ear and down the neck to the chest wall, where they are attached to the electrical pulse generator and battery.[45] (**Fig. 3**) The location of the stimulating electrode within the brain depends on which disease is being treated. Common targets include the subthalamic nucleus for Parkinson disease and obsessive-compulsive disorder, the ventral intermediate nucleas of the thalamus for essential tremor, and cingulate gyrus for medically refractory depression. For dystonia, the most common therapeutic target used is the internal nucleus of the globus pallidus (GPi), as shown in **Fig. 4**. Following implantation, the device is generally turned on 2 to 4 weeks after surgery and is pro-grammed by the patient's neurologist, titrating the stimulation to maximize therapeutic

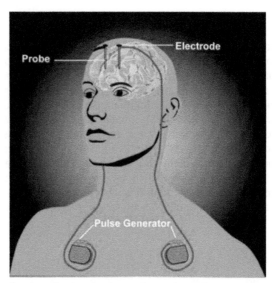

**Fig. 3.** Schematic of a deep brain stimulator. Electrode probes are inserted via stereotactic guidance into deep brain structures. The probes are connected to electrical leads under the scalp and tunneled to the combination pulse generator and battery, which is placed in the subcutaneous space of the chest wall. (*Courtesy of* National Institute of Mental Health, Bethesda, MD, USA; with permission.)

effect and avoid off-target adverse effects. The therapeutic mechanism of DBS remains under investigation, but is thought to be mediated by several changes that affect brain circuitry and function, such as network reorganization, neural plasticity induction, the disruption of pathologic neuronal oscillations, and alterations in neurotransmitter release.[46]

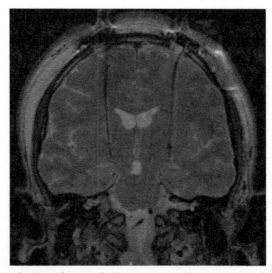

**Fig. 4.** Coronal MRI showing the standard trajectory and termination of bilateral electrodes targeting the GPi nucleus in a patient with primary generalized dystonia.

In the United States, DBS for dystonia is currently approved under a humanitarian device exemption for primary, generalized dystonia or cervical dystonia in patients over the age of 7, and its use in other forms of dystonia are considered off-label.[44] Surgery should only be offered to patients who have exhausted all medical therapies, but increasing evidence has been put forth for the use of DBS early in the treatment of primary dystonia attributable to certain genetic mutations, such as the DYT-1 gene mutation. These patients have been shown to be highly responsive to DBS.[47] The efficacy of DBS for certain dystonia subtypes has been well studied in a prospective and randomized fashion. In adult patients with primary general or segmental dystonia, a randomized, sham-controlled study demonstrated a highly significant effect of stimulation on movement parameters in a commonly used dystonia scale.[48] Patients continued to experience the benefits of stimulation in long-term follow-up studies.[49,50] Similar results were also achieved in a randomized, sham-controlled study of patients with cervical dystonia.[51] A consistent finding throughout many trials is that dystonias with certain underlying genetic mutations, especially DYT-1, are highly responsive to DBS.

The procedure is generally well-tolerated and has a risk of intracranial hemorrhage around 3% and 30-day mortality rate of 0.4%. Longer-term complications, including device malfunction or infection, can reach rates of 10%, with infection being the most common.[47] Notably, the use of infection avoidance protocols can lower this rate considerably.[52] Adverse effects related to stimulation include speech abnormalities, akinesias, and depression, but these can often be improved through adjustment of stimulation parameters. Of note, sudden interruption of stimulation in patients with severe dystonia can result in a medical emergency with re-emergence of life-threating dystonic symptoms, so batteries should be changed before they become completely depleted to avoid this complication.[50]

Although not yet supported by randomized trials, DBS for dystonia in children has been shown to be efficacious in several prospective case series, allowing for its use in children over the age of 7.[53] DBS has also been studied in small case series of children with secondary dystonias and has been found to be effective at symptom control, although the effect was more modest than that seen in primary dystonic conditions.[53] As a new technology, DBS continues to be studied in several other disease states associated with muscle hyperactivity. Small studies have tested DBS for the treatment of dystonia-choreoathetosis associated with CP, tarvide dystonia, and muscle hyperactivity associated with Lesch-Nyhan syndrome and have shown promising results.[44,54,55]

## SUMMARY

Neurosurgical interventions have an important role to play in the treatment of disorders of muscle hyperactivity. For patients with focal or multifocal spasticity, selective peripheral neurotomy should be considered, as it has been shown to efficacious in providing relief of isolated spasticity. A trial nerve block should always be performed prior to neurotomy to ensure that the patient will achieve the desired result of surgery. Also, an understanding of the peripheral nervous system and musculoskeletal anatomy are essential for patient evaluation and selection for this procedure. For patients with more generalized spasticity, such as those with spastic diplegia in the setting of cerebral palsy, selective dorsal rhizotomy is a viable option that has been validated in prospective controlled trials to improve spasticity and improve motor function in ambulatory patients, especially children. Often compared with intrathecal baclofen infusion, selective dorsal rhizotomy can offer a durable result with a more desirable outcome profile in properly selected patients without the need for further device-related interventions. Therefore, these 2 options should be weighed carefully for all potential patients. Dorsal root entry zone lesioning is less often performed because of its more destructive nature, but it does offer a good option for patients with severe spasticity of a nonfunctioning limb, especially when a component of pain is present. DBS, typically targeting the internal nucleus of the globus pallidus, has emerged as a highly effective therapy for patients with dystonia, especially primarily general, primarily segmental, or cervical dystonia. Genetic classification of dystonia has also become critical, as dystonia patients with certain genetic mutations, especially DYT-1, show excellent response to stimulation therapy. Indications for DBS will continue to grow as it is further studied in patients with disorders of muscle hyperactivity.

Ultimately, neurosurgeons will continue to offer valuable treatment options for patients with various disorders of muscle hyperactivity. Their involvement in the multidisciplinary decision-making process surrounding the care of these patients is essential, as the interventions they have to offer can make a lasting positive impact.

## REFERENCES

1. Boop FA. Evolution of the neurosurgical management of spasticity. J Child Neurol 2001;16(1):54–7.
2. Sindou M, Georgoulis G, Mertens P. Lesioning surgery for spasticity. In: Youmans and Winn RH neurological surgery. 7th edition. Philadelphia: Elsevier; 2017. p. 716–28.
3. Lorenz F. Uber chirurgische Behandlung der angeborenen spastischen Gliedstarre. Wien Klin Rdschr 1887;21:25–7.
4. Stoffel A. The treatment of spastic contractures. American Journal of Orthopaedic Surgery 1913;s2-10(4):611–44.
5. Sitthinamsuwan B, Nunta-Aree S. Ablative neurosurgery for movement disorders related to cerebral palsy. J Neurosurg Sci 2015;59(4):393–404.
6. Sindou MP, Simon F, Mertens P, et al. Selective peripheral neurotomy (SPN) for spasticity in childhood. Childs Nerv Syst 2007;23(9):957–70.
7. Lazorthes Y, Sol J-C, Sallerin B, et al. The surgical management of spasticity. Eur J Neurol 2002;9(s1):35–41.
8. Bollens B, Deltombe T, Detrembleur C, et al. Effects of selective tibial nerve neurotomy as a treatment for adults presenting with spastic equinovarus foot: a systematic review. J Rehabil Med 2011;43(4):277–82.
9. Sitthinamsuwan B, Chanvanitkulchai K, Phonwijit L, et al. Surgical outcomes of microsurgical selective peripheral neurotomy for intractable limb spasticity. Stereotact Funct Neurosurg 2013;91(4):248–57.
10. Buffenoir K, Rigoard P, Ferrand-Sorbets S, et al. Retrospective study of the long-term results of selective peripheral neurotomy for the treatment of spastic upper limb. Neurochirurgie 2009;55(Suppl 1):S150–60.
11. Puligopu AK, Purohit AK. Outcome of selective motor fasciculotomy in the treatment of upper limb spasticity. J Pediatr Neurosci 2011;6(Suppl 1):S118–25.
12. Bollens B, Gustin T, Stoquart G, et al. A randomized controlled trial of selective neurotomy versus botulinum toxin for spastic equinovarus foot after stroke. Neurorehabil Neural Repair 2013;27(8):695–703.
13. Foerster O. On the indications and results of the excision of posterior spinal nerve roots in men. Surg Gynecol Obstet 1913;16(5):463–74.

14. Grunt S, Fieggen AG, Vermeulen RJ, et al. Selection criteria for selective dorsal rhizotomy in children with spastic cerebral palsy: a systematic review of the literature. Dev Med Child Neurol 2014;56(4):302–12.

15. Health Quality Ontario. Lumbosacral dorsal rhizotomy for spastic cerebral palsy: a health technology assessment. Ont Health Technol Assess Ser 2017;17(10): 1–186.

16. McLaughlin J, Bjornson K, Temkin N, et al. Selective dorsal rhizotomy: meta-analysis of three randomized controlled trials. Dev Med Child Neurol 2002; 44(1):17–25.

17. Narayanan UG. Management of children with ambulatory cerebral palsy: an evidence-based review. J Pediatr Orthop 2012;32:S172–81.

18. Tilton A. Management of spasticity in children with cerebral palsy. Semin Pediatr Neurol 2009;16(2):82–9.

19. Park TS, Liu JL, Edwards C, et al. Functional Outcomes of Childhood Selective Dorsal Rhizotomy 20 to 28 Years Later. Cureus 2017;9(5):e1256.

20. Dudley RWR, Parolin M, Gagnon B, et al. Long-term functional benefits of selective dorsal rhizotomy for spastic cerebral palsy. J Neurosurg Pediatr 2013;12(2): 142–50.

21. Ailon T, Beauchamp R, Miller S, et al. Long-term outcome after selective dorsal rhizotomy in children with spastic cerebral palsy. Childs Nerv Syst 2015;31(3): 415–23.

22. Nordmark E, Josenby AL, Lagergren J, et al. Long-term outcomes five years after selective dorsal rhizotomy. BMC Pediatr 2008;8:54.

23. Josenby AL, Wagner P, Jarnlo G-B, et al. Motor function after selective dorsal rhizotomy: a 10-year practice-based follow-up study. Dev Med Child Neurol 2012; 54(5):429–35.

24. Steinbok P. Selection of treatment modalities in children with spastic cerebral palsy. Neurosurg Focus 2006;21(2):e4.

25. Rumberg F, Bakir MS, Taylor WR, et al. The effects of selective dorsal rhizotomy on balance and symmetry of gait in children with cerebral palsy. PLoS One 2016; 11(4):e0152930.

26. Bolster EAM, van Schie PEM, Becher JG, et al. Long-term effect of selective dorsal rhizotomy on gross motor function in ambulant children with spastic bilateral cerebral palsy, compared with reference centiles. Dev Med Child Neurol 2013; 55(7):610–6.

27. Craft S, Park TS, White DA, et al. Changes in cognitive performance in children with spastic diplegic cerebral palsy following selective dorsal rhizotomy. Pediatr Neurosurg 1995;23(2):68–74 [discussion: 75].

28. Gigante P, McDowell MM, Bruce SS, et al. Reduction in upper-extremity tone after lumbar selective dorsal rhizotomy in children with spastic cerebral palsy. J Neurosurg Pediatr 2013;12(6):588–94.

29. Reynolds RM, Morton RP, Walker ML, et al. Role of dorsal rhizotomy in spinal cord injury-induced spasticity. J Neurosurg Pediatr 2014;14(3):266–70.

30. Gump WC, Mutchnick IS, Moriarty TM. Selective dorsal rhizotomy for spasticity not associated with cerebral palsy: reconsideration of surgical inclusion criteria. Neurosurg Focus 2013;35(5):E6.

31. Funk JF, Panthen A, Bakir MS, et al. Predictors for the benefit of selective dorsal rhizotomy. Res Dev Disabil 2015;37:127–34.

32. Reynolds MR, Ray WZ, Strom RG, et al. Clinical outcomes after selective dorsal rhizotomy in an adult population. World Neurosurg 2011;75(1):138–44.

33. Kan P, Gooch J, Amini A, et al. Surgical treatment of spasticity in children: comparison of selective dorsal rhizotomy and intrathecal baclofen pump implantation. Childs Nerv Syst 2008;24(2):239–43.
34. Ingale H, Ughratdar I, Muquit S, et al. Selective dorsal rhizotomy as an alternative to intrathecal baclofen pump replacement in GMFCS grades 4 and 5 children. Childs Nerv Syst 2016;32(2):321–5.
35. D'Aquino D, Moussa AA, Ammar A, et al. Selective dorsal rhizotomy for the treatment of severe spastic cerebral palsy: efficacy and therapeutic durability in GMFCS grade IV and V children. Acta Neurochir (Wien) 2018;160(4): 811–21.
36. Steinbok P. Selective dorsal rhizotomy for spastic cerebral palsy: a review. Childs Nerv Syst 2007;23(9):981–90.
37. Mertens P, Sindou M. Microsurgical drezotomy for the treatment of spasticity of the lower limbs. Neurochirurgie 1998;44(3):209–18.
38. Sindou M, Quoex C, Baleydier C. Fiber organization at the posterior spinal cord-rootlet junction in man. J Comp Neurol 1974;153(1):15–26.
39. Sitthinamsuwan B, Phonwijit L, Khampalikit I, et al. Comparison of efficacy between dorsal root entry zone lesioning and selective dorsal rhizotomy for spasticity of cerebral origin. Acta Neurochir (Wien) 2017;159(12):2421–30.
40. Sindou M. Microsurgical DREZotomy (MDT) for pain, spasticity, and hyperactive bladder: a 20-year experience. Acta Neurochir (Wien) 1995;137(1–2):1–5.
41. Konrad P. Dorsal root entry zone lesion, midline myelotomy and anterolateral cordotomy. Neurosurg Clin N Am 2014;25(4):699–722.
42. Balint B, Bhatia KP. Dystonia: an update on phenomenology, classification, pathogenesis and treatment. Curr Opin Neurol 2014;27(4):468–76.
43. Bressman SB. Genetics of dystonia: an overview. Parkinsonism Relat Disord 2007;13(Suppl 3):S347–55.
44. Stone SSD, Alterman RL. Deep brain stimulation for dystonia. In: Youmans and Winn neurological surgery. 7th edition. Philadelphia: Elsevier; 2017. p. 627–34.
45. The National Institute of Mental Health. Deep brain stimulation. 2016. https://www.nimh.nih.gov/health/topics/brain-stimulation-therapies/brain-stimulation-therapies.shtml. Accessed December 5, 2017.
46. Herrington TM, Cheng JJ, Eskandar EN. Mechanisms of deep brain stimulation. J Neurophysiol 2016;115(1):19–38.
47. Fox MD, Alterman RL. Brain stimulation for torsion dystonia. JAMA Neurol 2015; 72(6):713–9.
48. Kupsch A, Benecke R, Müller J, et al. Pallidal deep-brain stimulation in primary generalized or segmental dystonia. N Engl J Med 2006;355(19):1978–90.
49. Volkmann J, Wolters A, Kupsch A, et al. Pallidal deep brain stimulation in patients with primary generalised or segmental dystonia: 5-year follow-up of a randomised trial. Lancet Neurol 2012;11(12):1029–38.
50. Tagliati M, Krack P, Volkmann J, et al. Long-term management of DBS in dystonia: response to stimulation, adverse events, battery changes, and special considerations. Mov Disord 2011;26(Suppl 1):S54–62.
51. Volkmann J, Mueller J, Deuschl G, et al. Pallidal neurostimulation in patients with medication-refractory cervical dystonia: a randomised, sham-controlled trial. Lancet Neurol 2014;13(9):875–84.
52. Halpern CH, Mitchell GW, Paul A, et al. Self-administered preoperative antiseptic wash to prevent postoperative infection after deep brain stimulation. Am J Infect Control 2012;40(5):431–3.

53. Alterman RL, Tagliati M. Deep brain stimulation for torsion dystonia in children. Childs Nerv Syst 2007;23(9):1033–40.
54. Sako W, Goto S, Shimazu H, et al. Bilateral deep brain stimulation of the globus pallidus internus in tardive dystonia. Mov Disord 2008;23(13):1929–31.
55. Lipsman N, Ellis M, Lozano AM. Current and future indications for deep brain stimulation in pediatric populations. Neurosurg Focus 2010;29(2):E2.

# The Neuro-Orthopaedic Approach

Matthew T. Winterton, MD[a], Keith Baldwin, MD, MPH, MSPT[b],*

## KEYWORDS

- Spasticity • Upper motor neuron disease • Neuro-orthopaedics • Contracture
- Deformity

## KEY POINTS

- Upper motor neuron injury or disease leads to muscle overactivity or nonfunction, leading to development of functional deficiencies, contractures, pain, and poor hygiene.
- A variety of nonsurgical and surgical management tools are used to improve function, alleviate pain, and improve hygiene and cosmesis.
- Preoperative assessment should determine contributing muscle forces to each deformity because spasticity may mask any underlying volitional muscle control.
- Surgical techniques include tendon lengthenings, releases, transfers, osteotomies, and bony fusions.

## GENERAL PRINCIPLES OF NEURO-ORTHOPAEDICS

Upper motor neuron disease or injury leads to a variety of both positive and negative signs, notably including muscle spasticity and weakness throughout the body. Patients with spasticity are at risk for development of a variety of deformities caused by these imbalances in muscle forces, leading to functional impairments, contractures, pain, and poor hygiene. The approach to neuro-orthopaedic patients is by necessity multidisciplinary, because a variety of nonsurgical and surgical options are available. In evaluating each patient, surgeons must consider the severity and direction of any deformity, potential for improvement in function, the ability to alleviate pain, and potential for improvement in hygiene and cosmesis. Similar to the physiatry analog of botulinum toxin versus oral spasticity agents, surgery can

Disclosure: The authors declare no commercial or financial conflicts of interest or funding sources for this article.
[a] Department of Orthopaedic Surgery, Children's Hospital of Philadelphia, 3737 Market Street, 6th Floor, Philadelphia, PA 19104, USA; [b] Department of Orthopaedic Surgery, Children's Hospital of Philadelphia, University of Pennsylvania, 2 Wood Center, 34th and Civic Center Boulevard, Philadelphia, PA 19104, USA
* Corresponding author.
E-mail address: Neurorthopod@gmail.com

Phys Med Rehabil Clin N Am 29 (2018) 567–591
https://doi.org/10.1016/j.pmr.2018.04.007
1047-9651/18/© 2018 Elsevier Inc. All rights reserved.

be local in the form of muscle releases, fusions, joint arthroplasty, and other procedures, or it can be more global and far reaching, such as nerve ablation or dorsal rhizotomy.

In the setting of acute injury, a nonsurgical approach may be best because patients with traumatic brain injury may continue to regain functionality up to 6 months after injury. Patients with stroke may continue to recover for up to 1 year. Intervention in the acute setting is aimed at interventions that provide symptomatic relief and reduce the severity of downstream deformities. Nonsurgical approaches in the neuro-orthopaedist's toolbox are varied and include antispasmodic medications, Botox administration, chemodenervation, serial casting, splinting, orthoses, and physical and occupational therapy.

Operative interventions may be considered thereafter when the extent of recovery has been maximized, or when significant obstruction to rehabilitation has been refractory to nonoperative means. Keeping in mind the natural history of neurologic recovery, it is important to keep the following overarching management principles in mind: (1) operate early, before deformities become fixed and rigid; (2) distinguish between the function of the limb and the function of the patient; (3) spastic muscles are weak muscles, and surgery necessarily weakens them further; (4) be sure to get the diagnosis right and optimize length-tension relationships.

Preoperative assessment should determine contributing muscle forces to each deformity. Often, the spasticity of antagonizing musculature masks any underlying volitional control of agonists across a joint. Dynamic electromyography (EMG) studies can determine the primary causes of deformity,[1–4] whereas selective anesthetic blockade of antagonistic musculature can determine the extent of any volitional control. In general, patients with volitional control benefit from selective lengthening of the deforming musculature or tendon transfers to optimize function. Those without voluntary control can undergo selective releases or bony fusion procedures to optimize hygiene and passive function.

## CONSIDERATIONS IN SPINAL CORD INJURY

In the United States, there are approximately 400,000 patients living with spinal cord injury (SCI), and about 11,000 new cases occur per year. Common causes of SCI vary from motor vehicle accidents and gunshot trauma to sports injuries and falls. In general, patients follow a bimodal distribution: younger patients sustain injuries from higher-energy trauma, and older patients with spinal stenosis have lower-energy trauma.

SCI is classified by the spinal cord level and number of affected extremities (paraplegic vs tetraplegic) and completeness of the injury (complete vs incomplete). The American Spinal Injury Association (ASIA) classification further characterizes the extent of injury. Several well-known patterns of SCI, such as Brown-Séquard, central cord, and anterior cord syndromes, occur depending on the location of injury within the spinal cord and can be elucidated by their characteristic physical examination findings.

In the setting of acute SCI, patients may show signs of spinal shock, a temporary loss of spinal cord function and reflex activity below the level of injury. Diagnosis of a complete SCI cannot be made until after the resolution of spinal shock, which is assessed by the return of the bulbocavernosus reflex, in which the contraction of the anal sphincter is felt while squeezing the glans penis or clitoris. Complete SCI results in a permanent disruption in the reflex arc and the bulbocavernosus reflex does not return. Resolution of spinal shock is variable but generally returns within 48 hours.

Spasticity, clonus, and hyperreflexia develop progressively over the ensuing days to weeks.

Early intervention is imperative and targeted at maintaining range of motion and contracture and pressure-sore prevention. Maintaining fitness in patients with SCI is essential as patients experience muscle weakness, diminished autonomic function, increasing secondary medical conditions, and worsening activity limitations.[5] Recent studies have shown improvements in muscle strength, walking scores, and cardiovascular fitness in certain patients through body weight–supported treadmill and overground training exercises,[6] robotic-assisted treadmill exercises,[7,8] and hand-cycles.[9,10] Current literature suggests that exercise capacity stabilizes between 1 and 5 years after discharge from inpatient rehabilitation.[11] However, patients may need structured interventions to promote a more active lifestyle, because one recent clinical trial reported that a self-management intervention was not effective in changing behavior toward a more active lifestyle.[12]

Patients who are wheelchair bound are at higher risk for shoulder girdle damage (including rotator cuff tears and osteoarthritis) from repetitive overhead activity,[13] and carpal tunnel syndrome.[14] Such patients may benefit from activity modifications, assistive devices, or surgical intervention.

In tetraplegic patients, several surgical interventions can help restore function and prevent deformity (**Table 1**), especially targeting the upper extremity to participate in activities of daily living and independence and improve patient satisfaction.[15,16] Home-based exercise programs also have been shown to reduce pain and improve function and quality of life.[17,18] Specialized centers may even be able to perform transfers to the phrenic nerve, allowing ventilator-free respiration in high spinal cord injuries.[19]

## CONSIDERATIONS IN TRAUMATIC BRAIN INJURY AND STROKE

Traumatic brain injury (TBI) is one of the most common causes of neuromuscular dysfunction. The incidence of TBI is estimated at more than 200 per 100,000 people annually around the world.[20] More than 50% of TBI can be attributed to road traffic accidents. Long-term sequelae of TBI include cognitive, psychosocial, behavioral, emotional, and physical impairments. Rehabilitation following TBI is a complex, multidisciplinary process. A recent review cited a paucity of evidence in supporting most rehabilitation protocols and therapies, because most literature has focused on randomized control trials, which are difficult to perform in this patient population.[21] From a neuro-orthopaedic perspective, patients with TBI are at increased risk for the development of heterotopic ossification, which is discussed later in this article, as well as spasticity, contractures, weakness, and dysfunction or nonfunction. The surgical principles and approaches described in this article can be used to address these sequelae.

Stroke, or cerebrovascular accident (CVA), is also one of the commonest causes of disability worldwide. More than 50% of patients who have a CVA survive, and 50% of patients with stroke are consequently hemiplegic. As in patients with TBI, from a musculoskeletal standpoint, patients with stroke are at increased risk for the development of heterotopic ossification as well as spasticity and its downstream effects. Shoulder pain is the second most common sequela of stroke after depression, with an estimated incidence of 24% to 84%.[22–25] Poststroke shoulder pain results from a variety of causes, including rotator cuff tears, adhesive capsulitis, subluxation, impingement, and spasticity, evaluation of which is discussed later in this article.

**Table 1**
**Summary of possible surgical procedures to achieve patients' ability goals**

| Ability Goal | Functional Goal | Procedure |
|---|---|---|
| Stabilizing elbow in space, reaching overhead objects, pushing wheelchair, stabilizing trunk | Elbow extension | Reconstruction of triceps function<br>Posterior deltoid-triceps<br>Biceps-triceps<br>Teres minor and/or posterior deltoid nerve transfer to triceps heads<br>Brachialis nerve transfer to triceps |
| Use of utensils, handwriting, pushing wheelchair | Grip | Reconstruction of grip<br>Reconstruction of passive key grip<br>BR-ECRB<br>Brachialis nerve transfer to ECRL (if BR absent)<br>FPL-distal radius tenodesis<br>CMC I arthrodesis<br>Split FPL-EPL tenodesis or ELK procedure<br>House tenodesis<br>Reconstruction of active key grip and finger flexion<br>BR-FPL<br>ECRL-FDP<br>Brachialis, supinator or ECRB nerve transfer to AIN<br>CMC I arthrodesis<br>Split FPL-EPL tenodesis or ELK procedure<br>House tenodesis |
| Reaching for objects (eg, cup or glass), positioning of thumb and fingers for improved grasp control | Opening of the hand | Reconstruction of thumb and finger extensors<br>Passive opening<br>CMC I arthrodesis<br>EPL-dorsal forearm fascia tenodesis<br>Active opening<br>PT-EDC and EPL/APL<br>Supinator nerve transfer to PIN<br>Thumb stabilization<br>CMC I arthrodesis, ELK procedure<br>Reconstruction of intrinsics<br>Zancolli lasso tenodesis<br>House tenodesis<br>EDM-APB |

Rehabilitation typically includes active training within 24 h postsurgery and orthosis during night and between training sessions for tendon transfers and 2 wk immobilization for nerve transfers.

*Abbreviations:* AIN, anterior interosseus nerve; APB, abductor pollicis brevis; APL, abductor pollicis longus; BR, brachioradialis; CMC, carpometacarpal; ECRB, extensor carpi radialis brevis; ECRL, extensor carpi radialis longus; EDC, extensor digitorum communis; EDM, extensor digiti minimi; ELK, extensor pollicis longus loop knot; EPL, extensor pollicis longus; FPL, flexor pollicis longus; PIN, posterior interosseus nerve; PT, pronator teres.

*From* Fridén J, Gohritz A. Tetraplegia management update. J Hand Surg 2015;40(12):2489–500; with permission.

## SURGICAL MANAGEMENT OF THE SPASTIC LOWER EXTREMITY
### Hip Adductor Spasticity

Hip adductor spasticity can lead to untoward effects. In less actively functional patients, it can result in hip adduction contracture, which makes perineal care exceptionally difficult. This condition leads to skin hygiene problems, breakdown, and infection. In more functional patients, limb scissoring is caused by spastic hip adductors, resulting in crossover of the advancing limb during terminal swing. This crossover can cause balance problems and falls. Phenol block of the obturator nerve can help to confirm the diagnosis, although this is rarely necessary because it is apparent on physical examination and observational gait analysis.

Patients with concomitant hip and knee flexion contractures should have those addressed at the time of surgery. In adult patients, particularly those with SCI or TBI with preexisting hip trauma, preoperative radiographs are indicated to assess for the presence of heterotopic ossification or other bony deformities that may alter surgical treatment.

### Obturator neurectomy
Transection of the anterior branches of the obturator nerve leads to denervation of the hip adductors, allowing the patient to stand with a broader base of support. A transverse incision is made directly over the groin crease. A longitudinal incision is then made over the adductor longus tendon. The adductor longus is released with electrocautery. The anterior branch of the obturator nerve can be found coursing over the adductor brevis and is cut. This procedure has fallen out of favor in treatment of cerebral palsy because it has occasionally been found to result in abduction contractures; however, this has not been noted to any significant extent in adults. Some physicians have resorted to phenol block or stunning the nerve by crushing it with forceps, which does not permanently denervate the muscle but weakens it significantly.

### Hip adductor tenotomy
Hip adductor tenotomy is indicated in ambulatory patients with limb scissoring or in nonambulatory patients with consequent deficiencies in nursing care or hygiene. In the supine position, the adductor longus is palpated and a transverse incision is made over the groin crease. Using electrocautery, the adductor longus, adductor brevis, and gracilis tendons are released. The anterior branches of the obturator nerve can be preserved if a contracture release is performed. Typically, in ambulatory patients most of the brevis is preserved. In more nonfunctional patients the interval between the brevis and the pectineus can be exploited to identify the distal attachment of the iliopsoas, which can be tenotomized through this approach. Performing this part of the procedure is not recommended in ambulatory patients because it results in significant hip flexion weakness. A drain can be placed to prevent hematoma formation. Postoperatively, the patient is maintained in hip adduction using an abduction pillow for 4 weeks. Physical therapy is typically allowed but gentle range of motion only until the wounds are healed because dehiscence is a risk.

### Hip Flexor Spasticity

Hip flexor spasticity commonly manifests in patients as a crouched or jump gait pattern but may also be present in patients with increased lumbar lordosis, which may be the cause of or a compensation for said lordosis. These gait patterns are inefficient and require significantly increased energy expenditure from the surrounding hip and knee musculature to keep the patient upright. In nonambulatory patients, hip and knee flexion contractures can contribute to increased pressure on the sacrum and heel pressure areas while in bed, which can lead to skin breakdown.

Hip flexor deformities often occur in concert with knee flexion deformities, and surgical management of both should occur simultaneously to prevent recurrence of contractures postoperatively.

### Hip flexor tenotomy
A transverse incision is made over the groin crease through a medial approach to the hip and the longus is released. The interval between the pectineus and brevis may be

entered and bluntly dissected to the lesser trochanter. The iliopsoas tendon is visualized at this point. The tendon is released from its insertion on the lesser trochanter. Long right-angle retractors are needed and the tendon should be released off the bone to avoid the medial circumflex femoral artery. Postoperatively, the patient is allowed to weight bear and range of motion as tolerated.

### Iliopsoas recession
In ambulatory patients, an over-the-brim approach is preferred. An anterior incision is made starting just below the anterior superior iliac spine traveling distally along the inguinal ligament. An incision is made in the fascia cranial to the inguinal ligament and tagged for later repair. The floor of the abdominal wall is then incised and the psoas muscle belly is identified. The femoral nerve is identified and protected as it courses over the muscle. The interval between the muscle and the iliopectineal fascia (containing the femoral artery and vein) is developed. Long right-angle retractors are placed and the tendon is identified posterior and deep to the femoral nerve. The tendon is confirmed by rolling the hip, which should roll the tendon not the nerve; muscle fibers are noted entering the tendon; and the tendon is stimulated with the cautery to confirm its identity. There is less danger to the femoral nerve with this approach because it is identified and visualized throughout the procedure. The fascia must be meticulously closed following the surgery to avoid a hernia.

### Hip Extensor Spasticity

Hip extensor deformities are common in anoxic brain injuries, in which extension contractures of the hip and knee can result in inability to sit, and occasionally even with fractures of the femur during range of motion. Proximal hamstring release can be performed to improve posture. If flexion of the hip results in obligate abduction, consideration is made for release of the gluteus maximus as well.

### Proximal hamstring release
In the prone position, a longitudinal incision is made from the gluteal fold and continuing distally over the posterior thigh. The distal gluteus maximus is retracted using large retractors to allow access to the hamstring muscles (semimembranosus, semitendinosus, and biceps femoris). The hamstrings are detached proximally from the ischial tuberosity. The sciatic nerve can be observed coursing lateral to the hamstring tendons as it finds the sciatic notch proximally. The nerve should be identified and gently retracted laterally to avoid thermal injury as the hamstring tendons are released off the bone. Postoperatively, the patient is allowed to perform passive range of motion of the hip. Sitting 6 hours or more should be encouraged.

The deformity of hip extension contracture is notoriously difficult to correct completely; in nonambulatory patients, if the soft tissue procedure fails, a hip flexion osteotomy or femoral head and neck resection can be considered to solve the problem.

### Knee Flexion Spasticity

In addition to the presence of heterotopic ossification (HO) as discussed previously, knee flexion deformities are caused by spastic hamstring muscles or contracted posterior capsule of the knee. The two entities can be distinguished under anesthesia by checking a popliteal angle with the hip in 90° of hip flexion (which constitutes the hamstring contracture), and then checking with the knee in full extension (which checks the capsular contracture). Distal hamstring lengthening is recommended when both the flexion contracture is less than 60° and the patient can actively fire the hamstrings.[26] In general, 50% correction is achieved through surgery and the remainder is gained through serial casting and/or physical therapy. Nonambulatory patients benefit from hamstrings releases.

Knee flexion contractures frequently occur in concert with hip flexion deformities, and both must be addressed simultaneously to prevent recurrent flexion contractures. Cipriano and Keenan[27] found that patients with severe hip and knee flexion deformities often are best treated with extensive hip releases and knee disarticulation. However, this approach should be thoroughly discussed with the patient and family because significant discussion may be necessary to approve this decision.

### Distal hamstrings fractional lengthening and release

Hamstring surgery can be performed either prone or supine. The authors prefer a supine approach because it allows access to other areas that might be receiving surgery concomitantly. In cases in which an open capsular release is performed, the authors perform this prone.

A longitudinal incision is made over the distal lateral thigh proximal to the knee joint. The biceps femoris is fractionally lengthened by dividing the tendinous region of the myotendinous junction of the biceps femoris obliquely. Care must be taken to dissect the tendon free from the muscle and gradually lengthen it while confirming that the common peroneal nerve is protected. Distally, the nerve is very close but proximally it is not as close and can be protected better. The iliotibial band is divided transversely posterior to the axis of knee flexion.

On the medial distal thigh, an incision is made over the gracilis tendon. The gracilis is lengthened by tenotomy. The semimembranosus is typically surrounded by an investing layer of tissue, and, when it is identified, it is fractionally lengthened (**Fig. 1**). The semitendinosus is always located just posterior to the semimembranosus at this level and is lengthened by tenotomy. The sartorius can be lengthened by myotomy in nonambulatory patients if it is tight.

Capsular releases are performed through a posterior approach (**Fig. 2**). A lazy S-shaped incision is made with the medial limb being proximal and the lateral limb being distal. The common peroneal nerve is carefully dissected out and traced back to the popliteal nerve. The artery is located just anterior and medial to this structure. The hamstring tendons are completely released. The gastrocnemius heads are released off the posterior capsule, and the posterior capsule of the knee is then completely released, both medially and laterally. It is usually necessary to work on

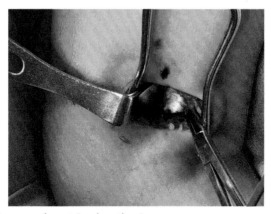

**Fig. 1.** Semimembranosus hamstring lengthening.

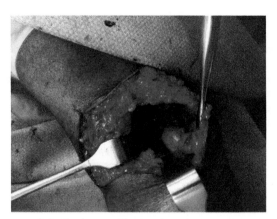

**Fig. 2.** Posterior approach to the knee with capsular release.

both sides of the neurovascular bundle. The posterior cruciate ligament can be released if it is tight. The limb is casted in a position that can be comfortably obtained so as to avoid vascular compromise. The authors recommend serial casting starting at week 1. Patient adherence is critical for this procedure to be a success.

### Knee disarticulation

Severe cases may be treated with knee disarticulation to allow comfortable sitting. Although a detailed treatise of this procedure is beyond the scope of this article, some highlights are included. Before incision, a posterior flap is planned to cover the knee. The patellar tendon is released from the tibial tubercle and proximal tibia dissected free from the surrounding soft tissues. The anterior and posterior cruciates are transected. The tibia is dislocated anteriorly. The posterior tibial vessels are ligated using silk ties. The posterior flap is pulled anteriorly. Closure is performed over large drains to prevent hematoma formation.

### Knee Extensor Spasticity

Patients with spasticity of the knee extensors have the inability to flex the knee. This inability becomes particularly problematic while walking and is known as stiff-knee gait. Stiff-knee gait is characterized by the inability to flex the knee during the swing phase of gait. Stiff-knee gait is dynamic and only occurs during gait; the patient has unrestricted passive knee motion at rest and the patient shows no difficulty with sitting. During the gait cycle, the patient acts as though there is a leg-length discrepancy with the stiff-knee limb functioning at a greater length; the patient compensates with any combination of circumduction of the affected limb, hiking of the pelvis, and contralateral limb vaulting.

Patients may benefit from a variety of different surgical options. The ideal surgical candidate should be able to ambulate and demonstrate minimal weakness in the hip flexors, which impart additional strength and momentum during the swing phase of gait. Patients may show an equinus deformity of the foot, which serves as an extension force while standing.

Preoperative evaluation should include dynamic EMG. Spasticity of the rectus femoris is the usual cause, although patients commonly show abnormal activity in the vastus musculature as well. Patients in whom a block of the rectus femoris results in improved knee flexion during gait have a more favorable surgical prognosis. Rectus femoris to gracilis transfer converts the spastic extension force into a flexion force.[28] Some have preferred a simple excision of the rectus femoris as a simpler surgical option that makes more intuitive sense in the setting of disease processes that cause crouch gait, such as cerebral palsy.[29]

Patients with spastic knee extensors may show an extension contracture. These patients usually have history of brainstem injury and may also demonstrate hip extension contractures in concert with knee flexion deformities resulting in difficulty with sitting. In such patients, selective quadriceps lengthening can alleviate the extension deformity and result in improved posture during sitting. Patients with severe extension contractures may require a V-Y lengthening of the quadriceps.

### Rectus femoris to the gracilis transfer and fractional quadriceps lengthening

The rectus femoris is a flexor of the hip and extensor of the knee. If acting dyssynergically during the swing phase of gait, it can cause the knee to remain in extension throughout swing. Transfer of the rectus femoris to the gracilis removes the rectus as a deforming extension force and converts it into a corrective flexion force during this portion of gait. Beginning in the anterior midthigh, a longitudinal incision is made distally over the rectus femoris and carried distally to the level of the midpatella. The rectus is dissected out from the other quadriceps muscles (**Fig. 3**). A cuff of periosteum is taken with the distal rectus muscle to gain additional length for the transfer. In cases of dyssynergic rectus and crouch gait, 2 to 3 cm is simply excised from the tendon. If a transfer is desirable, a locking suture (eg, Krakow) is placed in the distal tendon. Selective lengthening of the vasti can be performed at this time if dynamic EMG showed spasticity by transecting the tendinous fibers of the myotendinous junction.

Another incision is made over the posteromedial distal thigh and the gracilis tendon is identified and released proximally at the myotendinous junction. The rectus femoris tendon is tunneled subcutaneously to the second incision; the intermuscular septum needs to be incised to allow passage of the tendon. External rotation of the femur and knee flexion also facilitates passage. The gracilis and rectus tendons are sutured together in a Pulvertaft fashion.

Postoperatively, the patient is placed in a knee immobilizer to prevent flexion contracture. Weight bearing is commenced immediately and a continuous passive motion machine may be used immediately. The knee immobilizer is discontinued after

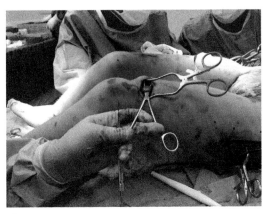

**Fig. 3.** Rectus femoris exposure.

1 to 2 weeks and passive range-of-motion exercises and quadriceps and hip flexor strengthening are begun.

### V-Y lengthening of the quadriceps
Beginning in the anterior midthigh, a longitudinal incision is made distally over the rectus femoris and carried distally to the level of the midpatella. The distal rectus tendon is cut in an inverted V shape. Slowly flexing the knee to allow lengthening of the tendon, the rectus tendon is then sutured together in V-Y fashion. Care must be taken to release fully along the retinaculum in order to prevent excessive force and distal femur fracture. In long-standing contractures with hyperextension, occasionally patellectomy is necessary, although this is rarely of functional consequence in a non-ambulatory individual.

### Foot and ankle
**Cavus deformity** Pes cavus deformity is characterized by an elevated longitudinal arch caused by spasticity of the extrinsic and intrinsic foot musculature. It is important to determine whether the patient has a flexible deformity as determined by the Coleman block test, which evaluates flexibility of the hindfoot. A block is placed under the lateral foot, which eliminates contribution of the first ray to the deformity; a flexed first ray can contribute to the deformity. If the deformity corrects to neutral, then the hindfoot is flexible and a soft tissue procedure is adequate for correction (**Fig. 4**). If the deformity persists, then the deformity is rigid and bony surgery must be performed in addition.[30] Several procedures can be performed to correct the cavus or cavovarus foot. The workhorses for correction are described in further detail later.

*Steindler release* Using a medial approach, a longitudinal incision is made on the foot. The plantar fascia is visualized and proximal insertion released. The abductor hallucis is released proximally off the medial tuberosity of the calcaneus, as well as the flexor digitorum brevis. The foot is casted in neutral. Postoperatively, the patient is allowed to weight bear as tolerated. Patients often require a SPLATT (split anterior tibial tendon) procedure simultaneously. A more plantar-based incision can also be used in situations in which no forefoot adduction is present and no access to the knot of Henry is needed.

*Dorsiflexion osteotomy of the first metatarsal* In the supine position, a 4-cm incision is made dorsally over the first tarsometatarsal joint extending distally over the metatarsal shaft, taking care to protect the dorsal medial cutaneous nerve to the hallux. The extensor hallucis longus (EHL) tendon is identified and retracted medial

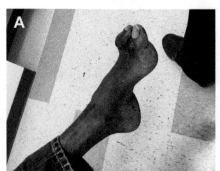
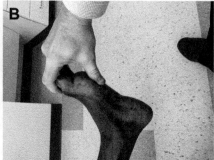

**Fig. 4.** Flexible cavovarus deformity. (*A*) Cavovarus deformity. (*B*) Demonstrating the flexible nature of the deformity displayed with passive manipulation.

or lateral. The osteotomy site is localized about 1.5 cm distal to the metatarsocunei-form joint. Using a microsagittal saw, a dorsal wedge osteotomy is made to correct the requisite amount of preoperative plantarflexion. A 3.5-mm screw or small locking plate is placed across the osteotomy site to secure it.

*Peroneus longus to brevis transfer* A curvilinear incision is made posterior to the lateral malleolus, extending distally to the interval between the peroneus longus and brevis. Taking care to identify and protect the sural nerve, the tendons are identified distal to the superior peroneal retinaculum. An incision is made in the tendon sheaths and the peroneus longus is transferred to the brevis in a side-to-side fashion.

*Jones transfer* A longitudinal incision is made over the distal first metatarsal. The EHL is identified and transected as distally as possible. A nonabsorbable suture is placed in the distal tendon. A drill hole is made in the metatarsal neck transversely from medial to lateral and the tendon is passed through the osseous tunnel from lateral to medial using a meniscal needle or similar. The tendon is sutured to itself using a Pulvertaft technique. The hallux interphalangeal (IP) joint can be fused in the modified Jones procedure.

**Equinus or equinovarus deformity** Acquired spastic equinovarus deformity is one of the most common musculoskeletal deformity after stroke or TBI (**Fig. 5**). Equinus deformity can be attributed to a fixed contracture (static) or results from overactivity of the gastrocnemius-soleus complex (dynamic). Patients experience difficulty with gait, because initial heel contact and clearance impede both the swing and stance phases of gait. Nonoperative management consists of physical therapy with emphasis on stretching, serial casting, dynamic splinting, phenol blocks and botulinum injections, and ankle-foot orthoses. Note that phenol and botulinum toxin only weaken the tone so the fixed shortening can be more easily stretched, and ankle-foot orthoses only substitute for strength or accommodate deformity, they do not correct it. Surgical lengthening may be considered if the ankle cannot be accommodated in a brace and nonoperative means have failed.

More proximal lengthening techniques, such as the Strayer or Baumann, are desirable because they do not weaken the muscles' power as much as more distal lengthening techniques such as the Hoke or even the Vulpius. The authors prefer an examination under anesthesia using a Silverskiold test. This test is performed by checking passive dorsiflexion with the heel in varus first with the knee in full extension (hence checking the contracture of the gastrocnemius), and then with the knee flexed to 90° (hence checking the soleus). If both are severely tight, a nonselective heel cord

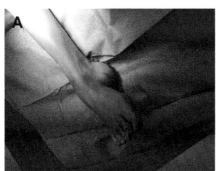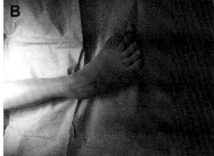

**Fig. 5.** Equinocavovarus foot. (*A*) Cavovarus deformity. (*B*) Demonstrating the flexible nature of the deformity displayed with passive manipulation.

lengthening, such as a Hoke or open heel cord lengthening, is necessary. If just the gastrocnemius is tight, a selective procedure such as a Strayer may be performed. If both are tight but the contracture is mild, a milder nonselective procedure such as a Vulpius may be selected. A fully dynamic contracture (ie, fully corrects under anesthesia) may be helped with a Baumann procedure.[31]

*Tendo-Achilles lengthening (hoke triple hemisection technique)* With the knee in full extension, the ankle is positioned in maximum dorsiflexion. Three percutaneous hemisections are made of the Achilles tendon. The first is made at the tendon insertion onto the calcaneus. The second tenotomy is made proximally just below the myotendinous junction (about 3–4 fingerbreadths proximally). The third is made midway between the first 2 cuts. If the heel is in varus, the first and third cuts are placed on the medial side and the middle cut is placed laterally. Hemisections with a valgus deformity of the heel are performed exactly opposite, with the first and third cuts placed laterally and the middle cut placed medially. The ankle is then gently dorsiflexed to the desired position. Postoperatively, the patient is placed in a short leg cast for 6 weeks, followed by an additional 6 weeks in an ankle-foot orthosis. A flexor digitorum longus (FDL) transfer to the heel can be considered in cases in which extreme lengthening can lead to a decrease in push-off power.

*Gastrocnemius recession (Strayer procedure)* A 3-cm incision is made medially at the intersection of the bulge of the calf and where the muscle of the calf becomes narrower. The fascia of the lower leg is incised. The plane between the gastrocnemius and soleus muscles is developed. The tendon of the gastrocnemius is released off the soleus fascia and allowed to slide proximally. The surgeon may elect to stitch the tendon in a more proximal position or allow it to be free to scar to a more proximal location following 4 weeks of casting.

Notably, a variety of other procedures to lengthen the triceps surae are available; however, these two are the workhorses for neuromuscular conditions of adult origin.

**Hindfoot varus** In acquired spastic muscle diseases, hindfoot varus foot deformity results variably from the relative overactivity of the tibialis anterior and tibialis posterior muscles, whereas in more hereditary situations, such as Charcot-Marie-Tooth, the varus may be driven by a forefoot supination or plantarflexion of the first ray. Other contributions may come from the EHL, flexor hallucis longus (FHL), FDL, and tibialis posterior muscles. Tendon transfers may be performed to balance the foot, and which procedure or combination of procedures depends on the origins of the deformity. Dynamic EMG may be performed to elucidate the contributing muscles. Following surgery, up to 70% of adult ambulatory patients can walk without an orthosis. Varus deformity is often seen in concert with equinus and claw toe deformities and both can be addressed during the same surgical procedure.

**Claw toe deformity** Claw toe deformity is characterized by metatarsophalangeal (MTP) hyperextension and consequent proximal IP (PIP) and distal IP (DIP) flexion. Neuromuscular diseases lead to intrinsic and extrinsic muscle imbalances and clawing of the 4 lesser toes; chronic MTP hyperextension leads to unopposed flexion of the DIP and PIP joints by the flexor digitorum tendons. Patients may develop metatarsalgia, pain, and/or ulceration at the tips of the toes or dorsal PIP joints from shoes. Claw toe deformity may worsen in patients undergoing tendo-Achilles lengthening; increased dorsiflexion places the toe flexors on stretch. Deformities are correctable with surgical release of the toe flexors. Transfer of the FDL tendon to the calcaneus can provide additional support to weakened calf muscles in patients with equinus or equinovarus deformities with concomitant claw toeing. Up to 70% of patients were able to ambulate without an ankle-foot orthosis following an FDL to calcaneus transfer.[32] This transfer should especially be considered in patients undergoing more distal lengthenings of the Achilles.

*Flexor digitorum longus/flexor digitorum brevis releases* Small longitudinal incisions are made on the plantar aspect of each the affected toe MTP joints. The scalpel is used to feel the edge of the flexor tendon, and the blade is then turned perpendicularly to release the tendon as the toe is passively extended.

*Flexor digitorum longus to calcaneus transfer* A curved incision is made on the medial foot and dissection carried deep to the FHL and FDL tendons at the master knot of Henry. These tendons are transected distally and separated. A second incision posterior to the medial malleolus is made. The FDL is identified and pulled through the incision. An absorbable suture is passed through the tendon end. A third incision is made medially over the calcaneal tuberosity, down to bone. A drill hole is made through the calcaneus from medial to lateral. The FDL tendon is tunneled subcutaneously toward the calcaneal incision. Using a meniscal needle or similar, the tendon is passed through the drill hole and secured with an interference screw or suture button technique while keeping the foot dorsiflexed.

*Flexor hallucis longus to lateral cuneiform transfer* Great toe hyperextension is common in patients with spastic equinovarus. The outflow of knee extension results in firing of the tibialis anterior, which can pull the foot into varus, and the EHL, which exacerbates the varus and also hyperextends the great toe. This condition can be observed clinically with a confusion test. In a seated position, the patient can flex and extend the knee several times. If the great toe hyperextends during this maneuver, an EHL transfer should be considered. The EHL is harvested distally at the level of the MTP, and the distal end is sutured into the tibialis anterior to prevent toe drooping. The proximal end is secured with a Krackow stitch and nonabsorbable suture. This tendon is then exposed over the lateral cuneiform. Care must be taken to retract the dorsalis pedis because it is close. A drill hole is placed in the lateral cuneiform and the tendon is secured in a 10° dorsiflexed position with a bioabsorbable interference screw.

**Valgus deformity** Spastic pes valgus is much less common than varus deformity and is attributed to spastic peroneal musculature. Dynamic EMG can elucidate the contributions of the peroneal longus and brevis musculature. Fractional lengthening of the peroneal muscles can be performed if the deformity is not overly severe, or a peroneal longus transfer to the navicular can be performed for severe deformity to support the longitudinal arch during stance. If the deformity is severe and paired with structural foot deformity, a lateral column lengthening osteotomy and a medial cuneiform plantarflexion osteotomy can be considered.

*Triple arthrodesis* A lateral incision is made over the foot from the tip of the distal fibula to the base of the fourth metatarsal. The personal tendons may be Z-lengthened from this approach if there is a planovalgus deformity; in cavus the dissection is performed dorsal to them. The talus may be dislocated off the navicular in more severe cases. The extensor digitorum brevis and fat pad are elevated, exposing the sinus tarsi, subtalar joint, calcaneocuboid joint, and lateral talonavicular. The sinus tarsi is cleared and the artery of the tarsal sinus ligated. A lamina spreader is inserted between the talus and calcaneus to expose the posterior facet. Using a combination of curettes, osteotomes, and burr, the subtalar, calcaneocuboid, and talonavicular joints are denuded of cartilage. Additional bone may be removed to correct deformity. A medial incision is made over the talonavicular joint to facilitate additional medial cartilage removal, and the tibialis posterior may be released off the navicular if the deformity is severe. Drill holes may be made in each joint surface to facilitate fusion. A variety of fixation options are available to maintain position during fusion (**Fig. 6**). The patient is placed in a short leg splint, which is converted to a cast in 2 weeks. Weight bearing is allowed in 6 weeks.

## SURGICAL MANAGEMENT OF THE SPASTIC UPPER EXTREMITY
### Shoulder Deformities

Functionally the shoulder has 2 tasks: the shoulder and elbow place the hand at an appropriate level, and the hand manipulates objects. From a practical standpoint, the upper extremity is more difficult to manage because patients use the hand for fine motor function and as such it is more difficult using surgery to achieve the goals of the upper extremity than it is to achieve similar lower extremity gross motor goals. However, passive function of the upper extremity is critical, because a typical flexion adduction contracture of an arm makes it difficult to dress and clean an individual.

The shoulder can be affected in a variety of ways in patients with upper motor neuron disease, including increased muscle tone of the shoulder girdle, HO, complex regional pain syndrome, brachial plexopathies, adhesive capsulitis, rotator cuff tears, shoulder subluxation, contractures, and fractures and dislocations.[33] Patients may

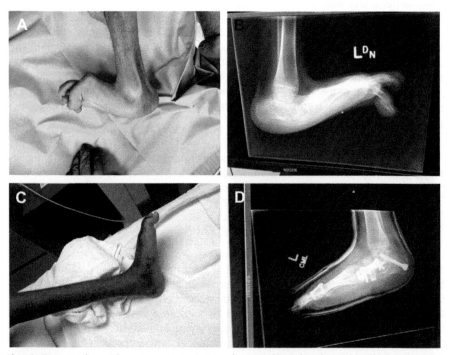

**Fig. 6.** Severe planovalgus reconstruction with a triple arthrodesis. (*A, B*) Preoperative photograph and radiograph, respectively. (*C, D*) Postoperative photograph and radiograph, respectively, demonstrating restoration of neutral alignment.

have active deficiencies or, if there is no active motion of the shoulder, may have difficulties with hygiene and activities of daily living.

### Adduction/Internal Rotation Contracture

The most common deformity observed in patients with upper extremity contractures in the shoulder are adduction/internal rotation contractures.[33] In patients with functionless limbs, release of the pectoralis major, latissimus dorsi, teres major, and subscapularis can result in superior motion and ease of care.[33–35] This release is performed through a slightly more medial approach than a standard deltopectoral incision. The incision is made approximately 1 fingerbreadth medial to a typical deltopectoral approach. The pectoralis major tendon is identified on the undersurface of the muscle and released off the lateral intertubercular groove. Patients should be advised that this may cause a bulge in the medial chest that may be noticeable if the patient is thin. The teres major and latissimus dorsi are released from the medial intertubercular groove. The subscapularis is released if external rotation and abduction are still limited to less than 70°. Note that the brachial plexus is encountered in this approach and must be gently retracted. In patients with functional upper extremities, fractional lengthening can be performed through the same approach, but the tendon lengthening should occur at the musculotendinous junction to preserve continuity of the muscle-tendon unit.[36] If dynamic EMG shows dyssynergy of the long head of the triceps, it may also be fractionally lengthened from this approach.

Patients with flaccid paralysis of the shoulder girdle can develop inferior subluxation of the shoulder and can be painful because of gravitational pull on the arm leading to stretching of the shoulder capsule, trapezius, or brachial plexus.[37] If reduction of the shoulder girdle alleviates the pain, then patients may benefit from surgical stabilization of the shoulder joint. The patient is offered a sling and, if the symptoms are relieved with the sling, a biceps suspension procedure is offered.[38] An incision is made in the standard deltopectoral interval and carried down to the long head of the biceps tendon. The tendon is freed from the surrounding muscle and released distally. Two drill holes are made in the bicipital groove in a longitudinal fashion. The tendon is then looped through these holes. The shoulder is manually reduced and the biceps is sutured to itself to secure the reduction. The arm is kept in a sling for 4 to 6 weeks, gentle passive range of motion is allowed, but the arm should be kept in a sling at all times when range of motion is not being performed. During range of motion it is important to support the arm.

### Elbow Spasticity: Flexion and Extension Deformities

Patients with elbow flexion deformities should be evaluated for volitional control of the elbow. If the patient has active movement, fractional myotendinous lengthening of the elbow flexors can be performed.[35,39] Dynamic EMG can evaluate for spasticity among the biceps, brachialis, brachioradialis, and triceps. Patients most commonly have spasticity of the biceps and brachioradialis.

Fractional lengthening of the long and short biceps is performed in the proximal arm, the brachialis at the elbow, and the brachioradialis in the forearm. The myotendinous junction of the biceps is released through a proximal anterior incision such as described earlier and the authors generally perform both procedures concomitantly. The brachialis is identified at the elbow through a sigmoid incision in which the proximal limb is lateral, the transverse limb is across the elbow crease, and the medial limb is distal. The interval between the brachioradialis and brachialis is developed, and the radial nerve identified deep between these two muscles. The tendon of the brachialis is broad and must be lengthened through its entire course. The medial extent of the lengthening comes close to the brachial neurovascular bundle so care must be taken to protect this. The brachioradialis is identified in the proximal forearm laterally. The tendon may be identified by the sensory branch of the radial nerve coursing on top of it. The tendon is fractionally lengthened after retracting the nerve out of the way (**Fig. 7**). Postoperatively the patient begins immediate active range of motion. At night, the patient is splinted in an extended position.

If the patient has no active movement with a fixed flexion deformity, release of the contracted elbow flexors is performed through a sigmoid incision as described earlier. As with other contractures, about 50% of the deformity is corrected surgically, and additional correction is achieved through serial casting and therapy. The lacertus fibrosus is released. The biceps tendon is either released or Z-lengthened depending on the situation. The brachialis and brachioradialis are completely released with care to preserve the radial nerve, which is between these two. The elbow capsule may be opened or weakened through this approach, although direct visualization is challenging. It is common for the radial nerve and brachial artery to be the tightest structure after surgery; as such, overextending the elbow following release is neither necessary nor desirable.

Patients with flexion deformities of the elbow can develop ulnar neuropathy secondary to constant traction on the nerve and compression in the cubital tunnel.[40] Patients may present with atrophy of the hand intrinsics and ulnar neuropathic symptoms. EMG confirms the diagnosis. Ulnar nerve transposition may be performed in addition to flexion contracture releases or lengthening.

Extension deformities are not common and are usually found in patients with brainstem insults. Triceps lengthening can be performed to gain elbow flexion and can be performed through a posterior approach.

### Forearm Spasticity

The forearms of patients with upper motor neuron syndromes can be affected with spasticity of the pronators or supinators. Pronation spasticity is more common than supination. Most patients have additional joint contractures that can all be addressed simultaneously.

In patients with spastic pronation, dynamic EMG can diagnose spasticity of the pronator teres, pronator quadratus, and biceps, because spastic elbow flexion is often seen in concert with pronation. Fractional lengthening of the pronators can be performed to improve pronation deformity. Pronator teres lengthening can be achieved

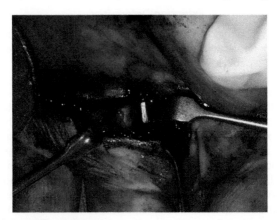

**Fig. 7.** Palmar interosseous exposure.

by identifying the tendon in the proximal forearm just lateral to the brachioradialis. The tendon is elevated off the radius and allowed to slide laterally, hence lengthening it. The pronator quadratus is elevated completely off the distal radius, hence weakening its pull. Static contracture of the intraosseous membrane may make complete correction of this deformity difficult.

Supination contractures can be addressed through rerouting the biceps tendon around the radius. A Z-plasty incision is made in the biceps tendon distally, and the distal segment is rerouted from the medial to the lateral side around the radial neck. With the arm held in neutral, the tendon is repaired and the arm is casted to protect the repair.

### Wrist Spasticity

Patients with upper motor neuron syndromes can have wrist spasticity presenting as flexion or extension deformities. These deformities are often accompanied by radial or ulnar deviations and clenched fists.

Flexion deformities are caused by spasticity of the wrist flexors, including the flexor carpi radialis and ulnaris, flexor digitorum superficialis (FDS), and flexor digitorum profundus (FDP). As usual, the approach to such deformities is to determine whether the patient has volitional control or not using dynamic EMG. If volitional control is present, selective fractional lengthening is performed. Patients without volitional control may benefit from tendon releases, proximal row carpectomy, wrist fusion, or superficialis to profundus (STP) transfer. Patients may also require carpal tunnel release because the volume of the carpal tunnel diminishes with extreme flexion or extension.[41]

Extension deformities are caused by spasticity of the extensor carpi radialis longus and brevis, and extensor carpi ulnaris. Similar to the wrist flexors, if volitional control is present, selective lengthening can be performed. Without volitional control, the wrist extensors are transected and a wrist fusion with or without proximal row carpectomy can be performed.

### Clenched-Fist and Thumb-in-Palm Deformities

Clenched-fist deformity is caused by spasticity of the FDS, FDP, flexor carpi ulnaris (FCU), and flexor carpi radialis (FCR) muscles. Dynamic EMG often shows the FDS as the principal cause. Patients often have a concomitant thumb-in-palm deformity from spasticity of the flexor pollicis longus (FPL) and thenar musculature, thumb adduction contractures secondary to spasticity of the adductor pollicis and first dorsal interosseous muscle, and contractures of the thumb web space or IP joint. FPL spasticity is suggested by resting thumb IP flexion. Affected patients may experience palmar skin breakdown from fingernails, difficulty with hygiene, recurrent nail bed infections, and compression of the median nerve if there is a wrist flexion contracture present.

Surgical management of the spastic clenched fist depends on the presence or absence of volitional control of the hand. If volitional control of the extrinsic flexors is appreciated on clinical examination and/or dynamic EMG, myotendinous lengthening of the wrist and finger flexors in the forearm may improve active hand function. Pronator teres and pronator quadratus may also be lengthened. In the nonfunctional hand, the flexor tendons cannot be adequately lengthened through fractional or myotendinous lengthening without causing discontinuity at the myotendinous junction, and an STP tendon transfer and wrist fusion are indicated.[42–46] If there are residual intrinsic hand deformities, additional surgery may be indicated, such as release of the intrinsics, the adductor pollicis, a Matev thenar slide, or even a Z-plasty of the skin with or without pinning of the involved joints.[43,47]

Surgical management can uncover intrinsic muscle spasticity postoperatively. Neurectomy of the ulnar motor nerve distal to the Guyon canal can prevent an intrinsic plus hand deformity secondary to hypertonicity of the lumbricals and interossei.[48] Thumb-in-palm deformity can manifest after the index STP procedure. Pappas and colleagues[49] showed relief of spasticity of the thenar musculature through recurrent median nerve neurectomy during the index STP procedure as an adjunct to ulnar motor nerve neurectomy. Given the increased morbidity of the Matev thenar slide (release of flexor pollicis brevis, adductor pollicis, and first dorsal interossei, with lengthy dissection and wound complications), recurrent median nerve neurectomy is a useful initial step for those patients with dynamic thumb-in-palm deformity. Matev thenar slide can then be considered if there is residual spasticity of the thumb-in-palm deformity after the initial release for dynamic deformity, either during the index procedure or a staged procedure in the case of a fixed deformity.

### Fractional lengthening of extrinsic finger flexors

A longitudinal incision is made on the volar forearm. The palmaris longus (PL) is identified and transected. The FDS, FDP, and FPL tendons are identified. A number 15 blade is used to incise only the tendinous portion of the myotendinous junction. The FCU and FCR tendons may also be lengthened if there is a wrist flexion deformity. Postoperatively, the patient is placed in a volar wrist splint, which is removed daily for active and active-assisted range-of-motion exercises. Such exercises contribute to the fractional lengthening of each tendon.

### Superficialis to profundus tendon transfer

A longitudinal incision is made volarly from the proximal forearm to the distal thenar crease. The PL, FCR, and FCU are identified and their tendons transected. The FDS tendons are sutured together distally and transected distal to the sutures. The FDP tendons are sutured together proximally and transected distal to the sutures. With the wrist and fingers in full extension, the FDS and FDP tendons are sutured together. Next, the FPL is transected proximally, transected, and sutured to the FDS-FDP mass while the thumb is held in extension.

Several additional procedures may be performed in the same setting to address concomitant deformities frequently seen. Carpal tunnel release is typically performed. If a neurectomy of the motor branch of the ulnar nerve is to be performed, the ulnar nerve is dissected distally through the Guyon canal. While protecting the superficial sensory branch, the deep motor branches and hypothenar branch are transected. Resection of a 1-cm segment reduces the risk of nerve regeneration. If a neurectomy of the recurrent median nerve is to be performed, the thenar musculature is dissected and the nerve identified and transected. Wrist arthrodesis in 10° to 15° of extension is performed using a dorsal wrist plate. Arthrodesis maintains the hand in a neutral position, improves cosmesis, and eliminates the need for a permanent splint.[50,51]

Postoperatively, the patient is placed in both dorsal and volar splints. The thumb and fingers are placed in full extension to the DIP joints. After 6 weeks, a removal volar wrist splint is used until the wrist fusion has healed, allowing the patient to come out of the splint for passive range of motion of the thumb and fingers.

### Thenar slide (Matev slide)

Thenar muscle slide, or Matev slide, is the recommended lengthening procedure in those patients with a fixed thumb-in-palm deformity or in those patients with dynamic deformity with persistent intrinsic thenar spasticity following recurrent median neurectomy as described previously. If a recurrent median neurectomy has not been previously performed, identification and protection of the nerve are essential. A longitudinal incision is made volarly along the thenar eminence. While extending the thumb, the origins of the thenar musculature are released off the palmar fascia and advanced radially. The adductor pollicis should be released off the third metacarpal, although this must be done with care because the radial artery passes between the transverse and oblique heads of this muscle and can be difficult to visualize.

Additional procedures may be indicated at the time of thenar slide. Concomitant spasticity of the FPL may be addressed through fractional lengthening in the forearm. Release of the adductor pollicis tendon or first dorsal interosseous muscle may also be indicated. Occasionally, for patients with advanced flexion contractures, fusion of the thumb IP joint may be necessary, which also serves to provide the patient with lateral pinch function. Z-plasty of the thumb web space may be performed for patients with persistent web space contractures following adequate muscle releases. Postoperatively, the patient is placed in a thumb spica splint for 3 weeks.

### Interosseous lengthening
Parallel longitudinal incisions are made over the palmar aspect of the distal metacarpals. The lumbricals are left intact because they have minimal muscle-tendon overlap. Deep to the lumbricals the bipennate palmar interossei are found and are fractionally lengthened (**Fig. 8**).

### Intrinsic release
The intrinsics can be released in patients without volitional control. A longitudinal incision is made in the midline over the proximal phalanx and dorsal metacarpophalangeal joint of each finger. On both the radial and ulnar aspects of the fingers, the lateral bands and oblique fibers of the extensor hood are released.

## APPROACH TO THE PATIENT WITH HETEROTOPIC OSSIFICATION

HO is the formation of bone in extraskeletal tissues. Typically, HO occurs between the muscle and the joint capsule and along tension vectors caused by spasticity.[52–55] It can form spontaneously or following traumatic injury. Following a neurologic insult, such as TBI or SCI, HO usually develops within 2 months.

Examination of the patient may reveal painless or painful loss of range of motion, joint contractures caused by tension on surrounding soft tissue, joint ankyloses, pathologic fractures, symptoms of chronic regional pain syndrome, limited functionality and inability to perform activities of daily living, decubitus ulcers from skin breakdown

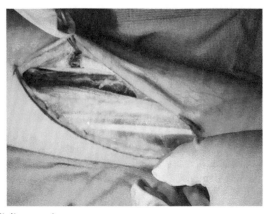

**Fig. 8.** Brachioradialis recession.

and/or poor hygiene, and peripheral neuropathy from impingement on surrounding neurologic structures. Notably, in the elbow in the absence of trauma, HO usually spares the radiocapitellar joint and forearm supination, and pronation is generally unaffected despite limited flexion and extension.

Patients with cerebral palsy often are found to have hip displacement, which is treated with proximal femoral resection, which is commonly associated with HO formation. Nonsteroidal antiinflammatory medications are commonly prescribed for prophylaxis in such surgeries, although recent literature suggests this intervention may not be effective.[56]

Plain radiographs reveal HO. Computed tomography scans can be performed for preoperative planning (**Fig. 9**A, B). Surgical treatment is considered when patients experience significant functional impairment, and several recent studies have shown improved clinical and functional outcomes from surgical resection.[57–67] **Table 2** evaluates common anatomic locations for HO and associated surgical approaches and considerations. Wide surgical exposure is essential to visualize important neurovascular structures that may be involved (**Fig. 9**C). Recurrence is common.

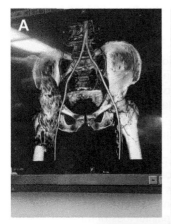
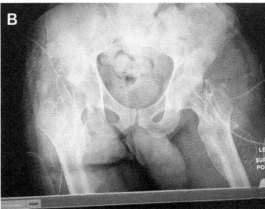
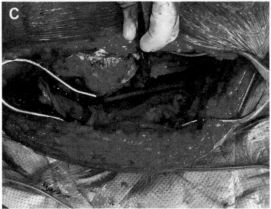

**Fig. 9.** Severe HO about the hip. (*A*) Preoperative computed tomography scan with three-dimensional reconstruction demonstrating the severe extent of HO involving the hip joint and extending to the iliac wing. (*B*) Postoperative radiograph. (*C*) Intraoperative view illustrating the need for wide exposure to visualize the neurovascular structures adequately because the HO often encases them.

**Table 2**
**Surgical approach to heterotopic ossification by anatomic location**

| Location | Description | Treatment |
|---|---|---|
| Hip[54] | | |
| Anterior | • Forms along regions of hip flexors, anterior superior iliac spine to proximal femur around lesser trochanter<br>• Follows iliopsoas muscle | • Anterior approach to hip<br>• Dissection of femoral triangle to identify all branches of femoral neurovascular bundle<br>• Femoral nerve is commonly encased |
| Posterior | • Forms along hip extensors, adjacent to posterior femoral head and neck<br>• Usually seen with hip flexion contractures | • Posterior approach to the hip<br>• Sciatic nerve commonly encased<br>• Sciatic nerve neurolysis may be indicated<br>• Anterior soft tissue release if persistent hip flexion contracture after HO excision |
| Medial | • Forms along hip adductors, inferomedial to the hip<br>• Can have associated anterior HO | • Medial approach to the hip<br>• Anterior approach to the hip as a separate incision if concomitant anterior HO exists<br>• Adductor release if contracted |
| Lateral | • Forms along hip abductors<br>• Usually occurs following trauma or surgery | • Direct lateral or posterior approach to the hip |
| Knee[61,68,69] | • Rare<br>• More common following SCI<br>• Medial aspect of the knee<br>• May be confused with Pellegrini-Stieda lesion<br>• Can cause knee flexion contracture<br>• Anterior HO beneath quadriceps with extensor spasticity<br>• Posterior HO rare with hamstring spasticity | • Approach depends on location of HO<br>• HO often extensive and multiple approaches may be warranted<br>• Medial approach to the knee<br>• Lateral approach to the knee<br>• Posterior approach to the knee |
| Shoulder[59] | • Rare<br>• 5% of patients with TBI<br>• Inferomedial to the glenohumeral joint | • Surgical management is uncommon<br>• Deltopectoral approach<br>• Posterior approach the shoulder<br>• Axillary nerve commonly encased |
| Elbow[70] | • Rare<br>• More common following TBI<br>• Occurs anteriorly and posteriorly<br>• Usually does not involve radiocapitellar joint in the absence of trauma | • Posterior approach to the elbow<br>• Medial or lateral approach to the elbow<br>• Anterior approach to the elbow<br>• Ulnar nerve commonly encased and neurolysis and transposition are recommended |

## SUMMARY

The neuro-orthopaedic approach to patients with upper motor neuron injury or syndromes can be challenging because a wide variety of nonoperative and operative interventions are available, as described here, and patients often have multiple deformities. Timing is critical; although the natural history of neurologic recovery may preclude early surgery, it is essential to continue nonoperative measures to prevent or lessen the severity of deformities. Operative measures should take place as early as is feasible to prevent fixed and rigid deformities. The patient's overarching functional status and the function of the limbs in question should be distinguished and thoroughly examined. In addition, a thorough discussion should be had with the patient and/or family regarding treatment options and setting expectations for surgical outcomes. Management of deformity takes time, participation, and concerted effort to achieve satisfactory outcomes.

## REFERENCES

1. Kozin SH, Keenan MA. Using dynamic electromyography to guide surgical treatment of the spastic upper extremity in the brain-injured patient. Clin Orthop Relat Res 1993;(288):109–17.

2. Keenan MA, Fuller DA, Whyte J, et al. The influence of dynamic polyelectromyography in formulating a surgical plan in treatment of spastic elbow flexion deformity. Arch Phys Med Rehabil 2003;84(2):291–6.

3. Keenan MA, Haider TT, Stone LR. Dynamic electromyography to assess elbow spasticity. J Hand Surg 1990;15(4):607–14.

4. Keenan MA, Romanelli RR, Lunsford BR. The use of dynamic electromyography to evaluate motor control in the hands of adults who have spasticity caused by brain injury. J Bone Joint Surg Am 1989;71(1):120–6.

5. Pershouse KJ, Barker RN, Kendall MB, et al. Investigating changes in quality of life and function along the lifespan for people with spinal cord injury. Arch Phys Med Rehabil 2012;93(3):413–9.

6. Senthilvelkumar T, Magimairaj H, Fletcher J, et al. Comparison of body weight-supported treadmill training versus body weight-supported overground training in people with incomplete tetraplegia: a pilot randomized trial. Clin Rehabil 2015;29(1):42–9.

7. Gorman PH, Scott W, York H, et al. Robotically assisted treadmill exercise training for improving peak fitness in chronic motor incomplete spinal cord injury: a randomized controlled trial. J Spinal Cord Med 2016;39(1):32–44.

8. Gorman PH, Geigle PR, Chen K, et al. Reliability and relatedness of peak VO2 assessments during body weight supported treadmill training and arm cycle ergometry in individuals with chronic motor incomplete spinal cord injury. Spinal Cord 2014;52(4):287–91.

9. Bakkum AJT, Paulson TAW, Bishop NC, et al. Effects of hybrid cycle and hand-cycle exercise on cardiovascular disease risk factors in people with spinal cord injury: a randomized controlled trial. J Rehabil Med 2015;47(6):523–30.

10. Bakkum AJT, de Groot S, Stolwijk-Swüste JM, et al. Effects of hybrid cycling versus handcycling on wheelchair-specific fitness and physical activity in people with long-term spinal cord injury: a 16-week randomized controlled trial. Spinal Cord 2015;53(5):395–401.

11. van Koppenhagen CF, de Groot S, Post MWM, et al. Wheelchair exercise capacity in spinal cord injury up to five years after discharge from inpatient rehabilitation. J Rehabil Med 2013;45(7):646–52.

12. Kooijmans H, Post MWM, Stam HJ, et al. Effectiveness of a self-management intervention to promote an active lifestyle in persons with long-term spinal cord injury: the HABITS randomized clinical trial. Neurorehabil Neural Repair 2017; 31(12):991–1004.

13. Akbar M, Balean G, Brunner M, et al. Prevalence of rotator cuff tear in paraplegic patients compared with controls. J Bone Joint Surg Am 2010;92(1):23–30.

14. Yang J, Boninger ML, Leath JD, et al. Carpal tunnel syndrome in manual wheelchair users with spinal cord injury: a cross-sectional multicenter study. Am J Phys Med Rehabil 2009;88(12):1007–16.
15. Bunketorp-Käll L, Reinholdt C, Fridén J, et al. Essential gains and health after upper-limb tetraplegia surgery identified by the International Classification of Functioning, Disability and Health (ICF). Spinal Cord 2017;55(9):857–63.
16. Wangdell J, Fridén J. Satisfaction and performance in patient selected goals after grip reconstruction in tetraplegia. J Hand Surg Eur Vol 2010;35(7):563–8.
17. Mulroy SJ, Thompson L, Kemp B, et al. Strengthening and Optimal Movements for Painful Shoulders (STOMPS) in chronic spinal cord injury: a randomized controlled trial. Phys Ther 2011;91(3):305–24.
18. Wangdell J, Carlsson G, Friden J. From regained function to daily use: experiences of surgical reconstruction of grip in people with tetraplegia. Disabil Rehabil 2014;36(8):678–84.
19. Nandra KS, Harari M, Price TP, et al. Successful reinnervation of the diaphragm after intercostal to phrenic nerve neurotization in patients with high spinal cord injury. Ann Plast Surg 2017;79(2):180–2.
20. The global burden of traumatic brain injury: preliminary results from the Global Burden of Disease Project | Injury Prevention. Available at: http://injuryprevention. bmj.com/content/16/Suppl_1/A17.2. Accessed December 28, 2017.
21. Maas AIR, Menon DK, Adelson PD, et al. Traumatic brain injury: integrated approaches to improve prevention, clinical care, and research. Lancet Neurol 2017;16(12):987–1048.
22. Adey-Wakeling Z, Liu E, Crotty M, et al. Hemiplegic shoulder pain reduces quality of life after acute stroke: a prospective population-based study. Am J Phys Med Rehabil 2016;95(10):758–63.
23. Chae J, Mascarenhas D, Yu DT, et al. Poststroke shoulder pain: its relationship to motor impairment, activity limitation, and quality of life. Arch Phys Med Rehabil 2007;88(3):298–301.
24. Lindgren I, Jönsson A-C, Norrving B, et al. Shoulder pain after stroke: a prospective population-based study. Stroke 2007;38(2):343–8.
25. Kendall R. Musculoskeletal problems in stroke survivors. Top Stroke Rehabil 2010. https://doi.org/10.1310/tsr1703-173.
26. Keenan MA, Ure K, Smith CW, et al. Hamstring release for knee flexion contracture in spastic adults. Clin Orthop 1988;236:221–6.
27. Cipriano C, Keenan MAE. Knee disarticulation and hip release for severe lower extremity contractures. Clin Orthop 2007;462:150–5.
28. Namdari S, Pill SG, Makani A, et al. Rectus femoris to gracilis muscle transfer with fractional lengthening of the vastus muscles: a treatment for adults with stiff knee gait. Phys Ther 2010;90(2):261–8.
29. Thawrani D, Haumont T, Church C, et al. Rectus femoris transfer improves stiff knee gait in children with spastic cerebral palsy. Clin Orthop 2012;470(5): 1303–11.
30. Maskill MP, Maskill JD, Pomeroy GC. Surgical management and treatment algorithm for the subtle cavovarus foot. Foot Ankle Int 2010;31(12):1057–63.
31. Shore BJ, White N, Kerr Graham H. Surgical correction of equinus deformity in children with cerebral palsy: a systematic review. J Child Orthop 2010;4(4): 277–90.
32. Keenan MA, Lee GA, Tuckman AS, et al. Improving calf muscle strength in patients with spastic equinovarus deformity by transfer of the long toe flexors to the os calcis. J Head Trauma Rehabil 1999;14(2):163–75.

33. Namdari S, Baldwin K, Horneff JG, et al. Orthopedic evaluation and surgical treatment of the spastic shoulder. Orthop Clin North Am 2013;44(4):605–14.

34. Namdari S, Alosh H, Baldwin K, et al. Shoulder tenotomies to improve passive motion and relieve pain in patients with spastic hemiplegia after upper motor neuron injury. J Shoulder Elbow Surg 2011;20(5):802–6.

35. Photopoulos CD, Namdari S, Baldwin KD, et al. Decision-making in the treatment of the spastic shoulder and elbow: tendon release versus tendon lengthening. JBJS Rev 2014;2(10). https://doi.org/10.2106/JBJS.RVW.M.00132.

36. Namdari S, Alosh H, Baldwin K, et al. Outcomes of tendon fractional lengthenings to improve shoulder function in patients with spastic hemiparesis. J Shoulder Elbow Surg 2012;21(5):691–8.

37. Dursun E, Dursun N, Ural CE, et al. Glenohumeral joint subluxation and reflex sympathetic dystrophy in hemiplegic patients. Arch Phys Med Rehabil 2000; 81(7):944–6.

38. Namdari S, Keenan MA. Outcomes of the biceps suspension procedure for painful inferior glenohumeral subluxation in hemiplegic patients. J Bone Joint Surg Am 2010;92(15):2589–97.

39. Namdari S, Horneff JG, Baldwin K, et al. Muscle releases to improve passive motion and relieve pain in patients with spastic hemiplegia and elbow flexion contractures. J Shoulder Elbow Surg 2012;21(10):1357–62.

40. Keenan MA, Kauffman DL, Garland DE, et al. Late ulnar neuropathy in the brain-injured adult. J Hand Surg 1988;13(1):120–4.

41. Orcutt SA, Kramer WG, Howard MW, et al. Carpal tunnel syndrome secondary to wrist and finger flexor spasticity. J Hand Surg 1990;15(6):940–4.

42. Botte MJ, Keenan MA, Gellman H, et al. Surgical management of spastic thumb-in-palm deformity in adults with brain injury. J Hand Surg 1989;14(2 Pt 1):174–82.

43. Heest AEV. Surgical technique for thumb-in-palm deformity in cerebral palsy. J Hand Surg 2011;36(9):1526–31.

44. Keenan MA, Korchek JI, Botte MJ, et al. Results of transfer of the flexor digitorum superficialis tendons to the flexor digitorum profundus tendons in adults with acquired spasticity of the hand. J Bone Joint Surg Am 1987;69(8):1127–32.

45. Botte MJ, Keenan MA, Korchek JI, et al. Modified technique for the superficialis-to-profundus transfer in the treatment of adults with spastic clenched fist deformity. J Hand Surg 1987;12(4):639–40.

46. Braun RM, Vise GT, Roper B. Preliminary experience with superficialis-to-profundus tendon transfer in the hemiplegic upper extremity. J Bone Joint Surg Am 1974;56(3):466–72.

47. Matev IB. Surgical treatment of flexion-adduction contracture of the thumb in cerebral palsy. Acta Orthop Scand 1970;41(4):439–45.

48. Pomerance JF, Keenan MA. Correction of severe spastic flexion contractures in the nonfunctional hand. J Hand Surg 1996;21(5):828–33.

49. Pappas N, Baldwin K, Keenan MA. Efficacy of median nerve recurrent branch neurectomy as an adjunct to ulnar motor nerve neurectomy and wrist arthrodesis at the time of superficialis to profundus transfer in prevention of intrinsic spastic thumb-in-palm deformity. J Hand Surg 2010;35(8):1310–6.

50. Rayan GM, Young BT. Arthrodesis of the spastic wrist. J Hand Surg 1999;24(5): 944–52.

51. Jebson PJ, Adams BD. Wrist arthrodesis: review of current techniques. J Am Acad Orthop Surg 2001;9(1):53–60.

52. Botte MJ, Keenan MA, Abrams RA, et al. Heterotopic ossification in neuromuscular disorders. Orthopedics 1997;20(4):335–41 [quiz: 342–3].

53. Chan K-T. Heterotopic ossification in traumatic brain injury. Am J Phys Med Rehabil 2005;84(2):145–6.
54. Cipriano CA, Pill SG, Keenan MA. Heterotopic ossification following traumatic brain injury and spinal cord injury. J Am Acad Orthop Surg 2009;17(11):689.
55. Dey D, Wheatley BM, Cholok D, et al. The traumatic bone: trauma-induced heterotopic ossification. Transl Res 2017;186:95–111.
56. Dartnell J, Paterson JMH, Magill N, et al. Proximal femoral resection for the painful dislocated hip in cerebral palsy: does indomethacin prevent heterotopic ossification? J Pediatr Orthop 2014;34(3):295–9.
57. Lee EK, Namdari S, Hosalkar HS, et al. Clinical results of the excision of heterotopic bone around the elbow: a systematic review. J Shoulder Elbow Surg 2013; 22(5):716–22.
58. Pansard E, Schnitzler A, Lautridou C, et al. Heterotopic ossification of the shoulder after central nervous system lesion: indications for surgery and results. J Shoulder Elbow Surg 2013;22(6):767–74.
59. Fuller DA, Mani US, Keenan MAE. Heterotopic ossification of the shoulder in patients with traumatic brain injury. J Shoulder Elbow Surg 2013;22(1):52–6.
60. Ippolito E, Formisano R, Farsetti P, et al. Excision for the treatment of periarticular ossification of the knee in patients who have a traumatic brain injury. J Bone Joint Surg Am 1999;81(6):783–9.
61. Fuller DA, Mark A, Keenan MAE. Excision of heterotopic ossification from the knee: a functional outcome study. Clin Orthop 2005;438:197–203.
62. Wangdell J, Fridén J. Activity gains after reconstructions of elbow extension in patients with tetraplegia. J Hand Surg 2012;37(5):1003–10.
63. Kozin SH. Biceps-to-triceps transfer for restoration of elbow extension in tetraplegia. Tech Hand Up Extrem Surg 2003;7(2):43–51.
64. Kozin SH, D'Addesi L, Chafetz RS, et al. Biceps-to-triceps transfer for elbow extension in persons with tetraplegia. J Hand Surg 2010;35(6):968–75.
65. Edwards P, Hsu J. SPLATT combined with tendo Achilles lengthening for spastic equinovarus in adults: results and predictors of surgical outcome. Foot Ankle 1993;14(6):335–8.
66. Fuller DA, McCarthy JJ, Keenan MA. The use of the absorbable interference screw for a split anterior tibial tendon (SPLATT) transfer procedure. Orthopedics 2004;27(4):372–4.
67. Hosalkar H, Goebel J, Reddy S, et al. Fixation techniques for split anterior tibialis transfer in spastic equinovarus feet. Clin Orthop 2008;466(10):2500–6.
68. Anderson MC, Lais RL. Excision of heterotopic ossification of the popliteal space following traumatic brain injury. J Orthop Trauma 2004;18(3):190–2.
69. Mitsionis GI, Lykissas MG, Kalos N, et al. Functional outcome after excision of heterotopic ossification about the knee in ICU patients. Int Orthop 2009;33(6): 1619–25.
70. Baldwin K, Hosalkar HS, Donegan DJ, et al. Surgical resection of heterotopic bone about the elbow: an institutional experience with traumatic and neurologic etiologies. J Hand Surg 2011;36(5):798–803.

# Upper Extremity Problem-Solving
## Challenging Cases

Nathaniel H. Mayer, MD[a,b],*

## KEYWORDS

- Upper motor neuron syndrome (UMNS) • Associated reactions
- Rheologic properties • Spastic cocontraction • UMNS weakness • Dynamic EMG
- Muscle selection for chemodenervation

## KEY POINTS

- One consequence of an upper motor neuron syndrome (UMNS) is weakness or paresis.
- Other consequences of UMNS are superimposed involuntary phenomena (spastic cocon-traction, spasticity, spastic dystonia, associated reactions, increased flexor reflex activity) that further impact voluntary movements and can also include superimposed viscoelastic and plastic (rheologic) changes in muscle.
- It is often difficult to sort out the degree to which observed motor behavior is neural volun-tary, neural involuntary, or non-neural rheologic; however, clinical differentiations will likely lead to a better treatment rationale.
- The cases presented describe spastic cocontraction, spastic dystonia, associated reactions, hyperextended wrist with finger flexor tenodesis, differentiating neural versus non-neural (rheologic) hypertonia, upper motor neuron weakness, the use of dynamic poly-electromyography to inform muscle selection for chemodenervation, and the use of electrical stimulation for muscle-specific targeting.

Holmes' companion, Dr John Watson, recently opened an upper limb practice for muscle overactivity in the upper motor neuron syndrome (UMNS). He publicly intro-duced his practice in the *London Gazette*, describing neurotoxin injections into mus-cles with focal UMNS hypertonia. However, Watson was bothered by John Hughlings Jackson's dictum that the brain was more concerned with movements than muscles.[1] This dictum is likely to be so, he mused, because more than one muscle crossed virtu-ally every upper limb joint and more than one muscle could be contracting when a particular joint moved. But which of those UMNS muscles had hypertonia? For example, elbow hypertonia could include biceps, brachialis, brachioradialis, pronator

Disclosure Statement: The author has nothing to disclose.
[a] Motor Control Analysis Laboratory, Department of PM&R, MossRehab, Einstein Healthcare Network, 60 Township Line Road, Elkins Park, PA 19027, USA; [b] Department of Rehabilitation Medicine, Temple University Health Sciences Center, 3500 North Broad Street, Philadelphia, PA 19140, USA
* 681 Broadmoor Drive, Blue Bell, PA 19422.
*E-mail address:* nmayer@einstein.edu

Phys Med Rehabil Clin N Am 29 (2018) 593–617
https://doi.org/10.1016/j.pmr.2018.04.003
1047-9651/18/© 2018 Elsevier Inc. All rights reserved.

pmr.theclinics.com

teres, and extensor carpi radialis (the last two flex when their distal ends are fixed). Should he inject all flexors, perhaps only 3 or just good old biceps? Should he decide by palpation? But how palpable is brachialis and deep muscles elsewhere? Muscle selection is something to ponder, thought Watson. Fortunately, technology-oriented Holmes dabbled with muscle identification using dynamic poly-electromyography (EMG). This tool combined with clinical skills and video recordings enabled Watson to describe some challenging cases later.

Before presenting them, Watson offered some clinical tips. Generally, the upper limb reaches and binds. Reaching transports the hand or object to a place in the environment. Commonly, reaching involves scapula protraction, shoulder flexion (with abduction/adduction and/or rotation), elbow extension, forearm overhand pronation/underhand supination, or midposition when holding a mug's handle. Patients with UMNS may have sufficient activation of agonists to generate movement, but antagonist overactivity and/or rheologic muscle stiffness may restrain movement.

Scapula protraction restraint affects the forward reach. Rhomboids and/or middle trapezius may be involved. Frank retraction is sometimes seen. Humeral flexion may be restrained by overactivity of teres major, latissimus dorsi, and/or long head triceps. Hand on head as in combing requires shoulder external rotation and flexion/abduction and is affected by restraint of internal rotator/adductor overactivity. Internal rotators/adductors may include pectoralis major, teres major, latissimus dorsi, and subscapularis. Selection, except for subscapularis, may be aided by palpation. In UMNS, it is hard to apply Gerber and Krushell's[2] lift-off test isolating subscapularis from other internal rotators. Yelnik and colleagues[3] rotated/abducted the shoulder passively to test subscapularis; but, in UMNS, this test does not differentiate other internal rotators/adductors. In their study, subscapularis alone was chemo-denervated. Finding good results, they concluded that subscapularis was the offending rotator. Muscle injection with follow-up assessment is one post hoc propter hoc method available to clinicians for determining selection of offending muscles. Local anesthetic blocks is another. Dynamic poly-EMG studies also inform decision-making for muscle selection.[4,5]

At the elbow, overactivity of brachioradialis, brachialis, pronator teres, and extensor carpi radialis may restrain active extension during reaching.[4] Biceps overactivity may also restrain extension; but, as a 2-joint muscle, biceps may be recruited to augment weak shoulder flexion. In this circumstance, chemodenervation may not be appropriate. However, biceps as a shoulder flexor works when elbow flexion is blocked, something patients with UMNS with paretic triceps may not be able to do. The elbow fixation principle is acknowledged in C5 quadriplegia when transferring brachioradialis to flexor pollicis longus (FPL) to create the thumb pinch, typically preceded by biceps-to-triceps transfer that provides an extensor force to counterbalance brachioradialis flexor force.[6]

Pronator teres and/or pronator quadratus overactivity restrains active supination.[7] Palpation may help identify pronator teres cocontraction. Pronator quadratus overactivity may be identified electromyographically (see later discussion). Otherwise, follow-up assessment after individual treatment provides long-term guidance for muscle selection.

One type of hand binding function is grasp, hold, release; a second is contact/articulation with surfaces and transmitting proximal forces (eg, door push); a third is manipulating objects. In UMNS, selective finger/thumb control and ability to manipulate objects is less seen in rehabilitation clinics that attract patients with severe lesions. Mass grasp, more commonly, holds objects; but hand opening is typically problematic. Finger extension orthoses are now available (see Kimberly Miczak and Joseph Padova's article "Muscle Overactivity in the Upper Motor Neuron Syndrome: Assessment and Problem Solving for Complex Cases: the Role of Physical and Occupational Therapy," in this issue) for web space opening and object entry. An extension assist orthosis also helps object release. Better finger extension may also result from fractional lengthening of finger flexors (see Matthew T. Winterton and Keith Baldwin's article "The Neuro-Orthopaedic Approach," in this issue).

Clenched fist and flexed wrist configurations do not necessarily signify paralysis of finger and wrist extensors. These configurations reflect a balance of forces that favors flexors. Sometimes extensors have severe volitional paresis, but they may also have reasonable volitional strength overwhelmed by cocontracting flexor forces. Unmasked wrist extension and intrinsic plus configurations can be seen after surgery, even chemodenervation. Dynamic EMG studies of wrist extensors and finger intrinsics can provide useful information before surgical intervention.[8] Sometimes weakening wrist flexors surgically or chemically unmasks wrist extension resulting in persistence of a clenched fist, promoted by finger flexor tenodesis.

Finally, a hyperextended wrist typically presents with a clenched fist because of tenodesis with or without underlying spastic/dystonic fingers. Treatment is aimed at wrist extensors, whereas treatment of finger flexors depends on whether they are demonstrably spastic. Injecting wrist flexors for a hyperextended wrist exacerbates clenching. The goal of treatment is to open the passive hand for hand-as-a-holder function, hygiene, and skin care. Chemodenervation of wrist extensors combined with control of wrist extension orthotically, as needed, works well. If spastic finger flexors are present (examine flexors with wrist in neutral), chemodenervation can lessen their clenching.

## THE CASE OF THE PICCADILLY PRONATORS

*History*: A 42-year-old woman sustained spastic right hemiparesis due to stroke at 39 years of age (**Fig. 1**). Among other complaints, she had difficulty turning her palm up.

*Examination*: The examination confirmed incomplete active supination when reaching underhand (see **Fig. 1**). Volitional supination was effortful and pronator restraint was suspected. Passive supination was complete. Resistance to passive stretch of pronators increased with increasing rates of stretch, indicating pronator spasticity. It was unclear clinically whether one or both pronators were spastic.

*Laboratory*: Dynamic poly-EMG of biceps, pronator teres, and pronator quadratus was performed. **Fig. 2** reveals that both pronators cocontracted during volitional effort

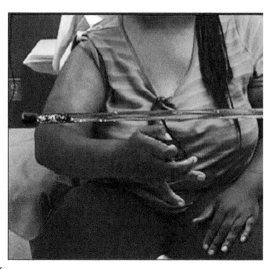

**Fig. 1.** Pronated forearm.

Reach for a Rod Underhand

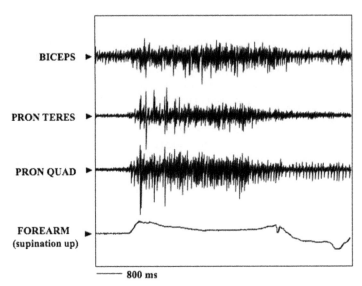

**Fig. 2.** Electromyographic co-contraction of pronators.

of reaching underhand. The movement trace revealed an initial supination movement that halted during pronator cocontraction, confirming the interpretation of pronator restraint of active supination.

*Commentary*: There are 2 pronator muscles that cannot be distinguished by clinical examination alone. If a clinician is considering chemodenervation, poly-EMG information regarding each pronator muscle can inform muscle selection for focal treatment. For purposes of focal chemodenervation, an individual muscle may be considered a unit of structure and function, a concept not applicable to oral antispastic medications that have a diffuse vascular distribution. A second point is that voluntary agonist-generated movement may be restrained by spastic cocontraction of antagonists.

## THE CASE OF THE AYLESBURY ADDUCTED/INTERNALLY ROTATED SHOULDER

*History*: A 56-year-old woman sustained a thalamic/internal capsule intracerebral hemorrhage with spastic right hemiparesis 5 months earlier (**Fig. 3**). She complained of being hampered by episodes of sudden elbow flexion and shoulder adduction. Episodes occurred when walking or doing ordinary daily activities. The limb was not used functionally.

*Examination*: The upper limb Fugl-Meyer score was 29%. Examination revealed spastic shoulder adductors including pectoralis major, teres major and latissimus dorsi. Other spastic groups included elbow, wrist and finger flexors, and flexor pollicis longus. Hemihypesthesia was present.

*Laboratory*: Dynamic EMG of pectoralis major, teres major, and latissimus dorsi was obtained to identify circumstances of muscle overactivity. Recordings were made when the patient laughed (see **Fig. 3**), coughed (**Fig. 4**), threw a ball with her unaffected arm (**Fig. 5**), and leaned on a cane with her unaffected hand to control balance (**Fig. 6**).

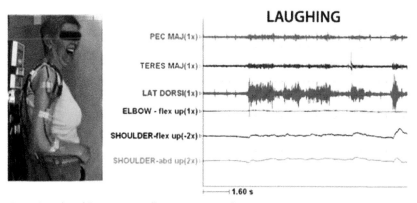

**Fig. 3.** Patient laughing. ELBOW flex up, ELBOW flexion is up; LAT DORSI, latissimus dorsi; PEC MAJ, pectoralis major; SHOULDER abd up, SHOULDER abduction is up; SHOULDER flex up, SHOULDER flexion is up; TERES MAJ, teres major. (*From* Mayer NH, Esquenazi A. Upper limb skin and musculoskeletal consequences of the upper motor neuron syndrome. In: Jankovic J, editor. Botulinum toxin therapeutic clinical practice & science. Philadelphia: Elsevier; 2009. p. 133; with permission.)

*Commentary*: Testing revealed several positive signs seen in UMNS, including spasticity and associated reactions. Associated reactions were first described by Walsh[9] in 1923 as "released postural reactions deprived of voluntary control."[9] Motor behavior including voluntary activity in one part of the body is accompanied by involuntary activity elsewhere, typically in UMNS limbs. Common behaviors, such as coughing, laughing, and cane use by the unaffected limb, can trigger associated reactions in an affected limb. **Figs. 3–6** show recorded activity of 3 shoulder adductor/rotators, and it is no surprise that the patient's clinical pattern was an adducted/internally rotated shoulder. Something to consider is that associated reactions, internally generated and linked with everyday behaviors, may play a greater role than spasticity, externally and passively generated, in reinforcing UMNS postural patterns.

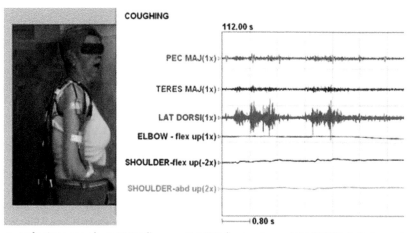

**Fig. 4.** Left view, cough. ELBOW flex up, ELBOW flexion is up; LAT DORSI, latissimus dorsi; PEC MAJ, pectoralis major; SHOULDER abd up, SHOULDER abduction is up; SHOULDER flex up, SHOULDER flexion is up; TERES MAJ, teres major.

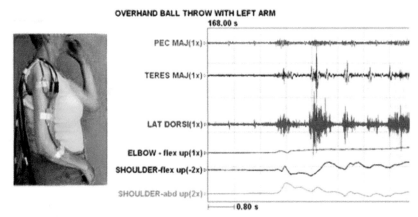

**Fig. 5.** Patient throwing ball with left arm. ELBOW flex up, ELBOW flexion is up; LAT DORSI, latissimus dorsi; PEC MAJ, pectoralis major; SHOULDER abd up, SHOULDER abduction is up; SHOULDER flex up, SHOULDER flexion is up; TERES MAJ, teres major.

### THE CASE OF THE COLCHESTER FINGER CAPER

*History*: A 31-year-old woman with polycythemia vera developed bilateral strokes at 28 years of age. She had good left upper limb recovery with usage, but she complained of a curled index finger (**Fig. 7**).

*Examination*: When she reached to grasp, the index finger curled, flexing the metacarpophalangeal (MCP), proximal interphalangeal (PIP), and distal interphalangeal (DIP) joints. The curled index finger reduced access into the hand, making object acquisition difficult. **Figs. 8–10** illustrate the curling sequence that led to finger knuckling against an object (soda can).

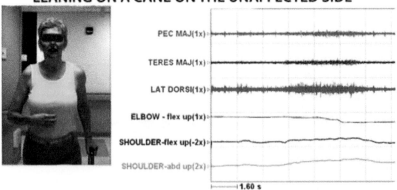

**Fig. 6.** Patient leaning on cane. ELBOW flex up, ELBOW flexion is up; LAT DORSI, latissimus dorsi; PEC MAJ, pectoralis major; SHOULDER abd up, SHOULDER abduction is up; SHOULDER flex up, SHOULDER flexion is up; TERES MAJ, teres major. (*From* Mayer NH, Esquenazi A. Upper limb skin and musculoskeletal consequences of the upper motor neuron syndrome. In: Jankovic J, editor. Botulinum toxin therapeutic clinical practice & science. Philadelphia: Elsevier; 2009. p. 133; with permission.)

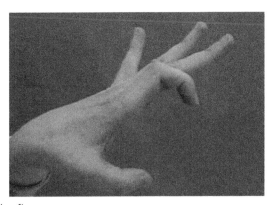

**Fig. 7.** Curled index finger.

*Treatment*: Treatment consisted of chemodenervation of the index finger flexor digitorum superficialis (FDS) and flexor digitorum profundus (FDP) with the rationale that converting extrinsic to intrinsic plus motor behavior would open the web space, facilitating object entry. Weakened grasp function secondary to blocked index extrinsics was considered less important than improving access for objects. **Fig. 11** shows the technique of FDS electrical stimulation through the injection needle. PIP joint flexion caused by electrical stimulation can be seen in **Fig. 11**. Once definitive flexion is obtained, neurotoxin injection is performed. Electrical stimulation was similarly performed to elicit DIP joint flexion before FDP injection. **Fig. 12** shows the

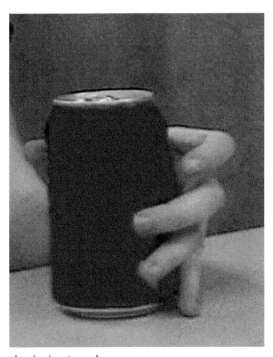

**Fig. 8.** Index finger beginning to curl.

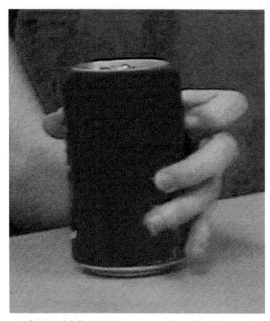

**Fig. 9.** Index finger making initial contact.

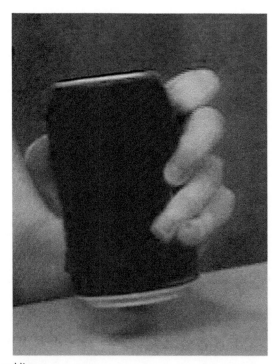

**Fig. 10.** Index knuckling.

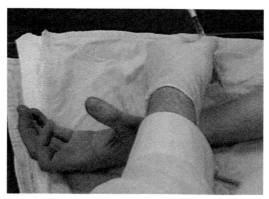

**Fig. 11.** Index FDS electrical stimulation technique.

chemodenervation result 3 weeks later. With the index finger out of the way, the soda can is grasped by the thumb and the long, ring, and little fingers. **Fig. 13** shows contact between the index finger and can as a result of tenodesis flexion generated by the patient's wrist extension (not seen in this view).

*Commentary*: Sometimes functional recovery from UMNS can be marred by a focal problem, such as a curled finger. Thumb and finger muscles are amenable to selective muscle chemodenervation using the technique of selective electrical stimulation. Ultrasound information may be helpful as well. UMNS commonly causes problems of access that interfere with object entry into the hand and holding function by the hand.

## A CASE OF DUNSTABLE ELBOW WITH SPASTIC DYSTONIA

*History*: A 45-year-old woman sustained spastic left hemiparesis due to a migraine stroke at 28 years of age. She presented with her typical daily posture of markedly

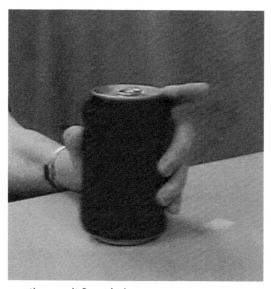

**Fig. 12.** Chemodenervation result 3 weeks later.

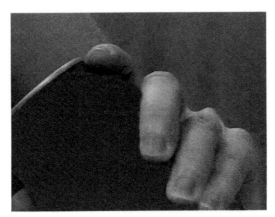

**Fig. 13.** Shows contact between index finger and soda can.

flexed elbow (**Fig. 14**). Some relaxation of the posture occurred when she was lying in bed at night.

*Examination*: Passive stretch of elbow flexors and elbow extensors was difficult to do, because there was increased resistance to passive movement in both directions.

*Laboratory*: Dynamic EMG of the elbow musculature (including extensor carpi radialis and anconeus) was performed. **Fig. 14** shows dystonic activity of all recorded muscles at rest, that is, when the patient and examiner did nothing to the arm.

*Commentary*: Dystonia after UMNS reflects the presence of muscle contraction in the absence of voluntary contraction, a triggered stretch reflex, or a nonstretch sensory trigger.[10] Dystonic activity is thought to result from an abnormal pattern of involuntary supraspinal drive, causing muscle activity at rest. In UMNS, dystonic muscles are often stretch sensitive, responding to the degree and duration of sustained stretch, hence, the term *spastic dystonia*. **Fig. 15** reveals the patient's spastic activity in biceps, brachioradialis, extensor carpi radialis, and pronator teres with low-grade activity in brachialis. Dystonic activity is observed in pronator teres, extensor carpi radialis, brachioradialis, and biceps before stretch onset and after stretch removal.

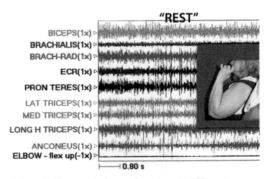

**Fig. 14.** Dystonic activity of all recorded muscles at rest. ECR, extensor carpi radialis; PRON TERES, pronator teres. (*From* Mayer NH, Esquenazi A. Upper limb skin and musculoskeletal consequences of the upper motor neuron syndrome. In: Jankovic J, editor. Botulinum toxin therapeutic clinical practice & science. Philadelphia: Elsevier; 2009. p. 137; with permission.)

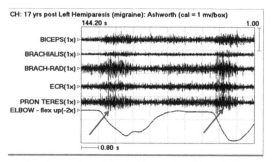

CH: 17 yrs post Left Hemiparesis (migraine): Ashworth (cal = 1 mv/box)

**Fig. 15.** Reveals the patient's spastic activity in biceps, brachioradialis, extensor carpi radialis, and pronator teres with low-grade activity in brachialis. The arrow points to spastic reactivity developing during muscle stretch. ECR, extensor carpi radialis.

## A CASE OF ROBIN HOOD'S RHEOLOGIC RESTRICTION

*History*: A 57-year-old man with right hemiparesis (cerebral palsy) complained he had difficulty opening his hand sufficiently to grasp, which was chronic since childhood. He had no sensory complaints.

*Examination*: His fingers extended more easily as wrist flexion increased (**Figs. 16** and **17**). As the examiner extended the wrist, active finger extension became slower and more effortful. Composite stretch of wrist and finger flexors was tight, range coming just to neutral and the finger, not the wrist, component was tight because full passive wrist extension was obtained when the patient's fingers were kept flexed. Clinical supposition suggested that spastic finger flexors were restraining active finger extension.

*Laboratory*: **Fig. 18** compares dynamic EMG of finger extensors and flexors performing alternating flexion/extension movements. There was no apparent increase of flexor EMG during the extension phase, ruling out spastic restraint of finger

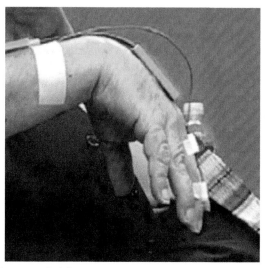

**Fig. 16.** Flexed wrist, extended fingers.

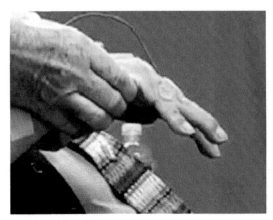

**Fig. 17.** Extended wrist, extended figures.

extension. Activity of the extensor digitorum communis (EDC) during the extension phase became strikingly more intense when the wrist was held extended by the examiner, indicating an increased load on EDC. Findings suggested that physical or rheologic tension of stretched finger flexors was restraining active finger extension.[11] Increased EDC activity with a more extended wrist reflects a need for greater activation of EDC to offset passive rheologic tension of finger flexors. Distinguishing between resistance due to spastic dystonia or tonic stretch reflex activity versus resistance due to rheologic properties of muscle is important because the distinction has therapeutic implications.[12] It would not be correct to treat such a patient with neurotoxin injection of finger flexors. Serial casting or fractional lengthening of the finger flexors may be considered.

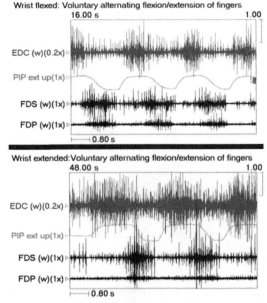

**Fig. 18.** Dynamic EMGs of finger extensors and flexors performing alternating flexion/extension movements. EDC, extensor digitorum communis.

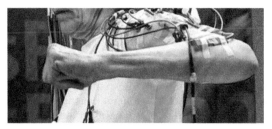

Fig. 19. Hyperextended wrist.

## A CASE OF TRAFALGAR SQUARE TENODESIS

*History*: A 64-year-old woman sustained a stroke with spastic left hemiparesis at 58 years of age (**Fig. 19**). She stated her chief complaint as "hard to pry open the left hand." Despite reduced sensation, she gave a positive history of hand usage, using visual guidance for hand-as-a-holder function. Nevertheless, clenched fingers restricted object size as the unaffected right hand attempted to push and wiggle objects into the left hand. She had some reaching ability and she was able to bring her hand to various parts of her body, but movements were effortful and slow. She could not work as a testing psychologist because of slow movement and restrictions on hand-as-a-holder function (**Fig. 20**). She underwent many treatments including constraint induced therapy, electrical stimulation and neurotoxin injections proximally and distally.

*Examination*: The examination revealed a Fugl-Meyer upper limb score of 32%. Her upper limb during walking revealed flexed elbow, hyperextended, radially deviated wrist, clenched fist and thumb-in-palm throughout swing and stance. Voluntary movements were slow and clumsy with motion appearing restrained at all joints. Her effort to reach forward revealed scapulothoracic protraction, glenohumeral flexion linked with some abduction, partial elbow extension, and a pronated forearm. She had no active forearm supination and poor control of active wrist

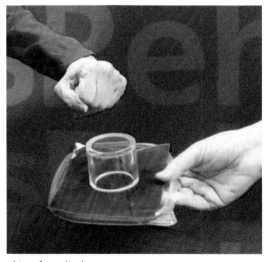

Fig. 20. Patient reaching for cylinder.

flexion and extension. There was a weak squeeze, more FDS than FDP, and no active finger extension. The thumb had weak IP joint volitional flexion and extension. Sensory examination showed diminished light touch (index, long, ring fingers) and diminished position sense (thumb).

Passive examination revealed a flexed elbow (**Fig. 21**), a hyperextended radially deviated wrist (see **Figs. 19–21**), and an FDS hand, that is, marked flexion of MCP and PIP joints with DIP joint extension. No finger or thumb joint contractures were present; but there were range limitations for hand intrinsics, extrinsic finger flexors, wrist flexors, forearm pronators, elbow flexors and extensors, shoulder adductors, extensors, and internal rotators. There was Ashworth 1 resistance of extrinsic finger flexors (wrist held neutral by the examiner). The finger intrinsics were very resistive to stretch (Ashworth technically not 4) (**Fig. 22**); thumb intrinsics (FPB mostly) had hypertonia (Ashworth 3), and FPL had minimal resistance (Ashworth 1). The wrist was extended at 40° in the rest position; the extrinsic finger flexors tightened strongly, consistent with tenodesis effect. The patient was observed inserting a series of calibrated cylinders with diameters of 0.5, 1.0, 1.5, 2.0, and 2.5 in into the affected clenched fist. She was only able to insert the 0.5-, 1.0-, and 1.5-in cylinders.

Clinical impression was binding dysfunction with tenodesis-driven clenched fist impairing access to the hand. Since the wrist and extrinsic and intrinsic finger and thumb muscles were involved, further clarification of muscle action was sought with poly-EMG. The authors generally record surface EMG; but, in this study, intramuscular wire electrodes were inserted into FDS, FDP, and EDC. Their location was confirmed by observing muscle contraction generated by electrical stimulation through the wire.

*Laboratory*: **Fig. 23** reveals weak recruitment of EDC activity during voluntary extension. But no finger extension was seen clinically. **Fig. 24** reveals activation of FDS and FDP during a task of volitional finger flexion. **Fig. 25** reveals low-grade spasticity to slow, moderate, and rapid passive stretch, FDS being more reactive than FDP. **Fig. 26** reveals considerable intrinsics spasticity except for first dorsal interosseous. At the wrist, **Fig. 27** reveals activation of wrist flexors but cocontraction of wrist

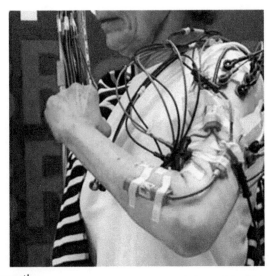

**Fig. 21.** Hand to mouth.

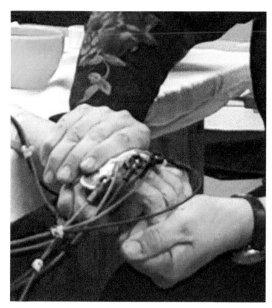

**Fig. 22.** Passive stretch of the finger intrinsics.

extensors restrains flexion movement (see wrist trace at bottom of **Fig. 27**). **Fig. 28** reveals spastic reactivity of the wrist extensors, especially ECR. **Fig. 29** displays voluntary alternating wrist flexion and extension movements. During the longer extension phase, wrist extensors were active but so were the cocontracting wrist flexors. The subsequent flexion phase was short and occurred by relaxation of all muscle groups. The wrist flexors were not reciprocally active during flexion. To achieve flexion, the patient allowed her wrist to drop passively rather than contract her wrist flexors actively. The net effect was to drive the wrist into greater hyperextension, one consequence being an enhancement of tenodesis finger flexion.

*Commentary*: **Fig. 30** reveals the tenodesis effect. Muscle-tendon tissue has physical or rheologic properties. When a muscle-tendon unit is stretched, it develops passive tension because of the inherent viscoelastic and plastic properties of tissue. When finger flexor tendons are stretched across the wrist joint during wrist extension,

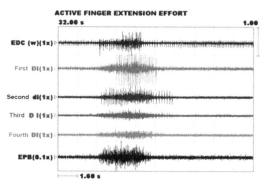

**Fig. 23.** Active finger extension effort. DI, dorsal interosseous; EDC, extensor digitorum communis; EPB, extensor pollicis brevis.

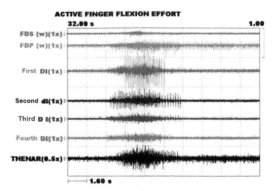

**Fig. 24.** Active finger flexion effort. DI, dorsal interosseous.

passive tension developing in the muscle/tendon unit exerts a flexion force acting on finger joints, flexing them as the wrist is extended. This effect is seen in the bottom hand of **Fig. 30**. The opposite effect of flexing the wrist puts the extrinsic finger flexors on slack while the finger extensors are stretched. Consequently, the patient's fingers extend, as seen in the top hand of **Fig. 30**.

Our patient's main problem was impaired hand opening. Dynamic EMG study revealed coactivation of EDC and the intrinsics during volitional extension effort (see **Fig. 23**). The intrinsics also had EMG features of spasticity and dystonia (see **Fig. 26**). An extended, radially deviated wrist was associated with extrinsic finger flexor tightness and a clenched fist configuration. Based on EMG findings, passive stretch of the finger flexors revealed only mild spastic reactivity so that finger flexion was interpreted as largely tenodesis driven. When she wanted to insert an object into her hand, she initially flexed her wrist with the unaffected hand in order to undo wrist hyperextension. Subsequently, she inserted the object with the wrist positioned about neutral. With the wrist in neutral, an intrinsic plus hand became manifest and because the intrinsics were spastic, object entry into the hand was constrained by an intrinsic plus hand. Changing the wrist angle shifted the clinical configuration from a clenched fist, tenodesis driven, to an intrinsic plus pattern, spastically/dystonically driven.

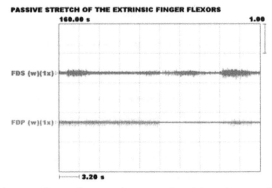

**Fig. 25.** Low-grade spasticity to slow, moderate, and rapid passive stretch; FDS being more reactive than FDP.

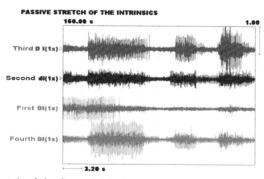

**Fig. 26.** Passive stretch of the finger intrinsics.

Because dynamic EMG revealed coactivation of EDC and the intrinsics (see **Fig. 23**), an ulnar nerve block was done at the wrist with lidocaine to see whether better finger extension could be unmasked if intrinsic antagonists, flexing the MCP joints, were weakened. In addition, blocking dystonic intrinsics might make object insertion easier. There was no improvement with an ulnar nerve block, the patient being unable to extend the fingers any better. No unmasking of EDC finger extension was seen. However, before and after videos of object insertion into the affected hand revealed quicker insertions and larger object sizes, likely reflecting reduced dystonic stiffness of the intrinsics.

Another key issue in the case was persistent wrist extension. During voluntary extension efforts (see **Fig. 29**), dynamic EMG revealed activation of wrist extensors together with wrist flexors (ie, spastic cocontraction). However, to flex the wrist, she did not activate wrist flexors but rather relaxed the extension effort, allowing the wrist to drop into (a small degree of) flexion. In the authors' view, spastic wrist extensors (see **Fig. 28**) and spastic cocontracting wrist flexors (see **Fig. 29**) combined with impaired flexor volition (while retaining extensor volition) promoted an extended wrist configuration that led to tenodesis-driven finger flexion rather than spastic finger flexion.

*Recommendations*: Although fractional lengthening of wrist extensors was a possibility, given the impaired volitional control of wrist flexors seen on dynamic EMG, the authors thought it would be difficult to achieve a balance between flexors and

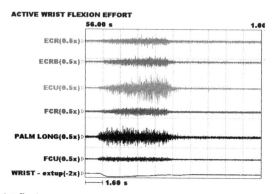

**Fig. 27.** Active wrist flexion.

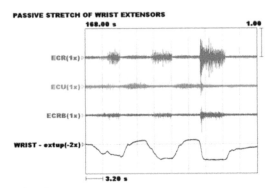

**Fig. 28.** Passive stretch wrist extensors.

extensors surgically. Therefore, a *wrist fusion* in neutral was recommended. The extrinsic finger flexors were not very tight with a neutral wrist; not being particularly spastic on dynamic EMG, the authors did not recommend fractional lengthening of the extrinsics. Tightness of finger flexors can be reassessed at the time of fusion surgery when anesthesia eliminates active muscle contraction completely. However, the authors did think lengthening the intrinsics was a consideration. If the intrinsics were lengthened and the wrist controlled by a fusion in neutral, the patient should be able to insert larger objects more easily into her hand, which was the patient's initially expressed functional goal.

## THE CASE OF PADDINGTON SHOULDER PARESIS

*History and brief examination*: A 38-year-old man sustained a bleeding aneurysm with left hemiparesis 8 months before the **Fig. 31** image. He was able to reach and place the hand in left, center, and right desk top spaces but complained of shoulder and arm weakness, particularly when holding his arm up during reach. Scapula protraction and 70° shoulder flexion was present when he reached forward. Elbow flexors exhibited spastic cocontraction, particularly brachioradialis, which popped up prominently during elbow extension. When performing alternating flexion/extension movements, extension phase was slower than flexion phase, suggesting restraint of extension by cocontracting flexors. He could open and close his hand for grasp and

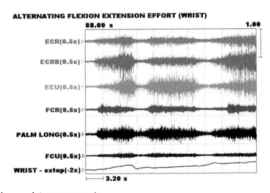

**Fig. 29.** Alternating wrist movements.

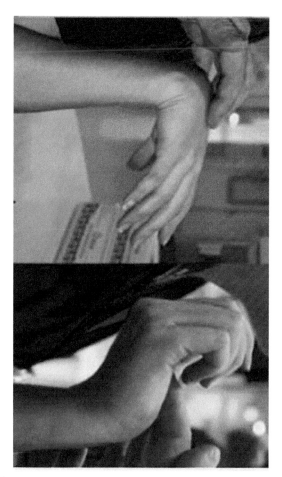

**Fig. 30.** Tenodesis.

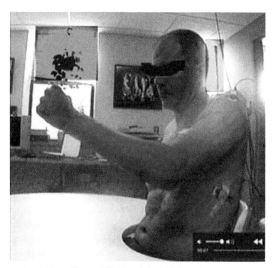

**Fig. 31.** Forward reach of the affected limb with 0-lb load.

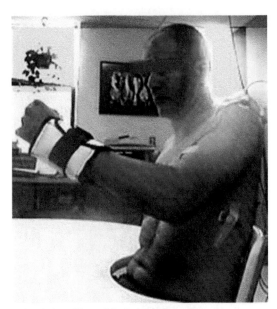

**Fig. 32.** Forward reach of the affected limb with 2-lb load.

release, but he did not have selective finger control. Finger extension was slower than flexion during alternating movements, suggesting extension restraint by cocontracting finger flexors.

*Laboratory*: Dynamic EMG of the upper, middle, and lower trapezii, latissimus dorsi, and serratus anterior was performed bilaterally. (Other muscles were recorded but not presented here.) Two conditions were imposed: reach forward with no weight and reach forward with a 2-lb weight on the wrist. **Figs. 31–34** reveal comparisons of left affected and right unaffected arm reaching. **Figs. 35–38** reveal dynamic EMG findings indicating that right upper and middle trapezius and serratus anterior on the unaffected side are active in the no load condition and become more active in the 2-lb load condition. On the affected side, left middle trapezius and serratus anterior recruit weakly in the no load condition and do not increase their activity in the 2-lb load condition. Note that the arm is held lower in the 2-lb condition on the affected side. Of

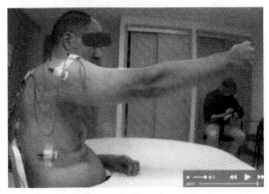

**Fig. 33.** Forward reach of the unaffected limb with 0-lb load.

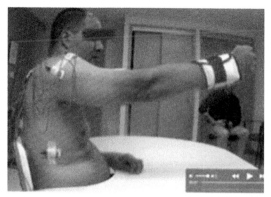

**Fig. 34.** Forward reach of the unaffected limb with 2-lb load.

interest is the large amount of left upper trapezius activity in the affected limb. This activity may represent compensatory activity of a muscle that was spared UMNS involvement.

*Comment*: What does weakness in the UMNS mean? The syntax of a voluntary act begins with an intention, for example, intention to eliminate morning breath. Intention activates a search for resources: toothpaste, toothbrush, cup, mouthwash, and so on. Acts (motor programs) are selected to use these resources. Movements and postures, such as reach, push, pull, and many others, make up

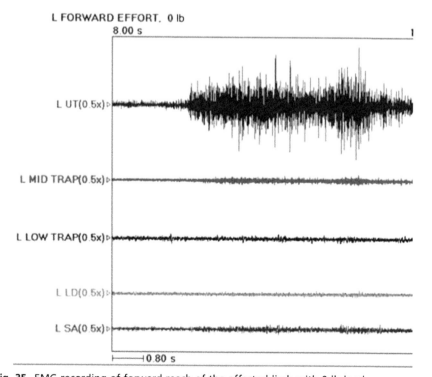

**Fig. 35.** EMG recording of forward reach of the affected limb with 0-lb load.

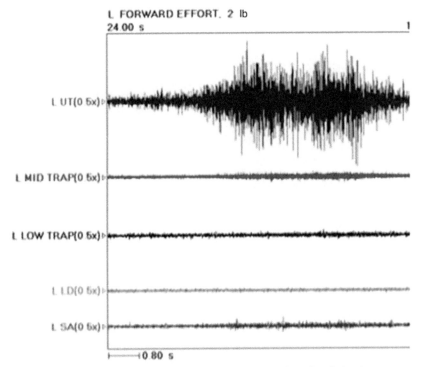

**Fig. 36.** EMG recording of forward reach of the affected limb with 2-lb load.

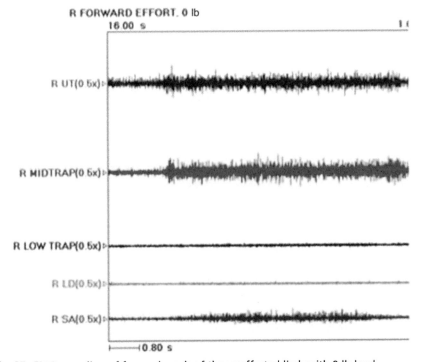

**Fig. 37.** EMG recording of forward reach of the unaffected limb with 0-lb load.

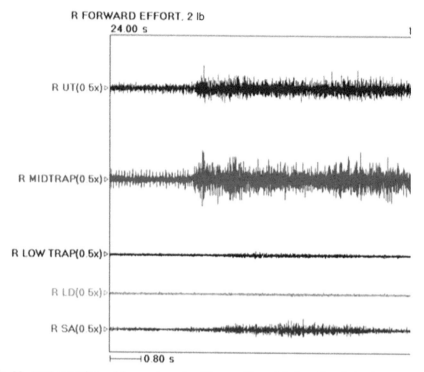

R FORWARD EFFORT, 2 lb
24.00 s

R UT(0 5x)▷

R MIDTRAP(0 5x)▷

R LOW TRAP(0 5x)▷

R LD(0 5x)▷

R SA(0 5x)▷

├────┤0.80 s

**Fig. 38.** EMG recording of forward reach of the unaffected limb with 2-lb load.

the components of acts. For a given intention (eg, elimination of morning breath) to achieve a specific (invariant) outcome (eg, freshened mouth), one or more acts with their component movements are assembled for production. Movements themselves (eg, reach, push, turn) are composed of muscle assemblies operated by motor programs. In the first half of the twentieth century, Lashley[13] had already pointed out that the same act could be executed by different effectors, a principle he called motor equivalence.[13–15] For example, one can write the letter B with one's arm on a blackboard or with one's leg on beach sand. It is as if the motor idea behind the act of writing the letter B floats free of a particular limb or muscle/joint assembly used to execute the act. The invariant outcome, namely, the written letter B, can be accomplished by different muscle synergies, that is, flexible combinations of muscle groups.[16,17] In UMNS, weakness reflects an impairment of specific muscle synergies required to carry out specific intentional acts. For example, reaching forward to grasp an object may partly require activation of the anterior, middle, and posterior deltoid in various degrees of contraction, more contraction of the anterior deltoid, less of the middle and posterior deltoid. If a corticospinal tract lesion interrupts descending signal transmissions to the anterior deltoid more than the middle and posterior deltoid, the net effect is likely to be a more abducted shoulder. Weakness reflects the degree to which signal transmission is impaired to each of the muscles assembled as a specific synergy for a specific voluntary movement. Because central lesions are typically variable, weakness of synergies will vary clinically; in particular, if a specific movement does not depend very much on a specific muscle, impaired transmission to that muscle will have less effect on an intended movement. This idea implies that the outcome or movement effect of some muscle synergies may be spared more than others. From this perspective, clinical manual muscle testing would not seem to be a helpful guide toward predicting what patients might be able to do in a different motor context. In the case presented in **Figs. 31–38**, reduced transmission to middle trapezius and serratus anterior on the affected side, reflected in reduced EMG activity, contributed to weakness of the shoulder (as experienced by the patient and revealed by video imaging). Increased activity of left upper trapezius may reflect motor equivalence, use of an available effector in a different way than on the unaffected side. The use of hip and trunk flexion compensation by a hemiparetic to advance the hand forward when reaching is another familiar example of motor equivalence.[18,19]

*Final comments*: The consequences of a UMNS include the following:

- Weakness: movement outcome resulting from the degree to which voluntary signal transmission is impaired to each of the muscles assembled and expressed as a specific synergy underlying a specific voluntary movement
- Involuntary phenomena (spastic cocontraction, spasticity, spastic dystonia, associated reactions, increased flexor reflex activity) superimposed on voluntary movement
- Rheologic (viscoelastic and plastic) changes in muscle superimposed on voluntary movement

It is often difficult to sort out the degree to which observed motor behavior is neural voluntary, neural involuntary, and/or non-neural rheologic. Nevertheless, the degree to which differentiation can be made clinically will likely lead to more rational treatment.

## REFERENCES

1. Phillips CG. Proceedings: Hughlings Jackson lecture. Cortical localization and "sensorimotor processes" at the "middle level" in primates. Proc R Soc Med 1973;66(10):987–1002.

2. Gerber C, Krushell RJ. Isolated rupture of the tendon of the subscapularis muscle. Clinical features in 16 cases. J Bone Joint Surg Br 1991;73(3):389–94.

3. Yelnik AP, Colle FM, Bonan IV, et al. Treatment of shoulder pain in spastic hemiplegia by reducing spasticity of the subscapular muscle: a randomised, double blind, placebo controlled study of botulinum toxin. J Neurol Neurosurg Psychiatry 2007;78:845–8.

4. Mayer NH, Esquenazi A. Muscle overactivity and movement dysfunction in the upper motoneuron syndrome. Phys Med Rehabil Clin N Am 2003;14:855–83.

5. Esquenazi A, Cioni M, Mayer NH. Assessment of muscle overactivity and spasticity with dynamic polyelectromyography and motion analysis. Open Rehabil J 2010;3:143–8.

6. Brys D, Waters RL. Effect of triceps function on the brachioradialis transfer in quadriplegia. J Hand Surg Am 1987;12(2):237–9.

7. Mayer N. Choosing upper limb muscles for focal intervention after traumatic brain injury. J Head Trauma Rehabil 2004;19(2):119–42.

8. Keenan MAE, Mayer NH, Esquenazi A, et al. Neuro-orthopaedic approach to the management of common patterns of upper motoneuron dysfunction after brain injury. Neuro Rehab 1999;12(2):119–44.

9. Walshe FMR. On certain tonic or postural reflexes in hemiplegia, with special reference to the so-called 'associated movements'. Brain 1923;46:1–37.

10. Sheean G, McGuire JR. Spastic hypertonia and movement disorders: pathophysiology, clinical presentation, and quantification. PM R 2009;1(9):827–33.
11. Mayer NH. Clinicophysiologic concepts of spasticity and motor dysfunction in adults with an upper motoneuron lesion. Muscle Nerve Suppl 1997;6:S1–13.
12. Hufschmidt A, Mauritz KH. Chronic transformation of muscle in spasticity: a peripheral contribution to increased tone. J Neurol Neurosurg Psychiatry 1985;48:676–85.
13. Lashley KS. Basic neural mechanisms in behavior. Psychol Rev 1930;37:1–24.
14. Marteniuk RG, Ivens CJ, Bertram CP. Evidence of motor equivalence in a pointing task involving locomotion. Motor Control 2000;4(2):165–84.
15. Kelso JA, Fuchs A, Lancaster R, et al. Dynamic cortical activity in the human brain reveals motor equivalence. Nature 1998;392(6678):814–8.
16. Tresch MC, Jarc A. The case for and against muscle synergies. Curr Opin Neurobiol 2009;19(6):601–12.
17. Rijntjes M, Dettmers C, Buchel C, et al. A blueprint for movement: functional and anatomical representations in the human motor system. J Neurosci 1999;19(18):8043–8.
18. Levin MF. Interjoint coordination during pointing movements is disrupted in spastic hemiparesis. Brain 1996;119(1):281–93.
19. Cirstea MC, Levin MF. Compensatory strategies for reaching in stroke. Brain 2000;123(5):940–53.

# Lower Extremity Problem-Solving: Challenging Cases

Daniel K. Moon, MD, MS[a],*, Ashley M.F. Johnson, MD[b]

## KEYWORDS

- Upper motor neuron syndrome • Muscle overactivity • Spasticity • Contracture
- Gait dysfunction • Equinovarus • Stiff knee deformity • Flexed knee deformity

## KEY POINTS

- Muscle overactivity, weakness, impaired motor control, and contracture can all play a role in lower limb dysfunction associated with upper motor neuron syndrome; however, muscle overactivity can also provide some benefits to the patient.
- Delineating the contribution of muscle overactivity from other factors, such as weakness or contracture, is the cornerstone of evaluation and management.
- Conservative treatment consists of identifying and addressing noxious stimuli, therapies, orthotics, and oral medications.
- Impairments due to focal muscle overactivity may be treated with chemodenervation or neurolysis to select muscles.
- Orthopedic surgery can correct underlying contracture not amenable to conservative management, as well as augment weakness via tendon transfers.

## INTRODUCTION

Increased tone and muscle overactivity in the lower limbs is a commonly encountered sequela of upper motor neuron syndrome that can have a significant impact on the patient's medical management, function, quality of life, and caregiver burden.[1] The most commonly described example of muscle overactivity is spasticity, which is velocity-dependent resistance to stretch.[2] Approximately one-eighth of traumatic brain injury, one-third of stroke, two-thirds of multiple sclerosis, and three-quarters of cerebral palsy patients will develop lower limb spasticity.[3] There is also a substantial financial

Disclosure: The authors have nothing to disclose.
[a] The Sheerr Gait and Motion Analysis Laboratory, The Motor Control Analysis Laboratory, Department of Physical Medicine and Rehabilitation, MossRehab, Einstein Healthcare Network, 60 Township Line Road, Elkins Park, PA 19027, USA; [b] Department of Physical Medicine and Rehabilitation, Temple University Hospital, 3401 North Broad Street, Philadelphia, PA 19140, USA
* Corresponding author. MossRehab, Department of Physical Medicine and Rehabilitation, 60 Township Line Road, Elkins Park, PA 19027.
E-mail address: moondani@einstein.edu

burden tied to spasticity. A Swedish study cited a 4-fold increase in direct cost of management of patients with spasticity in the first year after stroke compared with patients without spasticity.[4] Although evaluation and management of upper limb and lower limb spasticity share common principles, the potential for improving ambulation and transfers through a multimodal and multidisciplinary approach necessitates a separate dedicated review.

Spasticity is an often-used term to describe a collection of signs due to increased muscle tone and/or activity following injury to the central nervous system. However, there are other patterns of muscle overactivity encountered in patients with central nervous system disorders that are often confused with spasticity, including dystonia, clonus, myoclonus, flexor and extensor spasms, rigidity, and athetosis.[5] Before treating, the clinician should confirm that there is indeed underlying muscle overactivity. Otherwise, treatment may be misguided and the patient may be unnecessarily exposed to potential adverse effects such as sedation and increased weakness.[6] First, the clinician should consider if treatment is indicated because spasticity and other forms of muscle overactivity are clinical signs but may not necessarily be causing symptoms or interfering with function or care. Spasticity also provides numerous benefits. When these benefits can be isolated and exploited solely to the advantage of the patient and/or caregiver, both functional and clinical outcomes can be positively affected (**Table 1**). However, spasticity rarely presents without some troubling effects that cause symptoms or impede function (**Fig. 1**). Three main areas of concern to consider when defining treatment goals are symptom relief, passive function, and active function (**Fig. 2**). Symptoms are subjective observations by the patient that cannot be measured directly, such as pain. Symptoms also need to be correlated with clinical signs to ensure they are being addressed. Passive function is applied to or acted on the patient for care either by themselves or the caregiver, such as dressing and hygiene. Active function is initiated by the patient herself or himself, such as ambulation and transfers. These 3 areas are closely interrelated and addressing any aspect may affect another. The goals of treatment should be established before initiating treatment and after discussion between the treatment team, patient, and/or caregiver. The nature of these goals strongly affects the treatment approach for each patient, emphasizing the individualized nature of each patient care plan.

The treatment approach will vary depending on the stage of recovery and if the problem is focal versus systemic. The clinician may take a sequential approach, a synergistic approach, or a combination of the two when managing issues related to muscle overactivity. The sequential model of treatment is a step-wise approach to intervention that begins with the most conservative treatments and gradually incorporate more aggressive treatments as needed. This approach allows the clinician and treatment team to systematically assess the efficacy of treatment options, limit

| Table 1 |
| --- |
| **Potential benefits and consequences of muscle overactivity associated with the upper motor neuron syndrome** |

| Benefits | Consequences |
| --- | --- |
| • Prevention of deep vein thrombosis | • Skin breakdown |
| • Support of circulatory function | • Pain |
| • Maintain muscle tone | • Joint dislocations, subluxations, or fractures |
| • Assist in standing and/or transfers | • Masks volitional movement |
| | • Can impair respiratory function |
| | • Impedes balance and ambulation |
| | • Restrict joint motion and may lead to contracture |

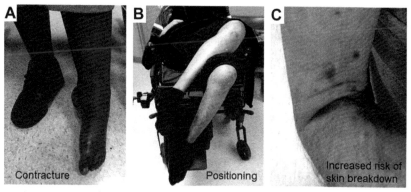

**Fig. 1.** Consequences of spasticity include (*A*) limitations in passive and active range of motion that can potentially lead to contracture, (*B*) abnormal positioning or seating and increased risk of pressure ulcer, and (*C*) reduced aeration leading to moisture buildup with risk of infection and skin breakdown.

confounding feedback, and escalate treatment from conservative to more aggressive measures only when deemed necessary. Whereas, the synergistic model of treatment allows the treatment team to utilize several modes of treatment simultaneously in attempt to address patient's symptoms and obtain goals as swiftly as possible. The sequential approach is appropriate when close monitoring may not be feasible, symptoms are relatively mild, or the patient is at high risk of adverse effects from treatment. The synergistic approach is often implemented in the inpatient setting where the patient is treated by a multidisciplinary clinical team and can be closely monitored; time

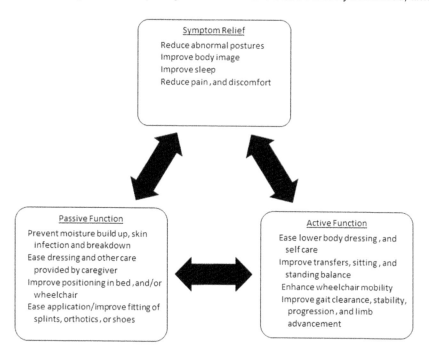

**Fig. 2.** Goals of treatment should address patient's symptoms, passive function, and active function, which are usually interrelated and can affect patient's quality of life.

is of the essence, especially if symptoms are severe. Regardless of approach, clinical decision-making should continually be guided by clearly delineated goals of treatment as established between the clinician, patient, and/or caregiver. This article describes 3 challenging patient cases and reviews approaches to assessment and treatment of issues due to lower limb spasticity.

## Case 1

The patient is an 18-year-old man involved in a motor vehicle accident 1 month prior, now currently in inpatient rehabilitation. He sustained hemorrhages to the right cerebellum, bilateral thalami, and basal ganglia, in addition to diffuse axonal injury. He is in a minimally conscious state and has increased tone in both lower extremities interfering with his care, especially perineal hygiene. He also has erythema at the right lateral foot over a bony protuberance. His physical examination demonstrates severe bilateral equinovarus deformities that are in approximately 50° plantarflexion and 30° of inversion with right claw toe deformity. With attempted passive dorsiflexion, the right ankle remains fixed at −50° but there is 10° of dorsiflexion on the left side to −40°. It is slightly easier to passively evert the ankles with the right ankle reaching −5° eversion and the left ankle reaching neutral. The tone of the ankles is rated 4 bilaterally on the Modified Ashworth Scale. The right hip and knee are maintained in extension and are also difficult to passively flex. The left hip and knee assume a flexed attitude with the hip adducted but the examiner can passively range the joint to neutral at the hip and knee. The tone is rated 3 on the Modified Ashworth Scale for the right hip and knee extensors, as well as the left hip adductors and knee flexors.

Prolonged hospitalization and bedrest, especially in the context of injury to the central nervous system, predisposes the patient to developing increased tension or tone in the lower limbs. However, it is important for the clinician to determine the cause of this increased tone because, although a patient may have an upper motor neuron syndrome, there may also be an underlying lower motor neuron pathologic condition and/or contracture contributing to the patient's presentation. Therefore, the first step in approaching management of this patient's increased tone is to determine the cause. The clinician should consider a broad differential. Potential causes of increased tone include the following: spasticity, dystonia, rigidity, contracture, bone, and/or joint deformity due to fracture or heterotopic ossification and volitional resistance to stretch. There are numerous treatment options for increased tone but initial evaluation and management should attempt to address potential nociceptive stimuli that may be exacerbating the underlying muscle overactivity and may even render subsequent treatments less effective (**Table 2**). In some cases, removal of noxious stimuli may sufficiently control symptoms alone.

**Table 2**
**Examples of nociceptive factors that could exacerbate muscle overactivity**

| Cause | Examples |
| --- | --- |
| Infectious | Pneumonia, viral illness, cellulitis, urinary tract infection |
| Gastroenterological | Constipation, fecal impaction, diet changes |
| Orthopedic | Fracture, sprains, heterotopic ossification |
| Integumentary | Pressure ulcers, ingrown toe nails |
| Vascular | Deep vein thrombosis |
| Genitourinary | Urinary retention, nephrolithiasis |

*Interim history*

Initial work up reveals a urinary tract infection and constipation. Radiological studies do not show any fracture. He is treated with antibiotics and placed on a bowel regimen after which the tone in the hip and knee flexors improves. Hip adductor tone remains problematic, especially with hygiene. This issue improves after he undergoes phenol neurolysis of the left obturator nerve. He continues to demonstrate severe equinovarus deformities at the ankle and there is concern for skin breakdown over the bony protuberance of his right lateral foot. He undergoes bilateral diagnostic tibial nerve blocks with lidocaine. The passive range of motion of the right ankle improves slightly from $-50°$ to $-40°$ dorsiflexion but does not change for the left ankle.

A diagnostic nerve block is a valuable tool in the clinician's armamentarium because it allows the clinician to determine if the joint deformity is due to abnormal neuromuscular activity or a fixed shortening of the muscle-tendon complex or other connective tissues.[7,8] Using anatomic or ultrasound guidance in conjunction with electrical stimulation, the nerve innervating the suspected antagonistic muscles is localized and injected with anesthetic to cause a temporary nerve block and reducing activity in the distal innervated muscles. If passive and/or active range of motion of the joint does not improve after the procedure, the clinician can more confidently conclude the increased tone is due to contracture and that treating the spasticity alone would not have a significant effect. However, this does not mean the underlying muscle overactivity does not need to be addressed because shortening of the muscle tendon complex will likely reduce the threshold for stretch reactivity, which may interfere with subsequent treatments such as splinting and casting. Underlying stretch reactivity of the muscle can be confirmed with surface or needle electromyography if questionable on physical examination.

Diagnostic nerve blocks not only differentiate the dynamic neurogenic component from the static soft tissue contracture component but can also determine potential benefits of treatment with chemodenervation or neurolysis, as well as identify potential undesirable outcomes such as excess weakness. Additionally, a temporary nerve block with a longer acting anesthetic, such as bupivacaine, may be useful to facilitate stretching and serial casting.

Therapeutic nerve and motor point blocks (chemical neurolysis) performed with an aqueous solution of phenol (5%–7%) or ethyl alcohol (50%–100%) can be very effective in the treatment of issues due to spasticity. The duration of efficacy can vary depending on the extent of neurolysis but has been reported to last anywhere from 3 months to several years.[9] Mixed sensory-motor nerves are typically avoided to prevent painful dysesthesias that may result from neurolysis of sensory nerves. The authors recommend using a needle connected to a syringe with tubing for maintenance of the position of the needle tip after localization for accuracy during injection and withdrawal and to avoid infiltrating a vessel because vascular thrombosis is a potential complication.[10] In large quantities, systemic exposure may cause seizures, central nervous system depression, respiratory issues, and cardiovascular collapse.[11] However, doses injected for neurolysis are a fraction of the lethal dose.

Other options to consider for management of increased tone in conjunction with physical modalities are enteral agents such as baclofen, tizanidine, valium, and dantrolene; however, the side effects may not be well-tolerated. Intrathecal baclofen therapy, though not typically recommended early in the period after brain injury recovery, has been shown to be effective in treating severe cases refractory to other modalities.[12]

*Further interim history*

The patient's arousal and participation in therapies continue to improve but he is unable to tolerate serial casting of bilateral ankles due to pain and discomfort, despite phenol motor point blocks to the gastrocnemius and soleus to reduce underlying spasticity. He is now able to stand for short periods with maximal assistance but progress is severely limited by equinovarus deformity of the ankles. He is referred to orthopedic surgery and undergoes bilateral split anterior tibialis tendon transfer (SPLATT), tendo-Achilles lengthening (TAL), and myotendinous lengthening of the tibialis posterior and right toe flexors. The patient completes inpatient rehabilitation and is then discharged home. He is seen in outpatient clinic 1 year later with a new complaint of toe discomfort with weightbearing on the left side. He is ambulating with only a single-point cane. On examination, passive range of motion of the ankles is improved with dorsiflexion to neutral on the right side and to 10° on the left side. Ankle clonus is elicited on the left side. Observation of barefoot walking reveals curling of the toes during left stance phase. He undergoes intramuscular botulinum toxin injections to the left flexor digitorum longus and flexor hallucis longus with subsequent improvement.

Equinovarus deformities are commonly observed in patients with upper motor neuron syndrome, especially following hospitalization with prolonged bedrest, in which the foot and ankle tend to rest in this position. In addition, the net balance of muscles acting at the ankle favor plantarflexion and inversion. In some cases, severe inversion may result in the formation of bony prominences that increase risk of skin breakdown over the lateral foot (**Fig. 3**). When attempting to walk, patients may complain of pain on the lateral forefoot due to abnormal weightbearing. Restricted ankle dorsiflexion also prevents forward progression during midstance and may impair limb clearance in the swing phase, especially if the hip flexors are also impaired. Mild cases may respond to implementation of an ankle-foot orthosis (AFO) with an

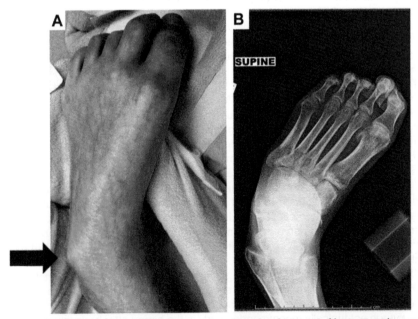

**Fig. 3.** (*A*) Severe equinovarus deformities can result in development of bony protuberances (*black arrow*), which can be prone to erythema and skin breakdown. (*B*) Associated radiograph of severe equinovarus deformity.

inversion control strap. A heel lift can be incorporated into the bracing system or shoe to accommodate the plantarflexion deformity and promote weightbearing through the heel.

Overactivity in most of these muscles could potentially be treated with neurolysis of the tibial nerve but, even if done correctly, there is a risk of dysesthesias. However, motor points for the gastrocnemius and soleus can be localized superficially and treated followed by serial casting to facilitate stretching of the plantarflexors. Spasticity of the gastrocnemius, soleus, tibialis posterior, flexor digitorum longus, flexor hallucis longus, and/or tibialis anterior can contribute to the equinovarus deformity and be targeted with focal chemodenervation.[13,14] In certain ambulatory patients, a flexed knee deformity from overactive or contracted hamstrings may also predispose a patient to bear weight on the forefoot and develop an equinus deformity.

Surgical interventions such as TAL; SPLATT; and myotendinous lengthening of the tibialis posterior, extensor hallucis longus, flexor hallucis longus, and flexor digitorum longus may be considered and can dramatically improve patient function by correcting the equinovarus contracture.[15–19] To supplement weak ankle plantar flexors, in addition to addressing toe curling, a release and transfer of the long toe flexors to the os calcaneus can be considered.[20]

Another consideration in this case is that surgical overcorrection of the equinovarus deformity could lead to excessive dorsiflexion and/or pronation of the ankle, which can cause excessive toe curling via tenodesis, especially if the toe flexors were not addressed surgically. Therefore, an AFO designed to limit dorsiflexion and valgus may subsequently help reduce toe curling.

## Case 2

A 60-year-old woman with right spastic hemiparesis resulting from a stroke 4 years ago presents to clinic with complaints of stiffness at the right knee and being unable to pick up her right leg when she walks. She is currently taking tizanidine and baclofen with some symptomatic improvement; however, she is unable to tolerate increased doses of these medications due to worsening sedation. She underwent a SPLATT, TAL, and lengthening of the tibialis posterior and toe flexors 1 year ago. She denies any trips or falls. On physical examination her right ankle is able to reach 5° passive dorsiflexion with the knee flexed and extended. An instrumented gait analysis is repeated along with dynamic surface electromyography of the muscles acting on the right hip and knee joint. Kinematic data reveals reduced right hip and knee flexion during swing phase (**Fig. 4**A). Dynamic electromyographic recordings demonstrate prolonged activity of the quadriceps muscles, hamstrings, and gluteus maximus. Based on these findings, she is offered 2 options to address the right stiff knee gait pattern: chemodenervation with botulinum toxin or surgical intervention. The patient ultimately undergoes a rectus femoris to gracilis transfer and demonstrates improved hip and knee flexion at her follow-up appointment 6 months later (**Figs. 4**B and **5**).

Observational gait analysis is commonly used but can be inadequate and vary from clinician to clinician. Instrumented gait analysis is a more objective method of evaluating a spastic gait dysfunction for treatment planning and can include temporal spatial parameters, joint kinematics, and kinetic and dynamic polyelectromyography.[21] The assessment should attempt to answer the following questions:

- Which muscles can the patient activate and to what degree?
- Which muscles are activated in response to stretch or are spastic?
- Which muscles are cocontracting as an antagonist during active movement?
- Does the joint have limitations due to a contracture?

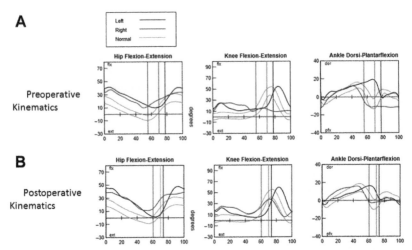

**Fig. 4.** Preoperative (*A*) and postoperative (*B*) kinematics obtained on patient presented in case 2. Note the improvement in peak knee flexion during swing phase in the right knee following a rectus femoris to gracilis transfer.

When instrumented gait analysis is not available, some of these questions can be answered with the use of video analysis and diagnostic nerve blocks, in addition to a detailed physical examination.

The stiff knee gait pattern typically results from a dynamic deformity created by abnormal muscle contraction and external joint moments, which can lead to impaired limb clearance and advancement. Abnormalities in both stance and swing phase can contribute to this gait dysfunction. Ankle equinus contributes to the stiff knee gait pattern by preventing forward progression of the tibia in stance, leading to hyperextension of the knee. Out-of-phase activation of the knee and hip extensor muscles in swing phase (cocontraction activity) may also be a culprit. Other considerations in the differential are slow walkers and patients with weak hip flexor muscles because they may not be able to generate enough forward momentum of the thigh to adequately flex the knee in swing phase. If the leg is maintained in external rotation, either to allow the hip adductors to advance the limb or to allow roll over a plantarflexed ankle, then the medial collateral ligament is preventing flexion of the knee in swing, resulting in a stiff knee gait pattern. Finally, a patient may generate an extensor moment at the knee in stance phase with forward trunk lean to compensate for weak calf muscles or hamstring overactivity to prevent buckling, which may subsequently carry over into swing phase. The development of genu recurvatum can also reinforce the stiff knee gait pattern because more work will be required from the hip flexors to overcome knee hyperextension. Contracture of the knee extensor complex and internal deformities should also be ruled out. Regardless of cause, shoe modifications such as contralateral lifts and ipsilateral toe sliders are recommended to assist with clearance and prevent trips and falls.

If stiff knee gait persists despite treatment of the ankle plantarflexors, a diagnostic block of the quadriceps and/or hamstrings will help not only determine the offending muscles but can also predict if treatment will result in knee instability. Based on the results, neurolysis or chemodenervation can be performed on select antagonistic muscles.[22,23] Surgical lengthening of the rectus femoris with or without

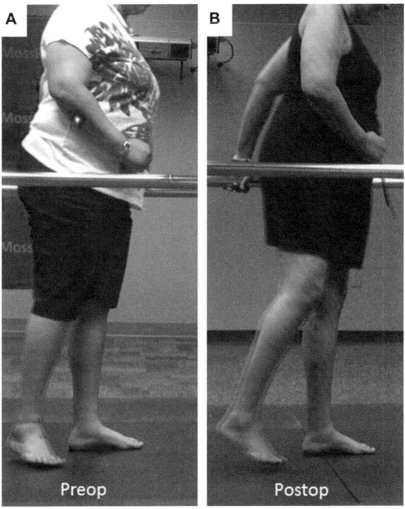

**Fig. 5.** Comparison of sagittal views of patient preoperative (*A*) and postoperative (*B*) during swing phase, demonstrating increased knee flexion and improved clearance following a rectus femoris to gracilis transfer.

the vastus intermedius can also be considered.[24–26] Alternatively, transfer of the rectus femoris to the semitendinosus, gracilis, sartorius, or iliotibial band may be done to augment weak hip flexors and may be more effective at improving swing phase knee flexion.[25–28]

### Case 3

A 36-year-old woman with history of right hemiparesis due to a stroke sustained as a complication of surgery over 30 years ago presents to outpatient clinic with complaints of right hip and buttock pain after slipping and falling on ice. She has history of derotational osteotomy of the femur, myotendinous lengthening of the hamstrings and rectus femoris, TAL, and SPLATT on the right side. She was previously ambulating with a platform rolling walker and a right-molded AFO. Her examination is limited by pain but her right hip is noted to be adducted and internally rotated with the knee flexed. Radiographs of her hip reveal chronic hip dysplasia, as well as a new supero-lateral subluxation of the right femoral head (**Fig. 6**). She undergoes a periacetabular osteotomy and is discharged to inpatient rehabilitation. She demonstrates right hip and knee flexion posturing limiting her ability to bear weight. With passive range of motion, her right knee lacks 20° extension but she experiences flexor spasms at end range. The examiner is unable to fully test hip range due to postoperative precautions. Spasms persist despite pain control and treatment of spasms with baclofen and valium. She is prescribed a right knee-AFO (KAFO) but she continues to report symp-toms of tightness and pain in the hamstrings.

This case illustrates some of the consequences of aging with a disability, especially when spasticity is involved. Ambulating with a spastic paretic limb or limbs and asso-ciated compensatory behaviors can exert abnormal stresses on the muscles and joints, leading to altered bone and joint development. Complications such as hip dysplasia, increased pelvic obliquity, and scoliosis, as well as accelerated joint degen-eration, can occur. It is not uncommon for patients who were doing reasonably well to have a sudden dramatic decline in function following an illness or injury due to either increased weakness, pain, and spasticity or to further loss in range of motion. These patients warrant close follow-up and, in some cases, a course of inpatient rehabilita-tion to aggressively manage their pain and spasticity and to maximize potential for re-turn to baseline function.

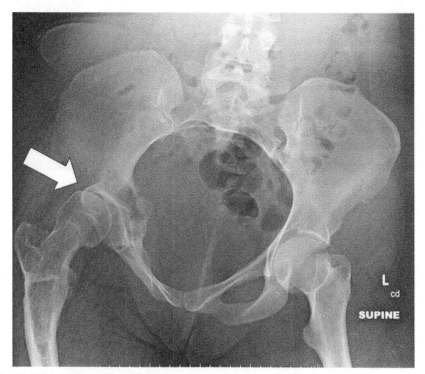

**Fig. 6.** Pelvic radiograph of patient with chronic hemiplegia since childhood showing dysplastic changes in the right acetabulum, as well as the superior subluxation of the femoral head (*white arrow*) following a fall.

### Interim history

She eventually undergoes chemodenervation of the medial and lateral hamstrings with botulinum toxin at outpatient follow-up. This not only results in reduction in knee flexor spasms but also allows the patient to trial ambulation with the KAFO's knee joint unlocked in physical therapy. She eventually is able to safely progress to a floor reaction AFO and a left forearm crutch for ambulation (**Fig. 7**).

The patient demonstrates hip and knee flexor spasticity exacerbated by postoperative pain. At first glance, it seems the hip flexor spasms are eliciting knee flexor spasms because these are often related owing to the biarticular action of the rectus femoris and hamstring muscles. However, on examination, isolated hamstring spasms are elicited with stretch with subsequent hip flexor spasms. If medications to control pain and spasticity are inadequate or poorly tolerated, neurolysis or chemodenervation should be considered. Direct neurolysis of the sciatic nerve would be discouraged owing to its large sensory component but motor point injections along the medial and lateral hamstrings can be helpful. However, chemodenervation with botulinum toxin to the hamstrings is preferred because this has reduced risk of dysesthesias and fibrosis, and is easier to perform. If hip flexion persists, the clinician should also consider treatment of the rectus femoris and iliopsoas. An intrathecal baclofen pump can be considered, especially if the pain and spasticity are interrelated, and would reduce the need for repeat injections. If contracture is significant, consider surgical lengthening of the hamstring muscles.[29] Also, the clinician should ensure the bowel and bladder regimen

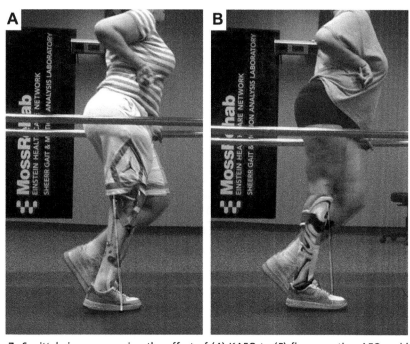

**Fig. 7.** Sagittal views comparing the effect of (*A*) KAFO to (*B*) floor reaction AFO and botulinum toxin injections to the hamstrings on patient's right midstance phase. (*A*) Note how the ground reaction force (*red line*) projects behind the knee with KAFO, exerting a flexor moment on the knee; however, (*B*) implementation of a floor reaction orthosis promotes projection of this force anterior to the knee joint center, thus exerting an extensor moment and providing further stabilization to the joint.

is optimized because constipation and retention can further exacerbate hip and knee flexor spasticity.

Patients should ideally have the least restrictive orthosis to maximize comfort and compliance, as well as minimize weight. A properly prescribed and fitted orthoses can compensate for neuromuscular and structural deficiencies. A KAFO with a locking knee joint is an effective mechanism for controlling severe knee instability due to quadriceps weakness or knee flexor spasms but can be heavy and difficult to manage. A floor reaction AFO is a rear entry brace designed to limit dorsiflexion at the ankle, which can prevent potential knee buckling, making it a good alternative to a KAFO in select patients.

## DISCUSSION

Patients with lower limb dysfunction resulting from spasticity and other patterns of muscle overactivity can be quite complex and require management with a multidisciplinary team consisting of a physiatrist, physical therapist, occupational therapist, orthotist, orthopedic surgeon, and/or neurosurgeon. A comprehensive team approach should be goal-directed and team members should be cognizant of each patient's unique needs to maximize the potential for functional gains, minimize caregiver burden, and ultimately improve quality of life. However, it is important to balance the patient and family's desire to return to premorbid status with realistic expectations while continuing to encourage and work toward progress.

## REFERENCES

1. Esquenazi A. The human and economic burden of poststroke spasticity and muscle overactivity. JCOM 2011;18(1):607–14.
2. Lance JW. Symposium synopsis. In: Feldman RG, Young RR, Koella WP, editors. Spasticity: disordered motor control. Chicago: Yearbook Medical; 1980. p. 485–94.
3. Martin A, Abogunrin S, Kurth H, et al. Epidemiological, humanistic, and economic burden of illness of lower limb spasticity in adults: a systematic review. Neuropsychiatr Dis Treat 2014;1:111–22.
4. Lundström E, Smits A, Borg J, et al. Four-fold increase in direct costs of stroke survivors with spasticity compared with stroke survivors without spasticity: the first year after the event. Stroke 2010;41:319–24.
5. Mayer NH, Herman RM. Phenomenology of muscle overactivity in the upper motor neuron syndrome. Eura Medicophys 2004;40(2):85–110.
6. Chang E, Ghosh N, Yanni D, et al. A review of spasticity treatments: pharmacological and interventional approaches. Crit Rev Phys Rehabil Med 2013;25(1–2):11–22.
7. Mayer N, Esquenazi A, Keenan MAE. Analysis and management of spasticity, contracture and impaired motor control. In: Horn L, Zasler N, editors. Medical rehabilitation of traumatic brain injury. Philadelphia: Henley & Belfus; 1996. p. 411–58.
8. Elovic EP, Esquenazi A, Alter KE, et al. Chemodenervation and nerve blocks in the diagnosis of spasticity and muscle overactivity. PM R 2009;1(9):842–51.
9. Horn L, Singh G, Dabrowski E. Chemoneurolysis with phenol and alcohol: a "Dying Art" that merits revival. In: Brashear A, Elovic E, editors. Spasticity diagnosis and management. New York: Demos Medical Publishing; 2011. p. 101–17.
10. Macek C. Venous thrombosis results from some phenol injections. JAMA 1983; 249(14):1807.

11. Gupta S, Ashrith G, Chandra D, et al. Acute phenol poisoning: a life-threatening hazard of chronic pain relief. Clin Toxicol (Phila) 2008;46(3):250–3.

12. Francisco GE, Hu MM, Boake C, et al. Efficacy of early use of intrathecal baclofen therapy for treating spastic hypertonia due to acquired brain injury. Brain Inj 2005;19(5):359–64.

13. Fietzek UM, Kossmehl P, Schelosky L, et al. Early botulinum toxin treatment for spastic pes equinovarus—a randomized double-blind placebo controlled study. Eur J Neurol 2014;21(8):1089–95.

14. Esquenazi A, Moon D, Wikoff A, et al. Hemiparetic gait and changes in functional performance due to OnabotulinumtoxinA injection to lower limb muscles. Toxicon 2015;107(Pt A):109–13.

15. Keenan MA, Creighton J, Garland DE, et al. Surgical correction of spastic equinovarus deformity in the adult head trauma patient. Foot Ankle 1984;5:35–41.

16. Fulford GE. Surgical management of ankle and foot deformities in cerebral palsy. Clin Orthop 1990;253:55–61.

17. Barnes MJ, Herring JA. Combined split anterior tibial-tendon transfer and intramuscular lengthening of the posterior tibial tendon: results in patients who have a varus deformity of the foot due to spastic cerebral palsy. J Bone Joint Surg Am 1991;73:734–8.

18. Vogt JC. Split anterior tibial transfer for spastic equinovarus foot deformity: retrospective study of 73 operated feet. J Foot Ankle Surg 1998;37:2–7.

19. Lawrence SJ, Botte MJ. Management of the adult, spastic, equinovarus foot deformity. Foot Ankle Int 1994;15:340–6.

20. Keenan MA, Lee GA, Tuckman SA, et al. Improving calf muscle strength in patients with spastic equinovarus deformity by transfer of the long toe flexors to the os calcis. J Head Trauma Rehabil 1999;14(2):163–75.

21. Moon D, Esquenazi A. Instrumented gait analysis: a tool in the treatment of spastic gait dysfunction. JBJS Rev 2016;4(6) [pii:01874474-201606000-00004].

22. Robertson JV, Pradon D, Bensmail D, et al. Relevance of botulinum toxin injection and nerve block of rectus femoris to kinematic and functional parameters of stiff knee gait in hemiplegic adults. Gait Posture 2009;29(1):108–12.

23. Tenniglo MJ, Nederhand MJ, Prinsen EC, et al. Effect of chemodenervation of the rectus femoris muscle in adults with a stiff knee gait due to spastic paresis: a systematic review with a meta-analysis in patients with stroke. Arch Phys Med Rehabil 2014;95(3):576–87.

24. Waters RL, Garland DE, Perry J, et al. Stiff-legged gait in hemiplegia: surgical correction. J Bone Joint Surg Am 1979;61(6A):927–33.

25. Sutherland DH, Santi M, Abel MF. Treatment of stiff-knee gait in cerebral palsy: a comparison by gait analysis of distal rectus femoris transfer versus proximal rectus release. J Pediatr Orthop 1990;10(4):433–41.

26. Ounpuu S, Muik E, Davis RB 3rd, et al. Rectus femoris surgery in children with cerebral palsy. Part II: a comparison between the effect of transfer and release of the distal rectus femoris on knee motion. J Pediatr Orthop 1993;13(3):331–5.

27. Ounpuu S, Muik E, Davis RB, et al. Rectus femoris surgery in children with cerebral palsy. Part 1: the effect of rectus femoris transfer location on knee motion. J Pediatr Orthop 1993;13(3):325–30.

28. Scully WF, McMulkin ML, Baird GO, et al. Outcomes of rectus femoris transfers in children with cerebral palsy: effect of transfer site. J Pediatr Orthop 2013;33(3):303–8.

29. Keenan MA, Ure K, Smith CW, et al. Hamstring release for knee flexion contracture in spastic adults. Clin Orthop Relat Res 1988;(236):221–6.

# Emerging Therapies for Spastic Movement Disorders

Preeti Raghavan, MD

## KEYWORDS

- Spasticity • Muscle stiffness • Peripheral mechanism • Stroke • Brain injury
- Hyaluronidase • Hyaluronic acid • Hyaluronan hypothesis

## KEY POINTS

- Neural mechanisms of spasticity do not fully explain the motor dysfunction in patients with spastic disorders.
- Peripheral non-neural mechanisms are not fully understood.
- The hyaluronan hypothesis postulates that the accumulation of hyaluronan, which functions as a lubricant in the extracellular matrix of muscle, may lead to the development of muscle stiffness.
- Hydrolysis of the accumulated hyaluronan may be safely achieved using local injections of the enzyme hyaluronidase to reduce muscle stiffness and increase both passive and active motion.
- Hyaluronidase is a potential emerging treatment for the management of patients with spastic movement disorder.

## INTRODUCTION

Muscle stiffness and spasticity cause severe disability in approximately 12 million people after neurologic injury of cerebral or spinal origin, such as stroke, cerebral palsy, spinal cord injury, and multiple sclerosis.[1] The prevalence of spasticity increases over weeks and months after the neurologic injury,[2] leading to muscle stiffness that persists for years, contributing to further disability and slowed recovery. Upper limb spasticity and muscle stiffness are associated with reduced functional independence and a fourfold increase in direct care costs during the first year after stroke alone.[3,4] They are challenging to treat, because the underlying mechanisms are not fully understood.[4,5]

Spasticity is classically defined as a velocity-dependent increase in tonic stretch reflexes resulting from hyperexcitability of the stretch reflex[6] because of decreased

Disclosures: New York University has filed a patent on the use of hyaluronidase for muscle stiffness. Dr P. Raghavan is cofounder of MovEase, Incorporated. This article discusses the off-label use of hyaluronidase for muscle stiffness.
Rusk Rehabilitation, NYU School of Medicine, 240 East 38th Street, 17th Floor, New York, NY 10016, USA
E-mail address: Preeti.Raghavan@nyumc.org

cortical influences on the inhibitory brainstem descending pathways to the spinal cord.[7] The imbalance between inhibitory cortical and brainstem pathways from the ventromedial reticular formation and the excitatory brainstem pathways from the bulbopontine tegmentum and the vestibular nucleus are thought to reduce pre-synaptic inhibition causing spasticity[8] (**Fig. 1**). However, hyperreflexia is only one component of the problem in patients with spasticity,[9–11] and the extent of hyper-reflexia may not be correlated with the extent of muscle stiffness.[12,13] Nevertheless, central nervous system (CNS) depressants (eg, benzodiazepines, baclofen, and tiza-nidine) are commonly used to treat muscle stiffness, but they also produce muscle weakness, fatigue, and sleepiness.[14] Botulinum toxin injections are effective in reducing muscle overactivity in patients with spasticity,[15] but it has long been known that muscles can be stiff even in the absence of electromyography (EMG) activation. Thus, although neural mechanisms may initiate spasticity, non-neural peripheral mechanisms clearly play a role in the development and exacerbation of muscle stiffness.[16,17]

Increased resistance to passive stretch can occur because of secondary non-neural changes in muscle fibers, collagen tissue, and tendon properties.[18,19] Early experiments on muscle properties[20] showed that the faster the change in muscle length, the greater is the passive tension generated in the muscle in the absence of muscle activation. This can be quantified with the length-tension curve, which shows a steeper slope in spastic compared with nonspastic muscles at equivalent speeds (**Fig. 2**). This non-neural, or passive stiffness, is distinct from the increase in EMG activity (neural response) when a muscle is stretched at faster speeds[21]

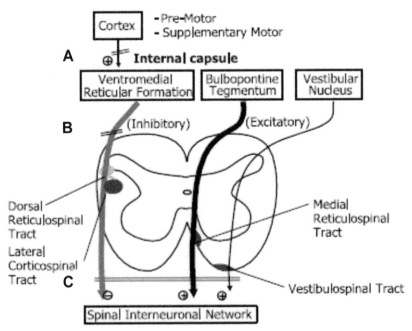

**Fig. 1.** CNS injury disrupts inhibitory descending pathways controlling spinal stretch reflex excitability. A = corticobulbar fibers; B = dorsal reticulospinal pathway; C = loss of all supra-spinal control. (*From* Sheean G. The pathophysiology of spasticity. Eur J Neurol 2002;9(Suppl 1):3–9; with permission.)

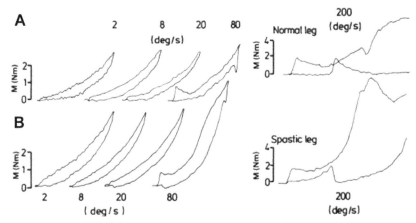

**Fig. 2.** Increased slope of the passive length-tension curve at faster speeds in spastic muscles (*B*) compared with nonspastic muscles on the unaffected side (*A*). (*From* Hufschmidt A, Mauritz KH. Chronic transformation of muscle in spasticity: a peripheral contribution to increased tone. J Neurol Neurosurg Psychiatry 1985;48(7):676–85; with permission.)

and can lead to the generation of increased torques despite the presence of weakness.[22,23] A previous hypothesis postulated that passive muscle stiffness may increase because of sarcomere shortening resulting from intracellular changes in the configuration of titin, the major passive load-bearing protein within the muscle fiber. However, subsequent studies found that the sarcomere is actually lengthened rather than shortened in patients with contracture.[24,25] Also, the titin isoform and passive mechanics of individual muscle fibers are unaltered in spastic muscles, although muscle fascicles are stiffer,[26] suggesting that passive stiffness may arise from alterations in the extracellular matrix (ECM).

The thickness of the ECM is increased in chronically spastic muscles, particularly the endomysium, perimysium, and epimysium, which are made up of collagen (types I and III)[27] (**Fig. 3**). Therefore, fibrosis and contracture were thought to produce muscle stiffness. If so, one would expect spastic muscle bundles to generate higher tension relative to normal muscle bundles. Surprisingly, spastic muscle bundles showed significantly lower tension (tangent modulus) than nonspastic muscle bundles.[28] Recent studies do not support a role for increased content and disorganization of collagen in muscle stiffness, although they have been the prime contenders for the development of passive muscle stiffness.[29,30] Thus, the precise non-neural mechanisms of muscle stiffness are still not fully understood.

## AN ALTERNATIVE EXPLANATION: THE HYALURONAN HYPOTHESIS

The author and colleagues proposed that hyaluronan, a nonsulfated high molecular weight glycosaminoglycan (GAG), and a major component of the ECM surrounding the endomysium, perimysium, and epimysium,[31] which normally provides lubrication to facilitate sliding and myofascial force transmission within and between muscles,[32] could potentially contribute to muscle stiffness after cerebral injury. This hypothesis was based on 3 main findings. First, muscle fiber atrophy after upper motor neuron injury in the context of paresis leads to a relative increase in the proportion of the ECM,[33,34] which could be occupied by hyaluronan.[35] Second, immobilization of

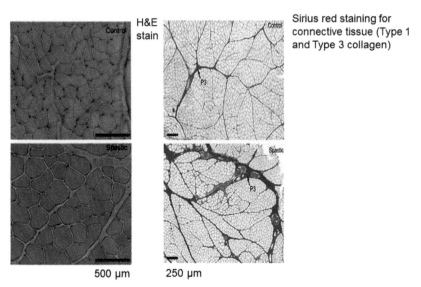

H&E stain

Sirius red staining for connective tissue (Type 1 and Type 3 collagen)

500 μm        250 μm

**Fig. 3.** Chronically spastic muscles show increased endomysial and perimysial thickness that stain for type 1 and type 3 collagen suggesting fibrosis. (*From* de Bruin M, Smeulders MJ, Kreulen M, et al. Intramuscular connective tissue differences in spastic and control muscle: a mechanical and histologic study. PLoS One 2014;9(6):e101038; with permission.)

the ankle joint in rats led to increased hyaluronan accumulation in the soleus muscle after 4 weeks (**Fig. 4**), around the endomysium and perimysium, which was hydrolyzed with *Streptomyces hyaluronidase*.[36] After 12 weeks, the endomysium also thickened (**Fig. 5**). Third, at high concentrations, hyaluronan and protein-crosslinked assemblies of hyaluronan aggregate[37] and dramatically increase the viscoelasticity of the ECM.[38] These large aggregated molecules cannot be cleared by the lymphatic system, particularly when movements are reduced. Thus, hyperviscous hyaluronan in the ECM can cause the muscle fibers and fascicles to stick to one another, reduce gliding during movement, and increase muscle stiffness (**Fig. 6**).

## PRELIMINARY EVIDENCE FOR THE HYALURONAN HYPOTHESIS AND AN EMERGING TREATMENT

Human recombinant hyaluronidase (Hylenex, Halozyme Therapeutics, Incorporated, San Diego, CA) is commercially available, safe in children and adults, and US Food and Drug Administration (FDA)-approved since 2005 for use as a tissue permeability modifier. It is currently indicated as an adjuvant in subcutaneous fluid administration for achieving hydration, to increase the dispersion and absorption of other injected drugs, and in subcutaneous urography for improving resorption of radiopaque agents.

In a recent retrospective case series,[39] 20 patients with unilateral upper limb spasticity of cerebral origin received off-label injections of human recombinant hyaluronidase in combination with preservative-free normal saline into 6 to 8 upper limb muscles at a single visit. All patients (mean age 41 plus or minus 22 years and mean time since injury 40.6 plus or minus 38.9 months) had moderately severe

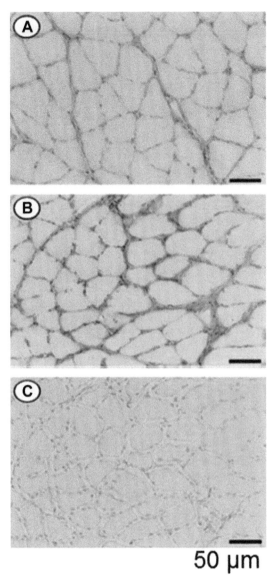

50 μm

**Fig. 4.** Sections of soleus muscle in 12-week-old rats showing accumulation of hyaluronan (stained brown with hyaluronic acid binding protein) compared with control animals (*A*) after 4 weeks of immobilization (*B*), which was hydrolyzed after treatment with *Streptomyces hyaluronidase* (*C*). (*From* Okita M, Yoshimura T, Nakano J, et al. Effects of reduced joint mobility on sarcomere length, collagen fibril arrangement in the endomysium, and hyaluronan in rat soleus muscle. J Muscle Res Cell Motil 2004;25(2):159–66; with permission.)

unilateral upper limb spasticity in more than 1 joint, defined by Modified Ashworth Scale (MAS) score of at least 2. The dose ranged from 450 to 600 units of hyaluronidase (3–4 vials of 150 units/mL) diluted with normal saline in a 1:1 ratio which was injected into multiple synergistically acting muscles (**Fig. 7**).

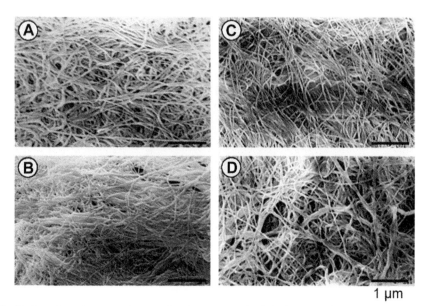

1 μm

**Fig. 5.** Scanning electron micrographs showing gradual thickening of soleus muscle endomysia compared with control animals (*A*) after 2 weeks of immobilization (*B*), after 4 weeks of immobilization (*C*) and particularly after 12 weeks of immobilization (*D*). (*From* Okita M, Yoshimura T, Nakano J, et al. Effects of reduced joint mobility on sarcomere length, collagen fibril arrangement in the endomysium, and hyaluronan in rat soleus muscle. J Muscle Res Cell Motil 2004;25(2):159–66; with permission.)

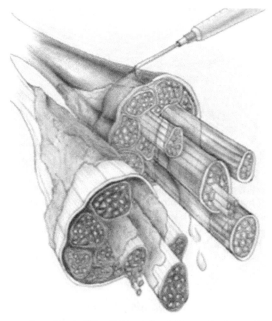

**Fig. 6.** The hyaluronan hypothesis. The dark patches represent aggregates of hyaluronan. Injection of the enzyme hyaluronidase can potentially hydrolyze the hyaluronan deposits and restore sliding of the muscle fibers and fascicles. (*Courtesy of* Dr Susie Kwon, MD, New York, NY.)

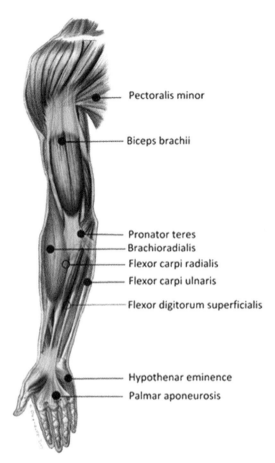

Fig. 7. Common sites of injection with hyaluronidase. (*From* Raghavan P, Lu Y, Mirchandani M, et al. Human recombinant hyaluronidase injections for upper limb muscle stiffness in individuals with cerebral injury: a case series. EBioMedicine 2016;9:306–13; with permission.)

There were no clinically significant adverse effects related to the treatment. Patients' passive and active range of motion was evaluated before and after injection to assess clinical response to treatment. Passive movement at all joints, and active movement at most joints increased within 2 weeks after injection (T1), and persisted at 4 to 6 weeks after injection (T2), and 3 to 5 months after injection (T3) for most joints (**Fig. 8**). There was a delayed increase in active elbow extension and forearm pronation, suggesting a possible interaction with neural mechanisms and motor learning. The percentage of joints with MAS = 3 decreased by 38.6% (from 44.4% at T0 to 5.8% at T1), and those with MAS = 0 increased by 46.9% (from 1.3% at T0 to 48.2% at T1) within 3 days to 2 weeks, suggesting that this was a clear effect of the injections (**Fig. 9**). The results persisted for at least 3 months. Most importantly, there were no adverse effects of muscle weakness or sedation. These results provide preliminary evidence that intramuscular hyaluronidase injections can reduce muscle stiffness and increase passive and active movement in multiple upper limb joints of patients with chronic spasticity.

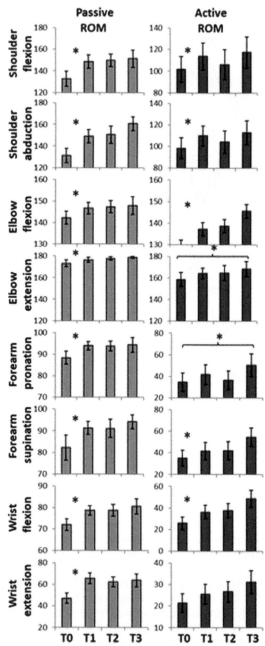

**Fig. 8.** Active and passive range of motion at T0 = before injection, T1 = within 2 weeks after injection, T2 = within 4 to 6 weeks after injection, and T3 = within 3 to 5 months after injection. * statistically significant differences at p<0.05. (*Data from* Raghavan P, Lu Y, Mirchandani M, et al. Human recombinant hyaluronidase injections for upper limb muscle stiffness in individuals with cerebral injury: a case series. EBioMedicine 2016;9:306–13; with permission.)

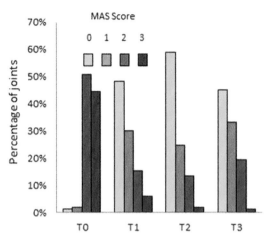

**Fig. 9.** MAS score across all the upper limb joints. (*Data from* Raghavan P, Lu Y, Mirchandani M, et al. Human recombinant hyaluronidase injections for upper limb muscle stiffness in individuals with cerebral injury: a case series. EBioMedicine 2016;9:306–13; with permission.)

## SUMMARY

Although spasticity develops as a result of neural mechanisms, muscle stiffness in spastic patients may occur as a result of peripheral non-neural mechanisms. The hyaluronan hypothesis postulates that the accumulation of hyaluronan within the ECM of muscle may lead to muscle stiffness. In a retrospective case series, the author and colleagues found that injections of hyaluronidase into upper limb muscles not only decreased muscle stiffness and increased passive movement, but also increased active movement,[39] providing preliminary evidence for the hyaluronan hypothesis. Increased levels of hyaluronan have also been shown to precede fibrosis in several organs[40–44]; therefore, hydrolysis of hyaluronan by hyaluronidase in muscle may potentially stop the progression to fibrosis, contracture, and disability. Confirmation of the findings and elucidation of the underlying mechanisms will result in a new treatment for a major disabling problem. A better understanding of the mechanisms underlying muscle stiffness, and the basis for treatment with hyaluronidase, can potentially transform clinical practice for the treatment of muscle stiffness after neurologic injury. Other treatments may also target this mechanism, and future studies may lead to elucidation of these treatments.

## ACKNOWLEDGMENTS

Many thanks to Dr Susie Kwon for the drawing representing the hyaluronan hypothesis and treatment with hyaluronidase.

## REFERENCES

1. Sommerfeld DK, Eek EU, Svensson AK, et al. Spasticity after stroke: its occurrence and association with motor impairments and activity limitations. Stroke 2004;35(1):134–9.
2. Watkins CL, Leathley MJ, Gregson JM, et al. Prevalence of spasticity post stroke. Clin Rehabil 2002;16(5):515–22.

3. Lundstrom E, Smits A, Borg J, et al. Four-fold increase in direct costs of stroke survivors with spasticity compared with stroke survivors without spasticity: the first year after the event. Stroke 2010;41(2):319–24.

4. Zorowitz RD, Gillard PJ, Brainin M. Poststroke spasticity: sequelae and burden on stroke survivors and caregivers. Neurology 2013;80(3 Suppl 2):S45–52.

5. Francisco GE, McGuire JR. Poststroke spasticity management. Stroke 2012; 43(11):3132–6.

6. Lance JW. The control of muscle tone, reflexes, and movement: Robert Wartenberg lecture. Neurology 1980;30(12):1303–13.

7. Sheean G, McGuire JR. Spastic hypertonia and movement disorders: pathophysiology, clinical presentation, and quantification. PM R 2009;1(9):827–33.

8. Sheean G. The pathophysiology of spasticity. Eur J Neurol 2002;9(Suppl 1):3–9 [discussion: 53–61].

9. Sinkjaer T, Toft E, Larsen K, et al. Non-reflex and reflex mediated ankle joint stiffness in multiple sclerosis patients with spasticity. Muscle Nerve 1993;16(1): 69–76.

10. Schindler-Ivens SM, Shields RK. Soleus H-reflex recruitment is not altered in persons with chronic spinal cord injury. Arch Phys Med Rehabil 2004;85(5):840–7.

11. Wilson LR, Gracies JM, Burke D, et al. Evidence for fusimotor drive in stroke patients based on muscle spindle thixotropy. Neurosci Lett 1999;264(1–3):109–12.

12. O'Dwyer NJ, Ada L. Reflex hyperexcitability and muscle contracture in relation to spastic hypertonia. Curr Opin Neurol 1996;9(6):451–5.

13. O'Dwyer NJ, Ada L, Neilson PD. Spasticity and muscle contracture following stroke. Brain 1996;119(Pt 5):1737–49.

14. McIntyre A, Lee T, Janzen S, et al. Systematic review of the effectiveness of pharmacological interventions in the treatment of spasticity of the hemiparetic lower extremity more than six months post stroke. Top Stroke Rehabil 2012;19(6): 479–90.

15. Gracies JM, Brashear A, Jech R, et al. Safety and efficacy of abobotulinumtoxin A for hemiparesis in adults with upper limb spasticity after stroke or traumatic brain injury: a double-blind randomised controlled trial. Lancet Neurol 2015;14(10): 992–1001.

16. Burke D, Wissel J, Donnan GA. Pathophysiology of spasticity in stroke. Neurology 2013;80(3 Suppl 2):S20–6.

17. Stecco A, Stecco C, Raghavan P. Peripheral mechanisms of spasticity and treatment implications. Curr Phys Med Rehabil Rep 2014. https://doi.org/10.1007/s40141-014-0052-3.

18. Foran JR, Steinman S, Barash I, et al. Structural and mechanical alterations in spastic skeletal muscle. Dev Med Child Neurol 2005;47(10):713–7.

19. Dietz V, Sinkjaer T. Spastic movement disorder: impaired reflex function and altered muscle mechanics. Lancet Neurol 2007;6(8):725–33.

20. Hill AV. First and last experiments in muscle mechanics. Cambridge (England): Cambridge University Press; 1970.

21. Ibrahim IK, Berger W, Trippel M, et al. Stretch-induced electromyographic activity and torque in spastic elbow muscles. Differential modulation of reflex activity in passive and active motor tasks. Brain 1993;116(Pt 4):971–89.

22. Hufschmidt A, Mauritz KH. Chronic transformation of muscle in spasticity: a peripheral contribution to increased tone. J Neurol Neurosurg Psychiatry 1985; 48(7):676–85.

23. Schmit BD, Dhaher Y, Dewald JP, et al. Reflex torque response to movement of the spastic elbow: theoretical analyses and implications for quantification of spasticity. Ann Biomed Eng 1999;27(6):815–29.

24. Lieber RL, Ponten E, Burkholder TJ, et al. Sarcomere length changes after flexor carpi ulnaris to extensor digitorum communis tendon transfer. J Hand Surg Am 1996;21(4):612–8.

25. Lieber RL, Friden J. Intraoperative measurement and biomechanical modeling of the flexor carpi ulnaris-to-extensor carpi radialis longus tendon transfer. J Biomech Eng 1997;119(4):386–91.

26. Smith LR, Lee KS, Ward SR, et al. Hamstring contractures in children with spastic cerebral palsy result from a stiffer extracellular matrix and increased in vivo sarcomere length. J Physiol 2011;589(Pt 10):2625–39.

27. de Bruin M, Smeulders MJ, Kreulen M, et al. Intramuscular connective tissue differences in spastic and control muscle: a mechanical and histological study. PLoS One 2014;9(6):e101038.

28. Lieber RL, Runesson E, Einarsson F, et al. Inferior mechanical properties of spastic muscle bundles due to hypertrophic but compromised extracellular matrix material. Muscle Nerve 2003;28(4):464–71.

29. Chapman MA, Pichika R, Lieber RL. Collagen crosslinking does not dictate stiffness in a transgenic mouse model of skeletal muscle fibrosis. J Biomech 2015; 48(2):375–8.

30. Smith LR, Barton ER. Collagen content does not alter the passive mechanical properties of fibrotic skeletal muscle in mdx mice. Am J Physiol Cell Physiol 2014;306(10):C889–98.

31. Piehl-Aulin K, Laurent C, Engstrom-Laurent A, et al. Hyaluronan in human skeletal muscle of lower extremity: concentration, distribution, and effect of exercise. J Appl Physiol (1985) 1991;71(6):2493–8.

32. Purslow PP, Trotter JA. The morphology and mechanical properties of endomysium in series-fibred muscles: variations with muscle length. J Muscle Res Cell Motil 1994;15(3):299–308.

33. Dietz V, Berger W. Cerebral palsy and muscle transformation. Dev Med Child Neurol 1995;37(2):180–4.

34. Springer J, Schust S, Peske K, et al. Catabolic signaling and muscle wasting after acute ischemic stroke in mice: indication for a stroke-specific sarcopenia. Stroke 2014;45(12):3675–83.

35. Girish KS, Kemparaju K. The magic glue hyaluronan and its eraser hyaluronidase: a biological overview. Life Sci 2007;80(21):1921–43.

36. Okita M, Yoshimura T, Nakano J, et al. Effects of reduced joint mobility on sarcomere length, collagen fibril arrangement in the endomysium, and hyaluronan in rat soleus muscle. J Muscle Res Cell Motil 2004;25(2):159–66.

37. Zhao M, Yoneda M, Ohashi Y, et al. Evidence for the covalent binding of SHAP, heavy chains of inter-alpha-trypsin inhibitor, to hyaluronan. J Biol Chem 1995; 270(44):26657–63.

38. Cowman MK, Schmidt TA, Raghavan P, et al. Viscoelastic properties of hyaluronan in physiological conditions. F1000Res 2015;4:622.

39. Raghavan P, Lu Y, Mirchandani M, et al. Human recombinant hyaluronidase injections for upper limb muscle stiffness in individuals with cerebral injury: a case series. EBioMedicine 2016;9:306–13.

40. Bensadoun ES, Burke AK, Hogg JC, et al. Proteoglycan deposition in pulmonary fibrosis. Am J Respir Crit Care Med 1996;154(6 Pt 1):1819–28.

41. Evanko SP, Potter-Perigo S, Petty LJ, et al. Hyaluronan controls the deposition of fibronectin and collagen and modulates TGF-beta1 induction of lung myofibroblasts. Matrix Biol 2015;42:74–92.

42. Jun Z, Hill PA, Lan HY, et al. CD44 and hyaluronan expression in the development of experimental crescentic glomerulonephritis. Clin Exp Immunol 1997;108(1): 69–77.

43. Hernnas J, Nettelbladt O, Bjermer L, et al. Alveolar accumulation of fibronectin and hyaluronan precedes bleomycin-induced pulmonary fibrosis in the rat. Eur Respir J 1992;5(4):404–10.

44. Halfon P, Bourliere M, Penaranda G, et al. Accuracy of hyaluronic acid level for predicting liver fibrosis stages in patients with hepatitis C virus. Comp Hepatol 2005;4:6.

# Moving?

## Make sure your subscription moves with you!

To notify us of your new address, find your **Clinics Account Number** (located on your mailing label above your name), and contact customer service at:

**Email: journalscustomerservice-usa@elsevier.com**

**800-654-2452** (subscribers in the U.S. & Canada)
**314-447-8871** (subscribers outside of the U.S. & Canada)

**Fax number: 314-447-8029**

**Elsevier Health Sciences Division**
**Subscription Customer Service**
**3251 Riverport Lane**
**Maryland Heights, MO 63043**

*To ensure uninterrupted delivery of your subscription, please notify us at least 4 weeks in advance of move.